CareWise
Suite 200
100 Railroad
Missoula, MT 59802

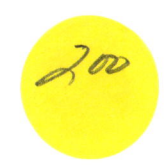

NECK PAIN

SAM W. WIESEL, M.D.
*Professor of Orthopaedic Surgery
The George Washington University
Medical Center
Washington, D.C.*

HENRY L. FEFFER, M.D.
*Director of Medical Research
Health Care Systems, Inc.
Professor Emeritus of Orthopaedic Surgery
The George Washington University
Medical Center
Washington, D.C.*

RICHARD H. ROTHMAN, M.D., PH.D.
*Professor and Chairman
Department of Orthopaedics
Jefferson Medical College
Philadelphia, Penna.*

THE MICHIE COMPANY
Law Publishers
CHARLOTTESVILLE, VIRGINIA

Copyright © 1986
BY
The Michie Company

Library of Congress Card Number: 86-62420
ISBN 0-87215-994-9

All rights reserved.

We dedicate this book to our Administrative Assistants, Diane Cooks and Qwetta Williams who are so helpful in every way.

TABLE OF CONTENTS

	Page
Dedication	iii
Preface	xix
Contributors	xxi

CHAPTER 1. NECK PAIN	1
§ 1-1. Scope of Problem	1
§ 1-2. Incidence	3
§ 1-3. Estimates of Whiplash Injuries in the United States	4
§ 1-4. Prevention of Injury	5
§ 1-5. Passenger Position in the Car	6
§ 1-6. Seat Belt and Shoulder Restraints	6
§ 1-7. Head Restraints	6
§ 1-8. Sex	8
§ 1-9. Age	8
§ 1-10. Other Factors	9
§ 1-11. Effect of Litigation	9
§ 1-12. Emotional Factors	10
§ 1-13. Implementation of an Organized Approach	11
§ 1-14. Economic Impact	14
§ 1-15. Summary	15
Bibliography	16

CHAPTER 2. ANATOMY AND PATHOPHYSIOLOGY OF NECK PAIN	19
§ 2-1. Introduction to Neck Anatomy	20
§ 2-1(A). Osseous Anatomy	21
§ 2-1(A)(1). Occiput	21
§ 2-1(A)(2). Atlas (C1)	21
§ 2-1(A)(3). Axis (C2)	22
§ 2-1(A)(4). Lower Cervical Vertebrae (C3-C7)	22
§ 2-1(B). Intervertebral Disc (IVD)	23
§ 2-1(C). Occipito-Atlanto-Axial Articulation	23
§ 2-1(D). Ligaments and Apophyseal Joints	23

TABLE OF CONTENTS

	Page
§ 2-1(E). Blood Supply	24
§ 2-1(F). Innervation	25
§ 2-1(G). Brachial Plexua	26
§ 2-1(H). Muscles	26
§ 2-2. Pathophysiology of Neck Pain	28
§ 2-3. Basic Scientific Knowledge of Cervical Spine	30
§ 2-3(A). Kinematics	30
§ 2-3(B). Biochemistry	31
§ 2-3(C). Biomechanics and Stability	33
§ 2-3(D). Nutrition	34
§ 2-3(E). Immunology	35
§ 2-3(F). Nociceptive Factors	36
§ 2-4. Clinical Condition	36
§ 2-4(A). Neck Sprain — Neckache	37
§ 2-4(B). Acute Herniated Disc	38
§ 2-4(C). Cervical Degenerative Disc Disease	43
§ 2-4(C)(1). Cervical Spondylosis (Cervical Spinal Stenosis)	44
§ 2-4(C)(2). Cervical Spondylosis With Myelopathy	46
§ 2-4(D). Rheumatoid Arthritis	48
Bibliography	51
Table I. Structures Causing Neck Pain	53
Table II. Causes of Neck and Neck Related Pain Syndromes	54
Table III. Mean Range of Cervical Motion of the Spine (Degrees)	55
Table IV. Physical Examination — Disc Herniation	56
Figure 1. The Atlas Viewed From Above and Below	58
Figure 2. The Axis	59
Figure 3. Typical Lower Cervical Vertebra	60
Figure 4. Three-Dimensional Anatomy of the Cup-Like Articulations of the Occipital-Atlantal Joints	61
Figure 5. The Cruciform and Tectorial Ligaments	62
Figure 6. Cervical Spine Viewed From the Side	63
Figure 7. Lower Cervical Spine in Neutral Position	64
Figure 8. Vertebral Artery	65
Figure 9. Sinuvertebral Nerve	66
Figure 10. Brachial Plexus and Lower Cervical Spine	67

TABLE OF CONTENTS

Page

CHAPTER 3. A STANDARDIZED APPROACH TO THE DIAGNOSIS AND TREATMENT OF NECK PAIN 69
§ 3-1. The Algorithm 70
§ 3-2. Cervical Spine Protocol 71
§ 3-3. Neck Pain Predominant 75
§ 3-4. Arm Pain Predominant (Brachialgia) 77
§ 3-5. Treatment Modalities 78
§ 3-6. Immobilization 78
§ 3-7. Drug Therapy 80
§ 3-8. Traction 81
§ 3-9. Trigger Point Injection 82
§ 3-10. Manipulation 82
§ 3-11. Exercises 83
Bibliography 83
Figure 1. Cervical Spine Algorithm 85
Figure 2. Differential Diagnosis of Neck Pain 86

CHAPTER 4. NON-MECHANICAL CAUSES OF NECK PAIN 87
§ 4-1. Introduction 92
§ 4-2. Rheumatologic Disorders of the Cervical Spine 94
  § 4-2(A). Introduction 94
  § 4-2(B). Rheumatoid Arthritis 96
    § 4-2(B)(1). Prevalence and Etiology 97
    § 4-2(B)(2). Clinical Symptoms 99
    § 4-2(B)(3). Physical Findings 100
    § 4-2(B)(4). Laboratory Findings 101
    § 4-2(B)(5). Radiographic Findings 102
    § 4-2(B)(6). Differential Diagnosis 103
    § 4-2(B)(7). Treatment 104
    § 4-2(B)(8). Prognosis and Course 106
  Bibliography 107
  § 4-2(C). Ankylosing Spondylitis 109
    § 4-2(C)(1). Prevalence and Etiology 110
    § 4-2(C)(2). Clinical Features 112

TABLE OF CONTENTS

	Page
§ 4-2(C)(3). Physical Examination	114
§ 4-2(C)(4). Laboratory Findings	114
§ 4-2(C)(5). Radiologic Findings	115
§ 4-2(C)(6). Differential Diagnosis	115
§ 4-2(C)(7). Treatment	116
§ 4-2(C)(8). Course and Outcome	117
Bibliography	118
§ 4-2(D). Reiter's Syndrome	120
§ 4-2(D)(1). Prevalence and Etiology	120
§ 4-2(D)(2). Clinical Findings	121
§ 4-2(D)(3). Physical Findings	122
§ 4-2(D)(4). Laboratory Findings	123
§ 4-2(D)(5). Radiologic Findings	123
§ 4-2(D)(6). Differential Diagnosis	124
§ 4-2(D)(7). Treatment	125
§ 4-2(D)(8). Course and Outcome	125
Bibliography	126
§ 4-2(E). Psoriatic Arthritis	128
§ 4-2(E)(1). Prevalence and Etiology	128
§ 4-2(E)(2). Clinical Features	130
§ 4-2(E)(3). Physical Findings	131
§ 4-2(E)(4). Laboratory Findings	131
§ 4-2(E)(5). Radiologic Findings	132
§ 4-2(E)(6). Differential Diagnosis	133
§ 4-2(E)(7). Treatment	134
§ 4-2(E)(8). Course and Outcome	135
Bibliography	135
§ 4-2(F). Enteropathic Arthritis	137
§ 4-2(F)(1). Prevalence and Etiology	138
§ 4-2(F)(2). Clinical Features	138
§ 4-2(F)(3). Physical Findings	140
§ 4-2(F)(4). Laboratory Findings	140
§ 4-2(F)(5). Radiographic Findings	140
§ 4-2(F)(6). Differential Diagnosis	141
§ 4-2(F)(7). Treatment	141
§ 4-2(F)(8). Course and Outcome	142

TABLE OF CONTENTS

	Page
Bibliography	143
§ 4-2(G). Diffuse Idiopathic Skeletal Hyperostosis (DISH)	144
§ 4-2(G)(1). Prevalence and Etiology	144
§ 4-2(G)(2). Clinical Findings	145
§ 4-2(G)(3). Physical Findings	145
§ 4-2(G)(4). Laboratory Findings	146
§ 4-2(G)(5). Radiographic Findings	146
§ 4-2(G)(6). Differential Diagnosis	146
§ 4-2(G)(7). Treatment	147
§ 4-2(G)(8). Course and Outcome	147
Bibliography	148
§ 4-2(H). Polymyalgia Rheumatica	149
§ 4-2(H)(1). Prevalence and Etiology	149
§ 4-2(H)(2). Clinical Findings	150
§ 4-2(H)(3). Physical Examination	150
§ 4-2(H)(4). Laboratory Findings	150
§ 4-2(H)(5). Radiologic Findings	151
§ 4-2(H)(6). Differential Diagnosis	151
§ 4-2(H)(7). Treatment	152
§ 4-2(H)(8). Course and Etiology	153
Bibliography	153
§ 4-2(I). Fibrositis	154
§ 4-2(I)(1). Prevalence and Etiology	154
§ 4-2(I)(2). Clinical Findings	155
§ 4-2(I)(3). Physical Examination	156
§ 4-2(I)(4). Laboratory Findings	156
§ 4-2(I)(5). Radiographic Findings	156
§ 4-2(I)(6). Differential Diagnosis	156
§ 4-2(I)(7). Treatment	157
§ 4-2(I)(8). Course and Outcome	159
Bibliography	159
Table I. Rheumatic Diseases Associated With Neck Pain	161
Table II. Non-Steroidal Anti-Inflammatory Drugs	163
§ 4-3. Infections of the Lumbosacral Spine	165
§ 4-3(A). Introduction	165

TABLE OF CONTENTS

	Page
§ 4-3(B). Vertebral Osteomyelitis	166
§ 4-3(B)(1). Prevalence and Etiology	167
§ 4-3(B)(2). Clinical Findings	169
§ 4-3(B)(3). Physical Findings	170
§ 4-3(B)(4). Laboratory Findings	170
§ 4-3(B)(5). Radiographic Findings	171
§ 4-3(B)(6). Differential Diagnosis	172
§ 4-3(B)(7). Treatment	173
§ 4-3(B)(8). Course and Outcome	174
Bibliography	175
§ 4-3(C). Meningitis	177
§ 4-3(C)(1). Prevalence and Etiology	178
§ 4-3(C)(2). Clinical Findings	178
§ 4-3(C)(3). Physical Findings	181
§ 4-3(C)(4). Laboratory Findings	181
§ 4-3(C)(5). Radiographic Findings	183
§ 4-3(C)(6). Differential Diagnosis	183
§ 4-3(C)(7). Treatment	183
§ 4-3(C)(8). Course and Outcome	184
Bibliography	185
§ 4-3(D). Paget's Disease of Bone	186
§ 4-3(D)(1). Prevalence and Etiology	187
§ 4-3(D)(2). Clinical Findings	188
§ 4-3(D)(3). Physical Findings	189
§ 4-3(D)(4). Laboratory Findings	190
§ 4-3(D)(5). Radiographic Findings	190
§ 4-3(D)(6). Differential Diagnosis	191
§ 4-3(D)(7). Treatment	192
§ 4-3(D)(8). Course and Outcome	193
Bibliography	193
§ 4-4. Tumors and Infiltrative Lesions of the Cervical Spine	195
§ 4-4(A). Introduction	195
§ 4-4(B). Osteoblastoma	196
§ 4-4(B)(1). Prevalence and Etiology	196
§ 4-4(B)(2). Clinical Findings	196

TABLE OF CONTENTS

	Page
§ 4-4(B)(3). Physical Findings	197
§ 4-4(B)(4). Laboratory Findings	197
§ 4-4(B)(5). Radiographic Findings	197
§ 4-4(B)(6). Differential Diagnosis	198
§ 4-4(B)(7). Treatment	198
§ 4-4(B)(8). Course and Outcome	199
Bibliography	199
§ 4-4(C). Giant Cell Tumor	200
§ 4-4(C)(1). Prevalence and Etiology	200
§ 4-4(C)(2). Clinical Findings	200
§ 4-4(C)(3). Physical Findings	201
§ 4-4(C)(4). Laboratory Findings	201
§ 4-4(C)(5). Radiographic Findings	202
§ 4-4(C)(6). Differential Diagnosis	202
§ 4-4(C)(7). Treatment	203
§ 4-4(C)(8). Course and Outcome	203
Bibliography	204
§ 4-4(D). Aneurysmal Bone Cyst	204
§ 4-4(D)(1). Prevalence and Etiology	205
§ 4-4(D)(2). Clinical Findings	205
§ 4-4(D)(3). Physical Findings	206
§ 4-4(D)(4). Laboratory Findings	206
§ 4-4(D)(5). Radiographic Findings	206
§ 4-4(D)(6). Differential Diagnosis	207
§ 4-4(D)(7). Treatment	207
§ 4-4(D)(8). Course and Outcome	207
Bibliography	208
§ 4-4(E). Hemangioma	208
§ 4-4(E)(1). Prevalence and Etiology	209
§ 4-4(E)(2). Clinical Findings	209
§ 4-4(E)(3). Physical Findings	210
§ 4-4(E)(4). Laboratory Findings	210
§ 4-4(E)(5). Radiographic Findings	210
§ 4-4(E)(6). Differential Diagnosis	211
§ 4-4(E)(7). Treatment	211
§ 4-4(E)(8). Course and Outcome	211

TABLE OF CONTENTS

	Page
Bibliography	212
§ 4-4(F). Eosinophilic Granuloma	213
§ 4-4(F)(1). Prevalence and Etiology	213
§ 4-4(F)(2). Clinical Findings	213
§ 4-4(F)(3). Physical Findings	214
§ 4-4(F)(4). Laboratory Findings	214
§ 4-4(F)(5). Radiographic Findings	214
§ 4-4(F)(6). Differential Diagnosis	215
§ 4-4(F)(7). Treatment	215
§ 4-4(F)(8). Course and Outcome	215
Bibliography	216
§ 4-4(G). Multiple Myeloma	216
§ 4-4(G)(1). Prevalence and Etiology	217
§ 4-4(G)(2). Clinical Findings	217
§ 4-4(G)(3). Physical Findings	218
§ 4-4(G)(4). Laboratory Findings	218
§ 4-4(G)(5). Radiographic Findings	220
§ 4-4(G)(6). Differential Diagnosis	221
§ 4-4(G)(7). Treatment	221
§ 4-4(G)(8). Course and Outcome	222
Bibliography	222
§ 4-4(H). Chordoma	224
§ 4-4(H)(1). Prevalence and Etiology	224
§ 4-4(H)(2). Clinical Findings	225
§ 4-4(H)(3). Physical Findings	225
§ 4-4(H)(4). Laboratory Findings	225
§ 4-4(H)(5). Radiographic Findings	226
§ 4-4(H)(6). Differential Diagnosis	226
§ 4-4(H)(7). Treatment	227
§ 4-4(H)(8). Course and Outcome	227
Bibliography	227
§ 4-4(I). Lymphomas	228
§ 4-4(I)(1). Prevalence and Etiology	228
§ 4-4(I)(2). Clinical Findings	229
§ 4-4(I)(3). Physical Findings	229
§ 4-4(I)(4). Laboratory Findings	229

TABLE OF CONTENTS

	Page
§ 4-4(I)(5). Radiographic Findings	230
§ 4-4(I)(6). Differential Diagnosis	230
§ 4-4(I)(7). Treatment	231
§ 4-4(I)(8). Course and Outcome	231
Bibliography	231
§ 4-4(J). Skeletal Metastases	232
§ 4-4(J)(1). Prevalence and Etiology	232
§ 4-4(J)(2). Clinical Findings	233
§ 4-4(J)(3). Physical Findings	234
§ 4-4(J)(4). Laboratory Findings	234
§ 4-4(J)(5). Radiographic Findings	235
§ 4-4(J)(6). Differential Diagnosis	236
§ 4-4(J)(7). Treatment	236
§ 4-4(J)(8). Course and Outcome	237
Bibliography	237
§ 4-4(K). Intraspinal Neoplasm	238
§ 4-4(K)(1). Prevalence and Etiology	239
§ 4-4(K)(2). Clinical Features	239
§ 4-4(K)(3). Physical Findings	240
§ 4-4(K)(4). Laboratory Findings	240
§ 4-4(K)(5). Radiographic Findings	241
§ 4-4(K)(6). Differential Diagnosis	242
§ 4-4(K)(7). Treatment	242
§ 4-4(K)(8). Course and Outcome	242
Bibliography	243
§ 4-5. Endocrinologic and Metabolic Disorders of the Cervical Spine	244
§ 4-6. Hematologic Disorders of the Cervical Spine	246
CHAPTER 5. CERVICAL HYPEREXTENSION INJURIES	249
§ 5-1. Introduction	249
§ 5-2. Pathophysiology	250
§ 5-3. Symptoms	252
§ 5-4. Management	253
§ 5-5. Treatment	254

TABLE OF CONTENTS

	Page
§ 5-6. Return to Work	257
Bibliography	258
Figure 1. Mechanism of Whiplash	259
Figure 2. Soft Tissue Injury in Whiplash	260

CHAPTER 6. ASSESSMENT AND RELATIVE IMPORTANCE OF PHYSICAL FINDINGS AND DIAGNOSTIC PROCEDURES 261

§ 6-1. History	262
§ 6-2. Physical Examination	263
§ 6-3. The Occipitocervical Segment	264
§ 6-4. Injury to the Upper Cervical Segment	265
§ 6-5. The Lower Cervical Segment	266
§ 6-6. Laboratory Tests	267
§ 6-7. X-Ray	267
§ 6-8. Myelography	269
§ 6-9. Electromyogram (EMG)	270
§ 6-10. Computerized Axial Tomography	270
§ 6-11. Thermography	271
§ 6-12. Discography	272
§ 6-13. Cervical Disc Distention Test	273
§ 6-14. Magnetic Resonance Imaging (MRI)	273
Bibliography	274

CHAPTER 7. INDICATIONS FOR CERVICAL SPINE SURGERY 275

§ 7-1. Introduction	276
§ 7-2. Surgical Indications for a Herniated Nucleus Pulposus	277
§ 7-2(A). Neck Pain	277
§ 7-2(B). Profound Spinal Cord Impingement	277
§ 7-2(C). Progressive Neurologic Deficit	278
§ 7-2(D). Unrelenting Radicular Arm Pain	280
§ 7-2(E). Recurrent Episodes of Arm Pain	280
§ 7-2(F). Patient Factors	281

TABLE OF CONTENTS

	Page
§ 7-2(G). Selection of the Operation for Acute Disc Herniation	283
§ 7-3. Indications for Surgery in Cervical Spinal Stenosis	284
§ 7-3(A). Selection of the Operation for Cervical Spinal Stenosis	286
§ 7-4. Indications for Cervical Spine Fusion	287
§ 7-4(A). Neck Pain Only	288
§ 7-4(B). Neck and Arm Pain	288
§ 7-4(C). Neck Pain and Myelopathy	289
§ 7-5. Results of Operative Treatment	289
§ 7-6. Complications of Cervical Spine Surgery	295
§ 7-6(A). Complications During the Operation	295
§ 7-6(A)(1). Complications as a Result of Position	295
§ 7-6(A)(2). Vascular Injuries	297
§ 7-6(A)(3). Visceral Injuries	298
§ 7-6(A)(4). Neural Element Injuries	299
§ 7-6(B). Immediate Postoperative Complications	302
§ 7-6(B)(1). Pulmonary Atelectasis	302
§ 7-6(B)(2). Urinary Retention	302
§ 7-6(B)(3). Intestinal Ileus	303
§ 7-6(B)(4). Thrombophlebitis and Pulmonary Embolus	303
§ 7-6(B)(5). Wound Problems	303
§ 7-6(B)(6). Spinal Cord Compression	304
§ 7-6(C). Technical Complications Resulting in Persistent Symptoms	305
§ 7-6(C)(1). Inadequate Nerve Root Decompression	305
§ 7-6(C)(2). Inadequate Spinal Cord Decompression	305
§ 7-6(C)(3). Disc Space Infection	306
§ 7-6(C)(4). Iliac Crest Pain	307
§ 7-6(C)(5). Late Instability and Degenerative Changes	307
§ 7-6(C)(6). Foreign Bodies	308
§ 7-7. Summary	308
Bibliography	309

TABLE OF CONTENTS

	Page
Figure 1. Removal of Osteophytic Spur	311

CHAPTER 8. PSYCHOSOCIAL PROSPECTIVES ON CHRONIC NECK PAIN ... 313

§ 8-1.	Introduction	313
§ 8-2.	Pain and the American Worker	314
§ 8-3.	Illness and Disease	316
§ 8-4.	Acute and Chronic Pain	319
§ 8-5.	What Is Chronic Pain?	320
§ 8-6.	Psychosocial Affects of Chronic Pain	322
§ 8-7.	"The Patient in Pain" Versus "The Pain Patient"	322
§ 8-8.	Is Chronic Pain Really a Variant of Depression?	323
§ 8-9.	Are Chronic Pain Patients Depressed?	325
§ 8-10.	The Complications of Treatment	326
§ 8-11.	The Failure of Traditional Treatment	326
§ 8-12.	The Adverse Effect of Pain Treatment on Pain Patients	329
§ 8-12(A).	Polypharmacy and the Overutilization of Analgesics	329
§ 8-12(B).	Loss of the Ability to Work	329
§ 8-12(C).	Experiencing the Loss of a Future Sense	330
§ 8-12(D).	Disruption of Social and Family Situations	331
§ 8-12(E).	Inappropriate Surgery and Hospitalization	331
§ 8-13.	Understanding the Pain Complaint	332
§ 8-14.	Pain as a Four Component System	333
§ 8-14(A).	Stage I: Nociception	334
§ 8-14(B).	Stage II: The Pain Message	334
§ 8-14(C).	Stage III: Suffering	336
§ 8-14(D).	Stage IV: Pain Behavior	336
§ 8-14(E).	Summary: Implications for the Treatment of Pain	337
§ 8-15.	The Importance of the Meaning of Pain	339
§ 8-16.	Doing and Not Doing	340
Bibliography		341

TABLE OF CONTENTS

Page

CHAPTER 9. PHYSICAL THERAPY, ERGONOMICS, AND REHABILITATION 345
§ 9-1. Introduction 346
§ 9-2. Modalities Used in Physical Therapy 346
 § 9-2(A). Heat 347
 § 9-2(B). Cold 348
 § 9-2(C). Electrical Stimulation 349
 § 9-2(D). Ultrasound 351
 § 9-2(E). Traction 352
 § 9-2(F). Joint Mobilization 355
§ 9-3. Impairment of Functional Ability 357
§ 9-4. Assessment of Cervical Musculoskeletal Disorders and Treatment Plan 359
 § 9-4(A). Assessment 359
 § 9-4(B). Treatment Plan 360
§ 9-5. Specific Cervical Pain Syndromes and Physical Therapy Treatments 362
 § 9-5(A). Whiplash 362
  § 9-5(A)(1). Ligament Sprain 364
  § 9-5(A)(2). Muscle Strain 366
 § 9-5(B). Spondylosis 369
 § 9-5(C). Nerve root (Radicular) Pain 370
 § 9-5(D). Postural Pain 371
  Figure 1. Posture 372
 § 9-5(E). Temporo-Mandibular Joint Dysfunction 374
§ 9-6. Cervical Collar 375
 Figure 2. Cervical Collar 376
§ 9-7. Exercise: Therapeutic, Postural, and Preventive . 377
 Figure 3. Therapeutic and Postural Exercises ... 378
 Figure 4. Postures for Preventing Neck Strain .. 387
§ 9-8. Ergonomics and Prevention 394
 Figure 5. Incidence of Impairments in the Neck Related to the Neck-head Angles of 57 Accounting Machine Operators 398
 Figure 6. Adjustment Features of an Ergonomic Work Seat 399

xvii

TABLE OF CONTENTS

	Page
Figure 7. Adjustment Features of an Ergonomic VDT Work Station	400
Figure 8. Recommended Approximate Dimensions (in centimeters)	400
Figure 9. The "Mean Body Posture" Under Practical Conditions at Preferred Settings of the VDT Work Station	401
§ 9-9. Returning the Injured Worker to the Job	402
§ 9-10. Summary	403
Bibliography	403
Table I. Limits and Representative Values of Range of Rotation	407
Table II. Mean Percentage	410
Table III. Approximate Percentage Restriction	412
Table IV. Flexion and Extension	413
Table V. Human Factors and Task Redesign	415
Table VI. Work Place Redesign Considerations	417
Table VII. Postural Efforts at VDT Work Stations	419
Table VIII. Medical Findings in a VDT Field Study	420
Table IX. Model for Prevention and Return to Work	421

CHAPTER 10. STANDARDIZED CERVICAL SPINE EVALUATION FOR IMPAIRMENT RATING 423
§ 10-1. The Cervical Spine Evaluation Problem 423
§ 10-2. Standardized Neck Evaluation Guidelines 425
Bibliography 428
Table I. Industrial Back Injury Work Restriction Classification 429
Table II. Disability Evaluation of the Cervical Spine 431

Index 435

PREFACE

Disorders of the spine are ubiquitous in today's society. A high percentage of these cases involve the lumbar spine and occur in the industrial setting. The topic of low back pain has been well addressed in *Industrial Low Back Pain.*

The cervical spine is just as complex as the lumbar spine. However, due to the lower overall incidence of cervical spine problems, not as much attention has been directed toward it. A large number of cervical spine injuries are secondary to automobile accidents. Many of the incidents result in soft tissue trauma where there are no objective findings to substantiate the patient's subjective complaints. This inevitably leads to litigation which can become quite costly and time-consuming.

Interaction among physicians, lawyers, insurance adjusters, and judges has to occur to assure quality medical care as well as due process of the law for the injured patient. Each of the above professionals has a different involvement in both the process and the outcome. This text has been created as a common resource which addresses the needs and concerns of the participants so that both the medical and legal solution can be achieved with understanding and appreciation by all concerned.

The text is organized so that each author can address his particular area of expertise and improve interdisciplinary communication. Since each section has been covered from a practical point of view based upon the most recent information available, it should prove both useful and informative. The book is structured so that it can serve as a source as well as a desk-top reference.

The editors are very pleased with the final text. We appreciate each of the contributions and are thankful for the time and effort each author spent. Finally, we would like to thank Fran Warren and Anna May Cutitta of The Michie Company who assembled the book and were a pleasure to work with.

CONTRIBUTORS

William I. Bauer, M.D.
Medical Director
Potomac Electric Power Company
Washington, D.C.

David G. Borenstein, M.D.
Rheumatologist
Associate Professor of Medicine
George Washington University Medical Center
Washington, D.C.

Rene Cailliet, M.D.
Professor of Physical Medicine and Rehabilitation
University of California
Director of Physical Medicine and Rehabilitation
Santa Monica Hospital
Los Angeles, Calif.

Henry L. Feffer, M.D.
Director of Medical Research
Health Care Systems, Inc.
Professor Emeritus of Orthopaedic Surgery
George Washington University
Washington, D.C.

Arthur I. Kobrine, M.D., Ph.D.
Professor of Neurological Surgery
George Washington University
Washington, D.C.

Michael W. Nabors, M.D.
Department of Neurological Surgery
George Washington University
Washington, D.C.

CONTRIBUTORS

Richard H. Rothman, M.D., Ph.D.
Professor and Chairman
Department of Orthopaedics
Jefferson Medical College
Philadelphia, Penna.

Brian Schulman, M.D.
Assistant Clinical Professor of Psychiatry
Georgetown University
Washington, D.C.

Jeffery L. Stambough, M.D.
Assistant Professor of Orthopaedics
University of Cincinnati Medical School
Cincinnati, Ohio

Thomas M. Welsh, R.P.T.
Chief, Physical Therapy
George Washington University Medical Center
Washington, D.C.

Sam W. Wiesel, M.D.
Professor of Orthopaedic Surgery
George Washington University Medical Center
Washington, D.C.

CHAPTER 1

NECK PAIN

William Bauer, M.D.

§ 1-1. Scope of Problem.
§ 1-2. Incidence.
§ 1-3. Estimates of Whiplash Injuries in the United States.
§ 1-4. Prevention of Injury.
§ 1-5. Passenger Position in the Car.
§ 1-6. Seat Belt and Shoulder Restraints.
§ 1-7. Head Restraints.
§ 1-8. Sex.
§ 1-9. Age.
§ 1-10. Other Factors.
§ 1-11. Effect of Litigation.
§ 1-12. Emotional Factors.
§ 1-13. Implementation of an Organized Approach.
§ 1-14. Economic Impact.
§ 1-15. Summary.
Bibliography.

§ 1-1. Scope of Problem.

Neck pain as a manifestation of illness or injury is a topic that is familiar to most individuals. It is commonly discussed by members of the legal and medical professions as well as the general public. It is frequently mentioned on radio and television as well as the daily newspapers and has caught the public's imagination. Despite the apparent universal interest in this topic there is a surprising lack of scientific medical information available. Even the medical nomenclature used to describe specific acute neck injuries is confusing. The medical and legal literature abound with terms such as acute neck sprain, acute cervical strain, cervical syndrome, hyperextension-hyperflexion neck injury, acceleration-deceleration neck injury, whiplash, and others.

Whiplash is a nonmedical term first used by Crowe in 1928 (see entry 6 in Bibliography at end of this chapter) to describe the hyperextension injury to the neck resulting from an indirect force usually a rear-end automobile collision. In this chapter I will use the term whiplash, in spite of its lack of scientific specificity, because of its common public usage, its apparent permanent ingrainment in the medical literature, its use as a codable injury diagnosis for hospital discharge and insurance reimbursement and because I find no better term available.

Whiplash injuries have been known since the first World War, when airplane pilots were often injured during catapult assisted takeoff when there was not adequate fixation of the cockpit seat. Following the early recognition and description of this condition which involved a limited number of individuals in a specialized occupational area, the magnitude of this type of injury has expanded until today, with rare exceptions, it is a frequently described injury almost universally associated with automobile accidents.

In an attempt to review the medical literature on this topic a Medline search of articles on acute neck injuries and whiplash dating back to 1966 was performed. This produced surprisingly few appropriate references. A significant percent of the references located related to infants impaired as a result of the battered child syndrome or cervical injuries at childbirth. A number of other archival retrieval sources were then investigated. The most productive of these was the TRIS (Transportation Research Information Service). This produced a number of good references not found in the usual medical literature. Therefore, while an attempt has been made to obtain reliable information, the sources of the following information are relatively limited and therefore the reliability must be considered open to some questioning.

Injuries to the neck after trauma produce a broad spectrum of disabling conditions ranging from minor neck discomfort to quadraplegia and even death. The consequences of these injuries are of great concern to many individuals — not only the individual injured but to members of the medical profession responsible for treatment, the patient's family, the employer, public insurers and lawyers. Society at large is often called upon to share the financial burdens of health care, disability, and unemployment that follows in the wake of these injuries. Because of the magnitude of the problem, automobile insurance rates have been adversely affected which therefore impacts on all insured drivers.

§ 1-2. Incidence.

While various types of trauma may result in neck pain the acute neck pain that results in the clinical syndrome referred to as whiplash are overwhelmingly the result of traffic accidents. It is this type of injury and the sequence of events that follow that frequently lead to prolonged periods of disability and litigation (entries 8, 10, 15). The precise number of neck injuries is difficult to determine. The best current information available comes primarily from the United States. However a limited amount of information is also available from Great Britain, Australia, and The Netherlands. While many estimates have been given concerning accidents and injuries the most accurate United States data appears to be that of the National Accident Sampling System which estimated that in 1979 there were over 530,000 cases of minor whiplash injury (entry 17).

§ 1-3. Estimates of Whiplash Injuries in the United States.

1979

Passenger Cars	Total Accidents	Whiplash	Percent
Towed	3,564,000	197,000	5.5
Not Towed	11,939,000	277,000	2.3
Other Vehicle	3,682,000	57,000	1.5
Total	19,185,000	531,000	2.8

This half-million people represent 2.8% of all occupants in police reported automobile accidents. In reviewing these data it is interesting to note that the gross number of whiplash injuries to individuals in automobiles that did not require towing from the scene of the accident was much higher than injuries to individuals in an accident where the vehicle required towing, and in fact, was higher than the combined total of towed vehicles and all other vehicle accidents. In addition, there is no correlation with the severity of damage to the automobile and the severity of the individuals' complaints of neck pain.

The National Safety Council has stated that 20% of all automobile accidents are rear-end impacts. It has been estimated that 85% of all neck injuries seen clinically result from automobile accidents. Of the automobile accidents that result in neck injuries 85% are rear-end impacts, the remaining 15% result from some other type of impact. (entries 11, 12, 19). McNab (entry 15) has estimated that one-fifth of exposed occupants sustained neck injuries.

While acute neck injuries do not rank as the major loss of time from work that is seen in acute low back pain, it still must be considered a significant industrial problem. There are no reliable figures available concerning whiplash injuries compared to type of employment but limited surveys of different work environments show that employers with employees who drive on public highways such as municipal transportation systems have the highest incidence of whiplash injuries while those with less public contact have lower rates. Shutt and Dohan (entry 18) in a study of industrial workers reported that the number of neck injuries sustained in automobile accidents was 14.5 per thousand employees.

When considering incidence figures one must also keep in mind the development of the "late whiplash syndrome." Late whiplash syndrome is a symptom complex which has been defined as a collection of symptoms and disabilities seen more than six months after a neck injury occurring as a result of a motor vehicle accident. The physical and emotional implications of this syndrome will be addressed in a later chapter. Balla (entries 1, 2) found a striking difference in the development of this syndrome when comparing individuals with acute neck injuries in Australia and Singapore. When he compared groups of similar patients with acute whiplash injuries in these two areas two years after the initial diagnosis none of the Singapore patients had symptoms of "late whiplash syndrome," however, it was a common finding among Australian patients with acute neck injuries. The significance and possible cause of this finding will also be reviewed later. From this and similar studies one certainly must conclude that the number of individuals suffering the "late whiplash syndrome" will show significant variations in different cultural environments.

§ 1-4. Prevention of Injury.

Since an overwhelming percentage of acute neck injuries are the result of rear-end automobile accidents it is appropriate to review certain factors concerning automobile accidents and automobile passengers which might influence the development of significant acute neck injuries. These include the wearing of seat belts and/or shoulder harnesses, the use of head restraints, the sitting location of the injured individual, whether the car was stationary or moving when hit as well as the age, sex, and size of the occupants.

§ 1-5. Passenger Position in the Car.

There is general agreement that neck injury is more frequent among front seat passengers than among rear seat passengers. (entries 14, 19). The individual most frequently injured is the front seat passenger. The number of injuries to the rear seat passenger and the vehicle driver are essentially the same.

§ 1-6. Seat Belt and Shoulder Restraints.

The influence of seat belts on acute neck injuries is dependent on other factors — the most important of which is the presence or absence of seat head restraints. If head restraints are present the use of seat belts alone result in fewer neck injuries. Without head restraints the use of seat belts alone appear to slightly increase the incidents of neck injuries. (entry 19). The combining of seat belts with a shoulder strap reduces the incidence of acute neck injuries with or without head restraints. The combined use of seat belt, shoulder strap, and head restraint significantly reduces the number of acute neck injuries.

§ 1-7. Head Restraints.

Various studies have been undertaken to evaluate the effectiveness of head restraints. Data from different sources have given figures which show a reduction in neck injuries from 10-40% with the use of head restraints. In one study (entry 13) adjustable head restraints were found to reduce injuries approximately 10%, while head restraints that were an integral part of the automobile reduced injuries 17%. This same study noted that 72% of the cars sold during 1960 to 1981 had adjustable restraints, while 25% had head restraints that were an integral part of the seat. Using this mix of adjustable and integral head restraints it was estimated that head restraints were responsible for the prevention of over 64,000 injuries per year. Other studies have estimated a significantly higher degree of protection for head restraints. While it is not possible to accurately project the reduction in acute neck injuries, it would appear that the best estimate available is that the use of head restraints has produced an approximate 20% reduction in the incidence of acute neck injuries in rear-end automobile accidents.

Studies have also shown that 75% of head restraints that are adjustable are in the lowest possible position. (entry 13). The head restraints are therefore, not placed in the appropriate position for the automobile occupant. A visual survey of drivers in 4,983 moving domestic passenger cars with adjustable head restraints in the Los Angeles and Washington, D.C. metropolitan areas indicated that in the Los Angeles area 74% of the male drivers and 57% of the female drivers had the head restraints improperly positioned. In the Washington, D.C. area 93% of the males and 80% of the females had the restraints improperly positioned. (entry 16). While this is a relatively small sample it is evident that a significant majority of the head restraints now in use in automobiles in the United States are not in the appropriate position to protect the automobile occupants. The proper placing of head restraints would undoubtedly increase their protective value significantly.

The possible use of head restraints in the rear seats of automobiles has been considered. There have been numerous studies which have shown that the use of head restraints in the rear seat of an automobile is not justified and would not significantly reduce the number of acute neck injuries.

§ 1-8. Sex.

There are conflicting data available concerning incidence of injuries in males compared to females. A majority of studies show an increased incidence of whiplash injuries in women when compared to men. Some studies have shown that neck injury frequency among women to be twice as high as among men (entry 14). Touissant and Fabeck found that significant injuries of the cervical spine were more common in men (in the ratio of 3 to 2), but whiplash injuries occurred more often in women (70%). This observation which is apparently contradictory has been confirmed by a number of other authors. (entries 5, 15, 9). The reason for this may be that women are traveling more often as passengers and the injury occurs while they are in a state of muscular relaxation. However, the driver, more often the male, may anticipate the impact and partially be able to neutralize the whiplash component by keeping his head flexed and by gripping the steering wheel. The studies which have concentrated on head-rest position have found that head rests are more protective for women than men. This is probably due to the head restraints being more often in the proper position for women.

§ 1-9. Age.

Age does not seem to be an important factor in acute neck injuries. It might be anticipated that with increasing age and the development of osteoarthritic changes in the cervical spine there would be an increased incidence of acute neck injuries with advancing age. This has not been the case. The usual age distribution for whiplash injuries has been found to be in individuals between the ages of 30 and 50.

§ 1-10. Other Factors.

Lightweight people appear to be more susceptible to acute neck injury than heavier individuals. There has also been found to be a correlation between height and neck injuries. (entry 19).

§ 1-11. Effect of Litigation.

The effect of litigation in acute neck injuries has received much attention (entries 5, 8, 12). Many articles with titles such as "The Whiplash; Tiny Impact, Tremendous Injury." (entry 3) or "Whiplash Injury of the Neck — Fact or Fancy" (entry 4) have been written. Anecdotal incidents such as the city bus filled with passengers which is rear-ended by a Volkswagen Beetle with no damage to the Volkswagen or the bus and the only injury being the bus driver who suffers an acute whiplash injury. This has led to speculation that litigation and compensation are the most important factors in the incidence and severity of whiplash injuries.

A unique factor in the type of accident which leads to whiplash injuries is that the striking vehicle is almost invariably at fault and therefore this removes the burden of proof of liability for the accident. In addition, since the injured individual rarely presents an objective demonstrable abnormality, one is left with a blameless victim incapacitated by subjective symptoms the existence of which are difficult to prove or disprove. This combination of accident events and subjective symptoms has led many individuals to see the accident and victim as a ready available candidate for legal intervention and disability remuneration.

How frequent do individuals with whiplash injuries seek monetary remuneration? This is difficult to determine because of the lack of follow-up and reporting of minor injuries and the current tendency to make out-of-court settlements. However, in a few controlled studies, well over 50% of the accident victims eventually receive some type of settlement (entry 16). A number of studies have been undertaken to determine if the awarding of a monetary settlement has resulted in significant improvement in the symptoms of injured individuals. It has been found that in individuals with only subjective complaints, over 50% improve significantly after litigation claims have been settled. In patients with objective findings, such as a reduced range of cervical movement or evidence of objective neurologic loss the percentage who improve after litigation is reduced below 25% after settlement of the insurance claim (entry 8).

§ 1-12. Emotional Factors.

One cannot overlook the presence in the whiplash injured individual of possible emotional factors which might contribute to the individual's symptoms and disability. These might be classified as either conscious malingering, or conscious exaggerating of underlying complaints or the subconscious exaggeration or modification of the underlying acute neck injury. In studies of other types of back injuries the conscious malingerer has been found to be relatively infrequent. The more usual circumstance appears to be the conscious exaggeration of an underlying complaint.

While it is sometimes difficult to separate the conscious from the subconscious exaggeration, under most circumstances this differentiation can be made fairly accurately by a careful examiner performing a detailed history and physical examination. We have found the typical conscious manipulator is the patient who arrives at the physician's office with extensive documentation of the accident or injury, demonstrates a persistently defensive attitude, is often overtly hostile, withholds information, actively involves his attorney to the degree that he may not answer relatively simple questions without consulting his lawyer, and shows variable and inconsistent hysterical symptoms. The patient with a subconscious emotional overlay often demonstrates a significantly different pattern. This individual often shows a lack of concern for documentation — while starting with a defensive attitude, this may decrease with only transient episodes of anger, and he does not knowingly withhold information. If hysterical symptoms are present they are usually constant. While these patients usually have an attorney they have a much more passive involvement with the lawyer.

While these are general descriptions which do not apply in all cases, this type of differentiation has served us well in managing the course of treatment and particularly in the use of independent medical examiners for employees suffering acute neck injuries.

§ 1-13. Implementation of an Organized Approach.

In 1980 this author undertook an evaluation of employees off work due to job related accidents in a public utility. Low back pain was found to be the predominant injury resulting in time away from work and therefore an organized approach to the treatment of individuals suffering low-back injuries was undertaken. With the implementation of this low-back program it soon became apparent that a similar approach could be used in other orthopaedic problems. Therefore, the algorithm developed by Wiesel, Feffer and Rothman (entry 20) was implemented for acute neck injuries. The medical aspects of this approach will be discussed in a later chapter, however, I will briefly review certain of the organizational aspects.

§ 1-13

The cervical spine algorithm was applied to employees with acute neck injuries at the Potomac Electric Power Company (PEPCO) from July 1, 1981 through June 30, 1982. Pepco is a public utility which supplies electric power to the Washington, D.C. area. It has 5,335 employees of whom 3,467 are blue collar workers. The Medical Department has a full-time Medical Director and all job-related injuries are evaluated by the Medical Department. If an employee is injured at work he may choose to see a private physician, but the Medical Department has the authority to follow the employee's care as it determines what is medically indicated.

Every patient with an acute cervical spine injury was evaluated within seven days of the time of the injury. The patients were then seen periodically, their treatment monitored as necessary, until their return to work. If during the course of treatment monitoring there was significant disagreement with the diagnosis or treatment recommendations of the attending physician, the attending physician was contacted for a discussion of the treatment differences. Under most circumstances this resulted in a better understanding of the treatment recommendations or a modification of the treatment program. If there was not significant agreement on the treatment being provided, a third physician was contacted for an independent medical opinion. The physicians monitoring the treatment were two university-based orthopaedic surgeons who were considered unbiased and were excluded from participation in active treatment of these employees in their offices. This enabled the Medical Department to provide employees with good orthopaedic care, free from any potential financial bias.

With this program we significantly reduced the time employees have been off of work or on light duty due to whiplash injuries. The lost time days were reduced by 65%

and the light duty days by 66%. The total number of acute neck injury accidents reported were also reduced by over 50% when compared with our baseline period in 1981. No other significant changes took place in the Company. The number and types of automobile accidents reported were essentially unchanged in the two-year periods.

One possible reason for this reduction in reported whiplash injuries is that the close monitoring of employee accidents became well known in the Company and may have resulted in fewer accident claims of injuries for individuals with minimal or non-existent injuries.

An important factor in the successful implementation of this program has been the availability of light and limited duty work. It is the Company's policy that if an individual is ready to return to work on a light or limited duty status, every attempt will be made to find work that fits within the specified limitations. That is, if the limitations placed on the employee by the Medical Department's physician are no prolonged standing, no overhead work, etc., the Company will make every effort to find a job that fits these limitations. In the past, there had been some reluctance on the part of managers to accept light and limited duty employees back on the job since they are added to their complement and yet, may be doing less work than a regular employee. This reluctance has been partially overcome by including the ability to find light and limited duty work for employees as part of the department manager's performance review when evaluating his effectiveness as a manager. This close monitoring of injured employees and the cooperation of a concerned management at all levels has been successful in the significant reduction in the time injured employees are off of work.

Another factor has been the careful follow-up of employees who have third-party suits. Employees who are injured as a result of an automobile accident in which there is a third-party payment to the employee, are carefully followed by the Company. If there is reimbursement to the employee based on time off of work, or medical costs, the Company insists on being reimbursed for these company incurred expenses. This fact is made known to the employee in a non-threatening way very early in the course of the accident treatment, so as to try and minimize the possible prolongation of disability to justify a higher settlement. How effective this has been in the total program is not known.

Employees involved in non-job related automobile accidents in which there is the possibility of a monetary settlement from a third party are also informed of this company policy. The employees involved in personal injury accidents are informed that medical expenses paid under the Company's self-insured medical and hospital benefit programs must be repaid if there is a third-party settlement.

§ 1-14. Economic Impact.

As a part of the review of this topic an attempt was made to obtain figures on the costs of medical care, hospital care, and monetary settlements for whiplash injuries. Despite a review of current medical literature we have been unable to find a reliable estimate of the general economic impact of this condition or the magnitude of the medical expenses or monetary settlements. This is in contradiction to low back pain accidents where estimates are available for items such as time away from work, medical and hospital costs, and other related costs. Since most of these accidents are not work related and therefore not covered by workers' compensation, there is no central source available for this information. In addition the majority of claims appear to be settled by out-of-court settlements which compound the problem of estimating total costs.

We have therefore attempted to estimate costs using the extremely limited data available and applying it to the national scene. Using as our base the National Accident Sampling System estimate of 531,000 whiplash injuries and utilizing our personal experience with a limited number of whiplash injuries followed in our orthopaedic clinic, we have projected the costs impact. Since few of these employees undergo surgery and their periods of hospitalization appear to be short, the major initial expenses incurred are physician, physical therapy, and appliances such as Tens units. The other major expenses involve time away from work and any final monetary settlement.

In a review of recent cases we found that the total cost of these items and the final settlement of the case averaged $10,000. If these figures are then applied to the total number of whiplash injuries an estimate of 5.3 billion dollars annually would be the cost of this injury in the United States. We understand the fallacies of this type of projection but have been unable to find a more reliable natural estimate.

§ 1-15. Summary.

Acute neck injuries are a significant medical problem in the United States. While not the most commonly occurring injury in industry — it is seen frequently enough to be of great concern to most employers, particularly those whose employees are involved in public transportation. Although data is limited, this clinical syndrome probably accounts for over five billion dollars per year in medical and other related expenses.

Acute neck injuries have resulted in a great deal of discussion but very little verifiable medical information. It is apparent that the major initiating factor is a rear-end automobile impact. It also appears clear that the number of resulting injuries could be significantly reduced by the proper use of seat belts, shoulder restraints, and the proper positioning of head restraints.

After the injury has occurred it has been shown that the implementation of an organized systematic approach to the treatment of these injuries, which includes careful evaluation, appropriate medical monitoring, and early return to light work has been successful in reducing disability by over 50%. The role of litigation in prolongation of disability appears to be significant. The need for research in all phases of this condition is apparent. Studies on prevention, diagnosis, treatment, and economic and social consequences need to receive increased emphasis if we expect to see a reduction in the frequency and severity of this condition.

BIBLIOGRAPHY

1. Balla, J.I. The late whiplash syndrome. Aust NZJ Surg 50(6):610-616, 1980.
2. Balla, J.I. The late whiplash syndrome: a study of an illness in Australia and Singapore. Cult. Med Psychiatry 6(2):191-210, 1982.
3. Bocchi, L., Osro, C.A. Whiplash injuries of the cervical spine. Italian J. Ortho. and Trauma. 9(Suppl): 171-181, 193.
4. Braaf, M.M., Rosner, S. Whiplash injury of the neck — fact or fancy? Int Surg Dig 46:176-182, 1966.
5. Cammark, K.V. Whiplash injuries to the neck. Am Jr Surg 93:663-666, 1957.
6. Crowe, H.E. Injuries to the cervical spine. Paper presented at the meeting of the Western Orthopaedic Association, San Francisco, 1928.
7. Gay, J.R., Abbott, K.H. Common whiplash injuries of the neck. JAMA 152:1698, 1983.
8. Gotten, N. Survey of one hundred cases of whiplash injury after settlement of litigation. JAMA 162:856-857, 1956.
9. Guy, J.E. The whiplash: tiny impact, tremendous injury. Ind Med and Surg 37(9):688-691, 1968.
10. Hohl, M. Soft-tissue injuries of the neck in automobile accidents: factors influencing prognosis. J. Bone Joint Surg (Am) 56-A:1675-82, 1974.

11. Jackson, R. The positive findings in alleged neck injuries. Am Jr Otho 6:178-187, 1964.
12. Jackson, R. Crashes cause most neck pain. Am Med News Dec. 5, 1966.
13. Kahane, C.J. An evaluation of head restraints. Federal Motor Vehicle Safety Standard 22. Tech Rpt Feb. 1982, 308-327.
14. Kihlberg, J.K. Flexion-torsion neck injury in rear end impacts. Proceedings of 13 annual conference of American Association for automotive Med Oct. 1969.
15. McNab, I. Acceleration injuries of the cervical spine. Jr Bone Joint Surg 46A:1797-1799, 1964.
16. O'Neill, B., Haddon, W., Kelley, A.B., Sorenson, W. Automobile head restraint — frequency of neck injury claims in relation to the presence of head restraints. Am Jr Pub Health 62:399-406, 1972.
17. Partyka, S. Whiplash and other inertial force neck injuries in traffic accidents. Paper for Mathematical Analysis Division, National Center for Statistics and Analysis. Dec. 1981.
18. Schutt, C.H., Dohan, F.C. Neck injury to women in auto accidents. A metropolitan plague. JAMA 206:2689-94, 1968.
19. States, J.D., Korn, M.W., Masengill, J.B. The enigma of whiplash injuries. N.Y. State J Med 70(24)2971-2978, 1970.
20. Wiesel, S.W., Feffer, H.L., Rothman, R.H. The development of a cervical spine algorithm and its prospective application to industrial patients. J.O.M. 27:4, 272-276, 1985.

CHAPTER 2

ANATOMY AND PATHOPHYSIOLOGY OF NECK PAIN

Jeffery L. Stambough, M.D.
Richard H. Rothman, M.D., Ph.D.

§ 2-1. Introduction to Neck Anatomy.
  § 2-1(A). Osseous Anatomy.
    § 2-1(A)(1). Occiput.
    § 2-1(A)(2). Atlas (C1).
    § 2-1(A)(3). Axis (C2).
    § 2-1(A)(4). Lower Cervical Vertebrae (C3-C7).
  § 2-1(B). Intervertebral Disc (IVD).
  § 2-1(C). Occipito-Atlanto-Axial Articulation.
  § 2-1(D). Ligaments and Apophyseal Joints.
  § 2-1(E). Blood Supply.
  § 2-1(F). Innervation.
  § 2-1(G). Brachial Plexua.
  § 2-1(H). Muscles.
§ 2-2. Pathophysiology of Neck Pain.
§ 2-3. Basic Scientific Knowledge of Cervical Spine.
  § 2-3(A). Kinematics.
  § 2-3(B). Biochemistry.
  § 2-3(C). Biomechanics and Stability.
  § 2-3(D). Nutrition.
  § 2-3(E). Immunology.
  § 2-3(F). Nociceptive Factors.
§ 2-4. Clinical Condition.
  § 2-4(A). Neck Sprain — Neckache.
  § 2-4(B). Acute Herniated Disc.
  § 2-4(C). Cervical Degenerative Disc Disease.
    § 2-4(C)(1). Cervical Spondylosis (Cervical Spinal Stenosis).
    § 2-4(C)(2). Cervical Spondylosis With Myelopathy.
  § 2-4(D). Rheumatoid Arthritis.
Bibliography.
Table I.   Structures Causing Neck Pain.
Table II. Causes of Neck and Neck Related Pain Syndromes.
Table III. Mean Range of Cervical Motion of the Spine (Degrees).

Table IV. Physical Examination — Disc Herniation.
Figure 1. The Atlas Viewed From Above and Below.
Figure 2. The Axis.
Figure 3. Typical Lower Cervical Vertebra.
Figure 4. Three-Dimensional Anatomy of the Cup-Like Articulations of the Occipital-Atlantal Joints.
Figure 5. The Cruciform and Tectorial Ligaments.
Figure 6. Cervical Spine Viewed From the Side.
Figure 7. Lower Cervical Spine in Neutral Position.
Figure 8. Vertebral Artery.
Figure 9. Sinuvertebral Nerve.
Figure 10. Brachial Plexus and Lower Cervical Spine.

§ 2-1. Introduction to Neck Anatomy.

The neck is a cylindrical structure connecting the head and trunk segments through which pass blood vessels, nerves, muscles, bones, joints, ligaments, intervertebral disc, and connective tissue. Any one of these structures may under pathologic circumstances cause neck pain, but it is only those causes related to the cervical spine and its supporting structures that are discussed in this chapter.

The neck is covered by skin which has a rich innervation and blood supply. The dorsal or posterior skin is thicker than the ventral or anterior. Tension lines representing skin folds perpendicular to the pull of the neck muscles run transversely about the neck. For this reason, anterior cervical skin incisions which are transverse give the best cosmetic scars. Immediately under the skin is a subcutaneous muscle, the platysma.

The normal anatomy of the bone, intervertebral disc, ligaments, joints, neck muscles, occipito-atlanto-axial articulation, blood and nervous supply, and the brachial plexus will be discussed in the following sections (§§ 2-1(A) to 2-1(G)) (entry 32).

§ 2-1(A). Osseous Anatomy.

The osseous anatomy of the cervical spine includes 7 cervical vertebrae and the occiput (base of the skull). The upper cervical vertebrae are peculiar while the lower cervical vertebrae (C3-C7) are similar. For purposes of this discussion, several generalizations are in order; all but two of the cervical vertebrae (C1 & C7) have spinous processes which are (1) bifid, (2) slant caudally, and (3) increase in size from cephalad to caudad. The bodies of the cervical vertebrae except for C1 and C2 are wider side to side than front to back. Additionally the body of the vertebrae tend to be taller in the front than in the back. Except for C7, all cervical vertebrae have openings in their transverse processes called transverse foramina and are the most characteristic aspect of the osseology. The overall shape of the C-spine reveals no normal lateral curvature and a gentle lordotic curve which has its apex at about C4-C5. The cervical spine is the most mobile of the spinal segments and the most susceptible to injury or degenerative processes which are known to associate with motion (e.g., cervical spondylosis).

§ 2-1(A)(1). Occiput.

The occiput or basiocciput represents the base of the skull. It has two downward projecting concave condyles which articulate with the C1 (atlas) lateral masses. The atlanto-occipital joint is a true synovial joint, which depends on its joint capsule for its primary support.

§ 2-1(A)(2). Atlas (C1).

The most atypical of all the cervical vertebrae is the atlas. The atlas is so named because it holds the head. It has no true vertebral body. The atlas is a ringed structure flanked laterally by two large bony prominences called lateral masses. The upper surface of the lateral mass is slightly convex to match the occipital condyles, while the inferior surface is slightly concave (see Figure 1).

§ 2-1(A)(3). Axis (C2).

The peculiar shape of the axis allows for 50% of the normal rotation motion in the neck. The axis has two major portions; a slender mushroom shaped odontoid process or dens and the vertebral body-arch complex. Embyologically the dens represent the body of C1 and articulates with the back edge of the C1 ring in a true synovial joint. This complex articulation is held together by a series of ligaments; a transverse ligament, two alar ligaments, an apical ligament, and cruciform ligaments. These ligaments are the key to the stability of this articulation. The axis body contains articular facets which are slightly convex superiorly and inferiorly. The axis has a well developed and prominent pars interarticularis which is commonly fractured in the so called traumatic spondylolithesis of the axis or hangman's fracture.

§ 2-1(A)(4). Lower Cervical Vertebrae (C3-C7).

These bony vertebrae have a similar shape and differ primarily by their posteriorly projecting spinous processes. The vertebral bodies are relatively small and trapezoidal. From the posterior superior border of the vertebral body projects the pedicle. These pedicles give rise to midline lamina (or act like shingles), and superior (joint faces to the front) and inferior (joint faces toward the back) articular processes. Out the midline of the lamina projects the spinous process. These bony components form a housing for the spinal cord and make lateral openings or foramina for the exit of spinal nerves beneath the pedicle. In the normal situation the spinal nerve occupies about 50% of this opening. Additional paired articulations along the body form postnatally as the uncovertebral joint. The superior border projects upward as an uncus or hook to articulate with the enchancrure or anvil of the vertebra above. These uncovertebral joints are unique to the mobile cervical spine (see Figure 3).

§ 2-1(B). Intervertebral Disc (IVD).

The intervertebral disc separates the bodies of the vertebrae from C2-T1. There is no intervertebral disc between the occiput, C1, and C2. The IVD is divided into an outer fibrous shell called the annulus fibrosis and a central semi-liquid material called the nucleus pulposus (entry 9). The normal IVD is slightly higher in front. The IVD is avascular both in utero and in the adult but receives a nerve and blood supply in the outer margins of the annulus.

§ 2-1(C). Occipito-Atlanto-Axial Articulation.

The atlanto-occipital and atlantoaxial joints are shown in Figures 4 and 5. The atlanto-occipital joint is primarily involved in flexion-extension and lateral flexion, whereas the atlantoaxial joint is involved in rotation of the head on the neck, and flexion and extension. The atlantoaxial articulation is the most complex and unique joint in the spine. The stability of the atlantoaxial articulation is provided entirely by ligaments where the transverse ligament is the most important stabilizer biomechanically.

§ 2-1(D). Ligaments and Apophyseal Joints.

The ligaments which surround the spinal column function as supporting structures and are divided into two major groups along with the apophyseal or synovial joint; the anterior complex and the posterior complex (see Figures 6 and 7). The anterior complex consists of the anterior and posterior longitudinal ligaments, uncovertebral joints, and the IVD. The posterior complex consists of the facet joints with their capsule, ligamentum flavum, interspinous ligaments, and a large supraspinous ligament called the ligamentum nuchae.

The apophyseal joints are true synovial joints containing hyaline articular cartilage which is bathed in synovial fluid secreted by the synovial cells lining the capsule. There are a total of four joints per articular segment from C2-C7. The atlanto-axial and atlanto-occipital joints have only two each, the dens — atlantal ring complex, and the atlas — basiocciput complex respectively. Since the facet or apophyseal joints are true synovial joints, they are subject to the same pathologic processes as other synovial joints (e.g., rheumatoid arthritis, osteoarthritis, etc.). The uncovertebral joints are not true synovial joints.

§ 2-1(E). Blood Supply.

The major arterial blood supply to the cervical spinal column and spinal cord is the vertebral artery (see Figure 8). The vertebral artery, a branch of the subclavian artery, enters the transverse foramina at C6 and ends after looping around the atlas as the basilar artery supplying the hindbrain. The artery gives off branches which supply the bone, joints, muscles, as well as the neural elements. As a consequence of its relationship at the superior edge of the atlas, it is vulnerable to injury in posterior surgery in the atlanto-occipital area.

The venous blood supply parallels the arterial in its anatomic design. The veins are valveless and thus communicate in both directions depending on pressure differentials. This explains why tumor or infection can spread from the pelvic area to the central nervous system without entering the systemic circulation.

§ 2-1(F). Innervation.

The nerve supply to the spinal column is derived from the spinal nerve root once it passes the neural foramina. The cervical nerve roots number eight in total with the first cervical nerve exiting between the atlas and the occiput. Subsequently, the cervical nerve roots C2-C8 exit from the neural foramina so that the lower cervical nerve root exits after crossing the intervertebral disc numbered one higher (e.g., C5 crosses the C4-5 disc).

The mixed spinal nerve contains motor fibers, sensory axons of the dorsal root ganglia, as well as preganglionics from the autonomonic nervous system. The main spinal nerve gives off three major branches before continuing into the brachial plexus; (1) primary dorsal rami; (2) primary anterior rami; and (3) the sinuvertebral nerve of Lushka (see Figure 9). The primary anterior and posterior rami supply the muscles about the spine and chest wall-abdomen. The sinuvertebral nerve contains only sensory and sympathetic fibers and each nerve branches to adjacent levels within the spinal canal. The nerve provides sensory ending for the entire spinal canal except for the nucleus pulposus and the ligamentum flavum. The sinuvertebral nerve is very sensitive to stretch and possibly ischemia. The facet joints are innervated by a branch of the primary dorsal rami and descends to at least one vertebral level below.

From the above discussion it is obvious that there are several possible sources of pain in and around the spinal column. The phenomena of referred pain or pain distance from the source follows the anatomic course of the given nerve. This helps to example why cervical spine disease is often referred to the scapular area, the shoulder, or the chest wall.

§ 2-1(G). Brachial Plexua.

The primary anterior rami of the fourth cervical nerve to the first thoracic nerve form an interconnection or plexus called the brachial plexus (see Figure 10). The cervical spinal cord actually is enlarged in this area due to the larger number of motor neurons needed to provide the motor axons for the brachial plexus. The brachial plexus form the major nerves that supply the muscles of the upper extremity.

These ramifications are important in our understanding of cervical disease and arm pain. Each of these contributing nerve roots supply a specific muscle or muscle group with an attendant reflex and sensory area.

§ 2-1(H). Muscles.

The muscles of the neck can be defined by anatomic limits, innervation, and function. Since the cervical spine is the most mobile section of the spine it contains the most elaborate and specialized muscle system of the spine.

The posterior muscles of the neck are divided into two groups; those which attach the upper extremity to the spine and those which act only on the spine. The trapezius muscle is the most superficial muscle of the posterior group and is innervated by the spinal accessory nerve; the 11th cranial nerve. The muscle originates from the spinous processes of C2-T12 and occiput to insert on the scapula, acromion, and clavicle. It functions to stabilize and elevate the scapula. Another muscle, the levator scapulae elevates the medial scapula as well as rotates it medially. It is intervated by the nerve to the levator scapulae and runs from the transverse process of the upper cervical spine to the superior medial scapula.

The deep muscles surrounding the spine are also called spinal intrinsic muscles and function primarily as spinal extensors. The muscles from superficial to deep are the splenius muscles, the spino-transversalis group and the transverospinalis group. They are all innervated segmentally by the branches of primary dorsal rami of one or more cervical nerves. This arrangement is related to the embryonic development and is termed segmental innervation.

The anterior cervical muscles function to flex the head and neck. The muscles are divided into two large triangles by the sternocleidomastoid muscle innervated by the spinal accessory nerve. The muscle arises from two heads; sternal and clavicular. Medial and deep to the sternocleidomastoid muscle is the carotid sheath containing the internal carotid artery, vagus nerve, and internal jugular vein. The so called strap muscles (attach to the hyoid, thyroid cartilage, and sternum) are medial to the sternocleidomastoid except for the posterior aspect of the omohyoid muscle and function to flex the neck. They are innervated by segmental branches of the cervical anterior primary rami. The muscles above the hyoid are innervated by the hypoglossal nerve and rarely encountered in anterior cervical spine surgery. Deep and medial to the carotid sheath is the anterior cervical spine vertebral bodies covered by a prevertebral fascia.

Immediately anterior to the cervical spine is the esophagus, trachea, and thyroid gland. These are covered by an intermediate fascial layer separate from the prevertebral fascia. Laterally along the transverse processes are the longus colli muscles. These muscles cover the vertebral artery in the transverse foramina and flex the neck. they are also innervated by local segmental primary anterior rami nerves. In the relatively avascular space between the anterior vertebral body and the carotid sheath pass several important nerves, arteries, and veins.The superior laryngeal nerve travels at the C3-4 level with the superior thyroid artery. Caudal to this at about the C6-7 level passes the inferior thyroid artery and vein. The recurrent laryngeal nerve, a branch of the vagus nerve, provides an essential innervation to the vocal cord. It crosses this plane at different levels on the left and right side. On the right the nerve loops around the subclavian artery before it enters the visceral fascia between the esophagus and trachea. Its course is somewhat variable. The left nerve loops around the arch of the aorta before entering the visceral fascia as on the right. Its course is more predictable and lower in the interval between the vertebrae and carotid sheath.

§ 2-2. Pathophysiology of Neck Pain.

The pathophysiology of neck pain attempts to provide the clinician with the understanding as to the cause of series of events leading to a particular clinical situation. To understand the origin of such pain, one must first ask, what structures can produce pain? The neck, bone, disc, ligaments, joints, muscles, fascia, and skin are innervated by pain fibers. Only the nucleus pulposus, inner layers of the annulus fibrosus, and the substance of the ligamentum flavum have no innervation. Thus, the origin of axial neck pain is potentially many.

Furthermore we must consider other problems; shoulder and arm pain, and referred pain. As discussed in this chapter, § 2-1, the cervical nerve roots C4-T1 form the brachial plexus which innervates the structures of the shoulder and arm. Nerve irritation in the neck either by stretch, inflammation, or vascular insufficiency can cause pain perceived as localized shoulder or arm. Referred pain is a well-known phenomenon in which pathology can be perceived as pain at a site away from its cause. For example, subdiaphragmatic processes such as cholecysitis can be referred to the right shoulder and neck as pain localized there. Structures causing neck and upper shoulder area pain other than those in the neck are listed in Table I.

The differential diagnosis of neck, shoulder, and arm pain is long including local and distance pathology. (See Table II).

How common is neck pain? While pain involving the low back affects almost everyone, neck pain is not as common. One possible explanation is that neck pain tends to be less debilitating than low back pain and has not been as much an occupational problem (entry 18). In one study in Sweden, 40% of the population complained of neck pain at one time or another. Unlike LBP, only a few studies discuss the epidemiology of neck pain but several important factors may be gleaned from the literature. Neck pain is associated with back pain but tends to occur between 5-10 years later. Therefore, most patients who present with neck pain tend to be older (fourth and fifth decades).

Prolapsed cervical intervertebral disc, the neck counterpart to the lumbar herniated disc, was studied by Kelsey et al., (entry 19). These authors found a male predominance with a peak incidence in the fourth decade. Three factors strongly correlated with this diagnosis; frequent lifting of heavy objects, frequent diving from a board, and cigarette smoking. Automobile driving and vibrating equipment contact was less strongly associated.

Degenerative disc disease or spondylosis is the most common cause of neck pain. The patient tends to be about a decade older than the patient with prolapsed disc and predominantly male. For a working population over the age of 50, over 50% of the people will have neck pain and stiffness. Of this group some 25-40 percent will have at least one episode of brachalgia or arm pain associated with their neck symptoms. Kellgren, in a study of persons living in Leigh, found 82% of patients over 55 to have X-ray evidence of cervical degenerative disc disease. Radiographic characterization of patients with neck pain revealed that only disc space narrowing was associated with this pain.

This study as well as that of Hitselberger and Witten (entry 15) indicate that radiograph or myelogram cannot solely explain the patient's neck or arm symptoms.

From these considerations, a typical patient presenting to the doctor would be a male about age 40 who was employed in a manual labor job possibly requiring driving a fork lift. He would smoke one to two packs of cigarettes per day. His exam would reveal loss of normal motion; pain radiating to the upper shoulders or upper thoracic area, and X-ray evidence of degenerative disc disease. He would have about a 33% chance of having arm pain, and be less likely to have neurologic dysfunction correlating with the arm pain.

§ 2-3. Basic Scientific Knowledge of Cervical Spine.

A great deal of basic science research involving the cervical spine has accumulated over the past several years. These effects have been interdisciplinary focusing attention to the following areas of clinical importance: biochemical, biomechanics, kinematics, nutrition, immunology, pain nociception, and psychosocial behavior. A brief review of these aspects of our basic knowledge is presented in the ensuing sections to serve as a foundation for our clinical management of problems of the neck and cervical spine.

§ 2-3(A). Kinematics.

Kinematics basically is the study of motion without the effects of muscles or other external forces. The cervical spine is the most mobile portion of the human spine and moves in the following manner: flexion, extension, lateral flexion, and rotation. These motions are dictated by (1) the geometry of the facet joints (2) intervertebral discs, and (3) the ligamentous support of the bony elements (entry 35).

The facet joints are angled 45 degrees downward and are parallel in the frontal plane. This factor accounts for primary motion patterns of the cervical spine. The atlantoaxial articulation is essentially a ring rotating around a peg (dens), and accounts for 50-60% of all neck rotation. Normal neck motions at the various levels are given in Table III. The normal neck moves as much as 130 degrees in flexion and extension, 75 degrees in lateral flexion, and 160 degrees in rotation (entry 35). These motions diminish to varying degrees with age.

§ 2-3(B). Biochemistry.

From the biochemical point of view, the intervertebral disc has been the most studied since it is the source of many clinical problems. The normal architecture of the intervertebral disc has been described. On the microscopic level, it consists of two adjacent hyaline cartilage end plates, and annulus fibrosus which is obliquely layered at angles between 40-80 degrees, and a nucleus pulposus consisting of an extracellular gelatinous matrix constituting a loosely arrayed network of collagen fibrils and a paucity of cells. The annulus fibrosus is thicker and stronger anteriorly and firmly attaches to the cartilage end plates and vertebral body. The annulus fibrosus contains the more liquid nucleus pulposus and gradually becomes thinner as it approaches the central nucleus pulposus.

One of the primary functions of the intervertebral disc is to stabilize the spine as well as allow for normal motion. To accomplish this, the normal intervertebral disc acts like a shock absorber by changing shape as the circumstances dictate. This property of the normal intervertebral disc depends primarily on its ability to bind or imbibe water. The water binding capacity of the intervertebral disc depends on two factors; the concentration of electrolytes and the concentration of proteoglycans in the nucleus pulposus. It has been demonstrated that with loading the normal disc loses water but increases its concentrations of salts. This in turn provides for an osmotic gradient to replenish the fluid once the disc is unloaded. Proteoglycan, the principal macromolecule of the nucleus pulposus, is a negatively charge protein which can attract water (hydrophilic). The water content of the intervertebral disc decreases with age which is particularly explained by a decrease in proteoglycan content (entry 16).

The intervertebral disc is a relatively avascular structure composed of 99% matrix and 1% cells. The cells survive by diffusion (entry 33). The matrix is composed of glycoproteins, collagen, proteoglycans, and other proteins. Collagen is the principal component of the annulus fibrosus. Of the four major subtypes of collagens, Type I (found in tendon, skin, knee, and ligaments) and Type II (found in hyaline cartilage) are found in the intervertebral disc. The outer layers of the annulus fibrosus contain primarily Type I collagen whereas the inner layers have more Type II. This differential is not apparent in the adolescent disc, but develops with increasing age (entry 5). This is thought to represent the response of the disc to repetitive forces and stresses since Type II (65% of a normal disc) has definite hydroscopic properties. Type I collagen is better able to handle tensile or stretching forces and has a restricted water content. Recently, elastin, a protein with elastic properties has also been identified in the intervertebral disc (entry 14). The noncollagen proteins of the intervertebral disc increase with age; nucleus pulposus 20 to 45%, and annulus fibrosus 5 to 25%.

Degenerative disc disease is a biologic process associated with aging. Several of the important age-related changes in the intervertebral disc have already been mentioned. To summarize, as the normal intervertebral disc ages, it gradually loses its ability to attract and hold water. This factor is explained by the changes in proteoglycans biochemistry as these macromolecules are found to have a diminished molecular weight, reduced ability to aggregate, and an increase in keratan sulfate content (entry 1). Furthermore, the annulus may undergo collagen degeneration as evidenced by an increase with age of noncollagenous proteins called betaproteins (10% at age 45 and 65% after age 45) (entry 26). These are relative changes believed to have significant secondary structural effects mainly in the facet joints and joint capsules posteriorly.

The ligaments of the spine (e.g., posterior and anterior longitudinal ligaments) contain predominantly Type I collagen with small amounts of Type III collagen (entry 36). These ligaments are important stabilizers of the cervical spine.

§ 2-3(C). Biomechanics and Stability.

Much of what is know about the normal biomechanics and pathomechanics of the cervical spine has been learned from static mechanical testing of cadaveric specimens in the laboratory. There is a wealth of information available discussing dynamic mechanics of all aspects of the spine. It is well established that forces and stresses can be applied to the spine in any combination of flexion, extension, rotation, and shear. These stresses affect the entire motion segment including the IVD, facet joints and capsules, anterior and posterior longitudinal ligaments, uncovertebral joints, and the other ligamentous structures. In real life, the muscles and the fascial attachments interact with the cervical spine to accommodate load, alter forces, as well as direct motion. Whereas the lumbar spine is well suited to accommodate heavy loads and provide stability, the cervical spine is better suited for mobility and is not required to transmit heavy loads. (Head weighs only 5-7 pounds.)

The biomechanical studies involving the cervical spine have concentrated on two major aspects (entry 1); kinematics (§ 2-3(A)), and clinical stability (entry 2). Stability as it applies to the spine may be defined as "the ability of the spine under physiologic loads to limit patterns of displacement so as not to damage or irritate the spinal cord or nerve roots and, in addition, to prevent incapacitating deformity or pain due to structural changes" (entry 35). While the issue of clinical spine stability is germane primarily in traumatic injuries of the cervical spine, the subject also applies to disorders of the neck as a consequence of rheumatoid arthritis.

§ 2-3(D). Nutrition.

The intervertebral disc has no intrinsic blood supply and hence, depends on the passive diffusion of small molecules for its nutrition. The blood supply to the intervertebral disc area is supplied by the segmental arteries which feed a structure, consisting of an arteriole, venule, and a glomerular tuft of capillaries ending near the vertebral end plate (entry 34). Recently, the importance of load in disc nutrition has been emphasized. In a manner similar to articular cartilage, the intervertebral disc diffusion is enhanced by a sponge-like action as the disc regains height once a load is removed. When the disc loses height, it does so by losing primarily water. This, in turn, creates a high salt concentration which produces an osmotic gradient favoring the reaccumulation of this water. Proteoglycans and other hydrophilic molecules will also favor this reaccumulation. With this exchange, the nutritive molecules like glucose, sulfate, etc., come into the disc and waste products can leave. This exchange of nutrients can occur through the cartilage end plates as well as through the annulus. The fact that intermittent loading has a beneficial effect on disc nutrition has clinical implications for the management of disc disease (entry 16). Also, cigarette smoking has been shown to significantly affect the nutrition of the disc by altering the already limited blood supply to the cartilage end plate (entry 17). Hypotheses have been suggested that the posterior annulus may have nutritional inadequacy accounting for the high incidence of disc herniations in this area.

§ 2-3(E). Immunology.

As previously stated, the normal intervertebral disc is avascular. As a consequence, the intervertebral disc and especially the nucleus pulposus seems to be an immunologically privileged site (entry 26). Naylor was the first to suggest than an autoimmune reaction may occur when degenerative changes within an intervertebral disc expose these proteins to the host's immune system. This autoimmune response in vitro has demonstrated a cell mediated mechanism of inflammation. In vitro evidence exists for this process, no definitive in vivo documentation has been found (entry 23). While this mechanism is attractive in explaining the inflammatory response in symptomatic radiculitis, other possibilities exist like ischemic neuropathy, defects in intraaxial transport or other local biochemical changes.

Rheumatoid arthritis is a systemic inflammatory disorder which can affect almost every organ of the body. The disorder has a propensity for the cervical spine and attacks the multiple synovial joints within the cervical spine. Rheumatoid arthritis is believed to an autoimmune disorder in which antigen-antibody complexes produces a humoral medicated inflammatory response in these synovial joints. The primary pathologic process is an erosive synovitis.This inflammatory reaction results in synovial proliferation, pannus formation, ligamentous destruction, and osteopenia (entry 21).

§ 2-3(F). Nociceptive Factors.

The underlying premise of this chapter is to identify the source of pain in and about the neck including arm pain so as to institute the appropriate treatment. The perspective of pain depends upon the peripheral sensation of pain (nociceptor) transmitted via a peripheral nerve to higher centers. The two nerves which meet this criterion for the cervical spine are the primary dorsal ramus, supplying sensation to the facet joints and posterior ligaments, and the sinuvertebral nerve as discussed previously. The sinuvertebral nerve can be stimulated by cervical disc injection producing pain in the neck as well as referred pain to the head, scapula, chest, shoulder, or arm depending on the level involved. The mechanism by which radicular pain is produced involves inflammation and has been hypothesized by some to involve scarring about the nerve root as a consequence of a herniated disc. Referred pain tends to be dull, nondermatomal and aching in quality compared to the lightning-like, sharp, or lacinating pain of true radicular arm pain (entries 13, 23).

Over the past decade, an increasing number of studies involving the central perception of pain have been published. The discovery of naturally occurring opiate-like compounds called enkephalins and endorphins have opened a vast door in the study of pain. These substances can be enhanced by exercise and depressed by exogenous narcotics (entry 7). Further research into this exciting field will hopefully aid in the management of acute as well as chronic pain processes.

§ 2-4. Clinical Condition.

There are many conditions which may present as neck pain with or without arm pain in any particular individual (see Table IV). However, the following five more common musculoskeletal problems will be presented in some detail: cervical sprain, acute herniated disc, cervical spondylosis (cervical spinal stenosis), cervical spondylosis with myelopathy, and rheumatoid arthritis.

§ 2-4(A). Neck Sprain — Neckache.

Neck sprain, while a misnomer, describes a clinical condition involving a non-radiating discomfort or pain about the neck area associated with a concomitant loss of neck motion (stiffness). While the clinical syndrome may present as a headache, most often the pain is located in the middle to lower part of the back of the neck. Unlike the hyperextension injury, a history of injury is rarely obtained but the pain may start after a night's rest or on simply turning the head. The source of the pain is most commonly believed to be the ligaments about the cervical spine and/or the surrounding muscles. The axial pain may also be produced by small annular tears without disc herniation, or from the facet joints (entry 32).

The pain associated with a neck sprain is most often a dull aching pain which is exacerbated by neck motion. The pain is usually abated by rest or immobilization. The pain may be referred to other mesenchymal structures derived from a similar sclerotome during embryogenesis. Common referred pain patterns included the scapular area, the posterior shoulder, the occipital area, or the anterior chest wall (cervical angina pectoris). These referred pain patterns do not connote a true radicular pain pattern and are not usually mechanical in origin.

Physical examination of patients with neckache usually reveals nothing more than a locally tender area(s) usually just lateral to the spine. The intensity of the pain is variable and the loss of cervical motion correlates directly with the pain intensity. The presence of true spasm defined as a continuous muscle contraction is rare except in severe cases where the head may be tilted to one side (torticollis).

Since the radiograph in cervical sprain is usually normal, a plain X-ray is usually not warranted on the first visit. If the pain continues for more than two weeks or the patient develops other physical findings, then an X-ray should be taken to rule out other more serious causes of the neck pain such as neoplasia or instability. The prognosis for these individuals is excellent since the natural history is one of complete resolution of the symptoms over several weeks. The mainstay of therapy includes rest and immobilization, usually in a soft cervical orthosis. Although medications such as anti-inflammatory agents or muscle relaxants may aid in the acute management of pain, they do not seem to alter the natural history of the disorder.

§ 2-4(B). Acute Herniated Disc.

A herniated disc is defined as the protrusion of the nucleus pulposus through the fibers of the annulus fibrosus (entry 31). Most acute disc herniations occur posterolaterally and in patients around the fourth decade of like when the nucleus is still gelatinous. The most common areas of disc herniation are: C6-7, C5-6, whereas C7-T1 and C3-4 are infrequent. Disc herniation of C2-3 is very, very rare. Unlike the lumbar herniated disc, the cervical herniated disc may cause myelopathy in addition to radicular pain due to the presence of the spinal cord in the cervical region (see Table IV).

The disc herniation usually affects the nerve root number lowest for the given disc level; for example, C3-4 disc affects the C4 nerve root, C4-5 the fifth cervical nerve root, C5-6 the sixth cervical root, C6-7 the seventh nerve root, and C7-T7 the eighth cervical nerve root. Unlike the lumbar region, the disc herniation does not involve other roots but more commonly presents some evidence of upper motor neuron findings secondary to spinal cord local pressure. McNab has stated that most cervical disc herniations have some element of long tract signs albeit usually mild and not clinically significant (entry 25).

Not every herniated disc is symptomatic. The presence of symptoms depends on the spinal reserve capacity, the presence of inflammation, size of the herniation, as well as the presence of concomitant disease such as uncovertebral joint osteophytes.

Clinically, the patient's major complaint is arm pain and not neck pain. The pain is often perceived as starting in the neck area but then radiates from this point down the shoulder, arm, forearm, and usually into the hand. The onset of the radicular pain often is gradual although there can be a sudden onset associated with a tearing or snapping sensation. As time passes, the magnitude of the arm pain will clearly exceed that of the neck or shoulder pain. The arm pain may also be variable in intensity precluding any use of the arm without severe pain to a dull cramping ache in the arm muscles with use of the arm. The pain is usually severe enough to awaken the patient at night.

Physical examination of the neck usually shows some limitation of motion and on occasion the patient may tilt the head in a cocked robin position (torticollis) toward the side of the herniated cervical disc. Extension of the spine will often exacerbate the pain as it further narrows the intervertebral foramina (Spurling's test). Axial compression, Valsalva maneuver, and coughing may also exacerbate or recreate the pain pattern.

The presence of a positive neurologic examination is the most helpful aspect of the diagnostic workup although the neurologic may remain normal despite a chronic radicular pattern. Even when a deficit exists it may not be temporarily related to the present symptoms but to a prior attack at a different level. To be significant, the neurologic must show objective signs of reflex diminution, motor weakness, or atrophy. The presence of subjective sensory changes are often difficult to interpret and require a coherent and cooperative patient to be of clinical value. The presence of sensory changes alone are usually not enough to make the diagnosis firm.

When the third cervical nerve root is compressed, no reflex change or motion weakness can be identified. The pain radiates to the back of the neck and toward the mastoid process and pinna of the ear.

Involvement of the fourth cervical nerve root again leads to no readily detectable reflex changes or motor weakness. The pain radiates into the back of the neck and into the superior aspect of the scapula. Occasionally, the pain will radiate into the anterior chest wall. The pain is often exacerbated by neck extension.

Unlike the third and fourth cervical root, the fifth through the eighth cervical roots have motor functions. Compression of the fifth cervical root is characterized by weakness of shoulder abduction usually above 90 degrees and weakness of shoulder extension. The biceps reflexes are often depressed and the pain radiates from the side of the neck to the top of the shoulder. Decreased sensation is often noted in the lateral aspect of the deltoid representing the autonomous innervation area of the axillary nerve.

Involvement of the sixth cervical nerve root produces biceps muscle weakness, as well as a diminished brachioradialis reflex. The pain again radiates from the neck down the lateral arm and forearm into the radial side of hand (index, long, and thumb). Numbness is occasionally found in the tip of the index finger, the autonomous area of the sixth nerve root.

Compression of the seventh cervical nerve roots produces reflexes changes in the triceps jerk with associated loss of strength in the triceps muscles which extends the elbow. The pain from this lesion radiates from the lateral neck down the middle of the area into the middle finger. Sensory changes are often found in the tip of the middle finger the autonomous area for the seventh nerve.

Lastly, involvement of the eighth cervical nerve by a herniated C7-T1 disc produces a significant weakness of the intrinsic musculature of the hand. This involvement can lead to a rapid atrophy of the interosseous muscle due to the small size of these muscles. Loss of the interossei lead to significant loss in fine hand motion. No reflexes are easily found, although the flexor carpi ulnaris reflex may be decreased. The radicular pain from the eighth cervical root radiates into the ulnar border of the hand and the ring and little fingers. The tip of the little finger often demonstrates a diminished sensation.

Nerve root sensitivity can be elicited by a method which increases the tension of the nerve root. Radicular arm pain is often increased by the Valsalva maneuver or by directly compressing the head. While these signs are helpful when present, the absence alone does not rule out radicular pain. As mentioned above, Spurling's test is where neck extension will often further narrow the involved neural foramen and recreate the patient's pain pattern. Conversely, a relief sign opposite to a stretch or tension sign called the shoulder abduction relief sign has been described (entry 8). The physical examination manuever involves raising the involved arm with the shoulder abducted to 90 degrees and the elbow flexed to 90 degrees. The patient with true radicular pain will report a relief of pain with this maneuver which favors a good surgical prognosis.

The provisional diagnosis of a herniated disc is made by the history and physical examination. The plain X-ray is usually nondiagnostic although occasionally disc space narrowing at the suspected interspace or foraminal narrowing on the oblique films will be seen. The value of the films are largely to exclude other causes of neck and arm pain. Tests such as an EMG or myelogram are confirmatory examinations and should not be used as screening tests since misinformation may ensue.

The treatment for most patients with a herniated disc is nonoperative since the majority of patients respond to conservative treatment over a period of months. The efficacy of the nonoperative approach, depends heavily on the doctor-patient relationship. If a patient is well informed, insightful, and willing to follow instructions, the chances for a successful nonoperative outcome are greatly improved.

The cornerstone to the management of a cervical herniated disc is rest and immobilization. The use of a cervical orthosis greatly increases the likelihood that the patient will rest. The patients should remain at home and at bedrest except for necessary trips to the bathroom. The bedrest should be maintained for at least two weeks and the patients should wear the cervical orthosis at all times. After the acute pain begins to abate, the patients should gradually increase their activity and wean off the orthosis. Most persons will be able to return to work in a month, at least under light duty.

Drug therapy is an important adjunct to rest and immobilization. Anti-inflammatory medications, analgesics, and muscle relaxants have historically been used in the acute management of these patients. Since it is commonly believed that the radicular pain is in part inflammatory, the use of aspirin or other non-steroidal anti-inflammatory medication seems to be appropriate. All these medications have gastrointestinal side-effects, but are generally well tolerated for brief periods. Oral systemic steroid administered in a tapering dosage for seven days may provide relief in more refractory cases, but should not be routinely used.

Analgesic medication is only rarely needed if the patient is compliant and approaches full bedrest with near total immobility; however, if the pain is severe enough, a brief course of oral codeine may be prescribed or in-hospital intramuscular narcotic may rarely be required. The use of muscle relaxants and the benzodiazepines are truly tranquilizers and central nervous system depressants. As such they have at best a limited role in the management of the acute herniated disc patient. While it is true that these medications help the patient relax and help ensue rest, the potential for additive effect on the patient's psychosocial problems are not worth the long-term risk for the short-term gain.

§ 2-4(C). Cervical Degenerative Disc Disease.

Acute cervical disc herniation is one aspect of cervical degenerative disc disease. Cervical degenerative disc disease also produces cervical spondylosis which may present in several ways (1) cervical spondylosis alone; (2) cervical spondylosis with radiculopathy; (3) cervical spondylosis with myelopathy; (4) cervical spondylosis with myeloradiculopathy; and (5) cervical spondylosis associated with visceral or vascular encroachment (esophagus or vertebral artery) (entry 10). Since we have already dealt with the manifestations of cervical radiculopathy due to soft HNP (§ 2-4(B)), the following two sections will focus on cervical spondylosis alone and with myelopathy (§ 2-4(E)). Radiculopathy due to cervical spondylosis will not be discussed further since it does not significantly differ from radiculopathy from soft HNP. Cervical spondylosis may have large anterior osteophytes which may infrequently irritate the esophagus anteriorly or vertebral artery in the transverse foramina producing symptoms of difficulty in swallowing or symptoms of vascular insufficiency.

§ 2-4(C)(1). Cervical Spondylosis (Cervical Spinal Stenosis).

What once was commonly referred to as cervical degenerative disc disease is more recently called cervical spondylosis. Cervical spondylosis is a chronic process defined as the development of osteophytes and other stigmata of degenerative arthritis as a consequence of age-related disc disease. This process may produce a wide range of symptoms and clinical presentations as discussed above. The following discussion will only apply to the clinical picture of cervical spondylosis without secondary spinal cord, nerve root, or visceral involvement.

The human neck pays the price for its mobility by degenerative disc disease. In cadaver studies, almost everyone over the age of 55 will show evidence of cervical spondylosis. Obviously not all of these patients are symptomatic. Friedenberg and colleagues (entry 12) have emphasized the lack of correlation between radiographs of the cervical spine and symptoms, not to mention the same lack of correlation with cervical myelography (entry 15). How then does the physician evaluate and treat a patient with suspected symptomatic cervical spondylosis? This question will be the subject of the remainder of this section.

Cervical spondylosis is believed to be the direct result of age-related changes in the intervertebral disc (see § 2-3(B)). These changes include dessication of the nucleus pulposus, loss of annular elasticity, and narrowing of the disc space or with disc protrusion or rupture. In turn, secondary changes include overriding of facets, increased motion in the spinal segments, osteophyte formation, inflammation of synovial joints, and even microfractures. These macro- and microscopic changes can result in various clinical syndromes (spondylosis, anklyosis, central or foraminal spinal stenosis, radiculopathy, myelopathy, or spinal segmental instability). The uncovertebral joints or joints of Lushka are subject to similar changes as the facet joints.

The usual patient with symptomatic cervical spondylosis is over the age of 40 complaining of neckache. Not infrequently though, these patients will have very little neck symptoms but present with referred pain patterns; shoulder area, suboccipital area, occipital headaches, intrascapular areas, anterior chest wall, or other vague symptoms suggestive of anatomic disturbances like blurring of vision, tinnitus, etc. These pain patterns are truly referred in a scleromatic pattern as shown by discography or supraspinous ligament saline injections (entry 4). In patients with predominantly referred pain, a past history for neck pain is usually offered.

Physical examination of the patient with cervical spondylosis is often associated with a dearth of objective findings. The patient will usually have some limitation of neck motion associated with midline tenderness. Not infrequently, palpation of the referred pain areas will also produce local tenderness and should not be confused with local disease. The neurologic examination is normal. Radiographs (AP, lateral, oblique) of the cervical spine in cervical spondylosis show varying degrees of changes. These include disc space narrowing, osteophytosis, foraminal narrowing, degenerative changes of the facets, or instability. As previously discussed, these findings do not correlate with symptoms. In large part, the radiograph serves to rule out other more serious causes of neck and referred pain such as tumors. Further diagnostic testing is usually not warranted.

Cervical spondylosis alone is treated by nonoperative measures. The mainstay of treatment for the acute pain superimposed on the chronic problem is rest and immobilization. In addition, oral anti-inflammatory medications like aspirin will be of benefit. Often these medications will need to be administered on a chronic basis or at least intermittently. Trigger point injections with local anesthetics (lidocaine) and corticosteroids (triamcinolone) may be therapeutic as well as diagnostic. Once the pain abates, the immobilization (usually a soft cervical collar) should be discontinued and the patient maintained on a series of cervical isometric exercises. Further counseling in regard to sleeping position, automobile driving, and work is in order. Manipulation and traction are rarely needed and may in fact be deleterious to the patient (entry 22).

§ 2-4(C)(2). Cervical Spondylosis With Myelopathy.

When the secondary bony changes of cervical spondylosis encroach on the spinal cord, a pathology process called myelopathy develops. When this involves both the spinal cord and nerve roots, it is called myeloradiculopathy. Radiculopathy regardless of its cause, causes shoulder or arm pain as described in § 2-4(B).

Myelopathy is the most serious and most difficult sequale of cervical spondylosis to treat effectively. Less than 5% of patients with cervical spondylosis develop myelopathy and are usually between 40-60 years of age. The changes of myelopathy are most often gradual and associated with posterior osteophyte formation (called spondylitic bone or hard disc) and spinal canal narrowing (spinal stenosis). Acute myelopathy is most often the result of a central soft disc herniation producing a high grade block by myelography. Edward and LaRocca has shown that spinal stenosis from cervical spondylosis is almost certain with mid cervical canal diameters less than 10 mm, at risk (premyelopathic) 10-13 mm, myelopathic prone 13-17 mm, and rarely with diameters greater than 17 mm (entry 11).

The characteristic stooped, wide based and somewhat jerky gait of the aged summarizes the chronic effects of cervical spondylosis with myelopathy. The spinal cord changes may develop from single or multiple level disease and as such may not present in a singular or standard manner. A typical clinical presentation of chronic myelopathy begins with the gradual notice of a peculiar sensation in the hands, associated with clumsiness and weakness. The patient will also note lower extremity symptoms which may antedate the upper extremity finding including: difficulty walking (initially at night), peculiar sensations, leg weakness, hyperreflexia, spasticity, and clonus. The upper extremity finding may start out unilaterally and include hyperreflexia, brisk Hoffman's sign, and muscle atrophy (especially the hand muscles). The finger escape sign may also be present. Neck pain per se is not a prominent feature of myelopathy. Sensory changes can involve at these levels and are often a less reliable index of spinal cord disease.

These include (1) the spinothalmic tract in the anteriolateral portion of cord for pain and temperature; (2) dorsal columns for position and vibratory sensation; and (3) the dorsal division of the nerve root which may produce unusual dermatomal sensory changes.

Radiographs of the cervical spine in these patients will often reveal advanced degenerative disease including: spinal canal narrowing by prominent posterior osteophytosis, variable foraminal narrowing, disc space narrowing, facet joint arthrosis, and instability. The myelogram is the diagnostic test of choice exhibiting a wash board appearance to the dye column with multiple anterior and posterior defects. The posterior defects are secondary to facet arthrosis and buckling of the ligamentum flavum.

In general, myelopathy is a surgical disease. Myelopathy is not an absolute indication for surgical decompression. Conservative therapy consisting of immobilization and rest with a soft cervical orthosis offers the myelopathic patient, who is not a good operative risk, a viable option. Lees and Turner, Nurick, Bradshaw, and Roberts (entries 3, 20, 27, 30) have reported clinical trials on the conservative management of myelopathy. In over 100 cases, the combined literature reported that 36% were improved, 38% remained the same, and 26% were worse. This is not significantly different from some clinical series. The goals of surgery in the myelopathic patient are to decompress the spinal canal to prevent further spinal cord compression and vascular compromise. If the myelopathy is progressive despite a trial of conservative treatment, surgery is clearly indicated. These indications may vary slightly from surgeon to surgeon because of the lack of absolute or definite clinical data.

§ 2-4(D). Rheumatoid Arthritis.

Rheumatoid arthritis affects 2-3% of the population. About 60% of patients with rheumatoid arthritis will exhibit signs and symptoms of cervical spine involvement whereas up to 86% will have radiographic evidence of cervical disease (entry 21). Cervical spine involvement secondary to the erosive, inflammatory changes of rheumatoid arthritis (synovitis) are divided into three categories: (1) atlantoaxial instability, (2) basilar invagination and (3) subaxial instability. Atlantoaxial instability is the most common and most serious of the instability pattern affecting 20-34% of hospitalized patients. Risk factors include: (1) steroid use, (2) long duration of the disease, (3) older patients and (4) erosive peripheral joint involvement. Actual mortality figures for these cervical instabilities are lacking. The natural history of the atlantoaxial instability of rheumatoid arthritis is controversial. In a study by Mathews, 33% of patients with AAI and 50% of patients with basilar invagination had evidence of long tract signs (entry 24). These three instability patterns above tend to occur together as shown by Ranawat; of 33 patients treated surgically for cervical spine involvement, 60% had atlantoaxial instability, 16% basilar invagination and 60% had

ANATOMY AND PATHOPHYSIOLOGY OF NECK PAIN § 2-4(D)

subaxial instabilities (entry 28). The clinical presentation of rheumatoid cervical spine disease falls into one of three categories (not mutually exclusive): (1) local arthritis, mechanical instability, and pain, (2) neurologic dysfunction of brainstem, spinal cord, or peripheral nerve, and (3) vertebral artery insufficiency (loss of balance, vertigo, diplopia, other visual disturbances). The evaluation of a patient with rheumatoid arthritis is difficult due to the multiple system involvement. The physical examination should start with a careful neurologic evaluation to rule out upper motor neuron disease before moving to neck range of motion or other vigorous maneuvers which may harm the patient.

The patient with cervical spine involvement from rheumatoid arthritis most often has neck pain, located in the middle posterior neck and occipital area. The range of motion is decreased and crepitance or a feeling of instability may be noted. The clunk or Sharp-Purser test should be done only with great caution or not at all. The neurologic changes can be variable and others difficult to elicit in the context of diffuse rheumatoid changes. Pyramidal tract involvement produces upper motor neuron signs (hyperreflexia, spasticity) and pathologic reflexes (Babinski and Hoffman's signs). Subjective sensory changes such as lightning like radiations into the legs (Lhermitte's sign), numbness, or other paresthesia may be noted. Brainstem involvement from basilar invagination of the odontoid produces symptoms of vertebrobasilar insufficiency or posterior internal cerebral or artery occlusion (Wallenberg syndrome). Urinary retention or incontinence may be noted as well as gait changes.

The evaluation of the patient with cervical rheumatoid arthritis begins with plain radiographs of the neck which reveal osteopenia, facet erosion, disc space narrowing, subluxation of the lower cervical spine (stepladder appearance). To determine atlantoaxial disease dynamic flexion extension views of the lateral upper cervical spine are often required. Atlantoaxial subluxations of more than 3.5 mm are abnormal with most authors suggesting translation of more than 7-8 mm be present before surgical intervention is suggested. Basilar invagination is defined as upper migration of the odontoid projecting into the foramen magnum. This is identified by MacGregor's line (a line drawn from the hand palate to occiput) where the tip of the odontoid is 8 mm or 9.7 mm above this line in females and males, respectively. The addition of CT scan with or without contrast material in the upper cervical spine has given valuable information as to the relationship of the bony elements to the spinal cord. Subaxial subluxations are identified by dynamic flexion-extension films and are defined as significant if the bodies translate 3.5 mm or more, or disc space angulation of more than 11 degrees occurs (entry 2).

The majority of these patients despite rather dramatic disease patterns can be successfully managed nonoperatively. While the natural history of rheumatoid arthritis predicts a high incidence of involvement of the cervical spine, it is estimated that only a few patients die from medullary compression with significant atlantoaxial disease and that atlantoaxial disease worsens with time with only 2-14% exhibiting neurologic progression (entry 21).

The mainstay in nonoperative therapy is the cervical orthosis (Philadelphia collar). Although this does not fully immobilize the atlantoaxial interval, it does produce symptomatic relief. Some authors have advocated intermittent home traction, but it must be used only with great caution under a physician's direction. Medications have a definite role in the nonoperative management of the rheumatoid disease. Initial management includes aspirin in high dosages monitored by serum drug levels. Secondary agents like methotrexate, chloroquine, or oral steroids are best administered under the direction of a rheumatologist.

BIBLIOGRAPHY

1. Akeson, et al. Biomechanics and biochemistry of the intervertebral disc. CORR 129:133-140, 1977.
2. Bailey, R.W. Instability of the cervical spine. Instructional Course Lectures, Vol. 27, pg 159, 1978.
3. Bradshaw, P. Some aspects of cervical spondylosis. Quarterly Medical Journal 616:832-909, 1957.
4. Bradshaw, P. Pain caused by cervical rheumatism. Spondylosis, 17:2-7, 1961.
5. Brickley, Parsons D., Glincher, M.J. Is the chemistry of collagen in intervertebral disc an expression of Wolff's law? Spine 9:184-188, 1984.
6. Bushell, G.R. Proteoglycon chemistry of the intervertebral disc. CORR 129:115-123, 1977.
7. Colt, E.W.D., et al. The effect of running on plasma beta endorphins. Life Sciences Vol. 28, 1637-1640, 1981.
8. Davidson, R.S., et al. The shoulder abduction test in the diagnosis of radicular pain in cervical extradural compressive monoradiculopathies. Spine 6:441-446, 1981.
9. DePalma, A.P., Rothman, R.H. *The Intervertebral Disc.* Philadelphia, W.B. Saunder Company, 1970.
10. DePalma, A.P., et al. The natural history of severe cervical disc degeneration. Acta Orthopaedic Scand 43:392-396, 1972.
11. Edward, W.C., LaRocca, S.H. The developmental segmental sagittal diameter in combined cervical and lumbar spondylosis. Spine 10:43-49, 1985.
12. Friedenberg, Z.B., Miller, W.T. Degeneration disc disease of the cervical spine. JBJS 45A, 1171-1178, 1963.
13. Frykholm, R., Hyde, J., Norlen, G., Skoglund, C.R. On pain sensations produced by stimulation of ventral roots in man. Acta Phys Scand Suppl 106:455-469, 1953.
14. Ghosh, et al. Collagens elastin and noncollagenous protein of the IVD. CORR 129:124-132, 1977.
15. Hitselberger, W.E., Witten, R.M. Abnormal myelograms in asymptomatic patients. J. Neurosurgery 28:204-206, 1968.
16. Holm, S., Nachemson, A. Variations in the nutrition of canine intervertebral disc induced by motion. Spine 3:866-874, 1983.

17. Holm, S., Nachemson, A. Nutrition of the intervertebral disc: acute effects of cigarette smoking. Int J Micro 3:406, 1984.
18. Holt, S., Yates, P.O. Cervical spondylosis and nerve root lesions. JBJS 43B:407-432, 1966.
19. Kelsey, J.L., et al. An epidemeological study of acute prolapsed cervical IVD. JBJS 66A:907-914, 1984.
20. Lees, F., Turner, J.W.A. Natural history and prognosis of cervical spondylosis. Brit Med J 2:1607-1610, 1963.
21. Lipson, S.J. Rheumatoid arthritis of the cervical spine. CORR 182:143-149, 1984.
22. Livingston, M.C.P. Spinal manipulation causing injury. (A Three-Year Study) CORR 81:82-86, 1971.
23. Marshall, L.L., et al. Chemical radiculitis: a clinical, physiological and immunological study. CORR 129:61-67, 1977.
24. Mathews, J.A. Atlantoaxial subluxation in rheumatoid arthritis. Ann Rheumat. Dis 28:260-266, 1969.
25. McNab, I. *The Cervical Spine.* Philadelphia, J.P. Lippincott Company, 1983.
26. Naylor, A. The biophysical and biochemical aspects of the intervertebral disc herniation and degeneration. Ann Roy Coll Surg 31:91, 1962.
27. Nurick, S. The natural history and the results of surgical treatment of the spinal cord disorder associated with cervical spondylosis. Brain 95:101-108, 1972.
28. Ranawat, C.S., et al. Cervical spine fusion in rheumatoid arthritis. JBJS 61A:1003-1010, 1979.
29. Riley, L.H. Various pain syndromes which may result from osteoarthritis of the cervical spine. Maryland State Med. Journal, May 103-105, 1969.
30. Roberts, A.H. Myelopathy due to cervical spondylosis treated by collar immobilization. Neurology 16:951-959, 1966.
31. Rothman, R.H., Marvel, J.P. The acute cervical disc. CORR 129:59-68, 1975.
32. Rothman, R.H., Simeone, F.A. *The Spine.* Philadelphia, W.B. Saunders Company, 1982, 1-53, 67-93, Neck; 440-499, C-Spine.
33. Urban, J.P.G., et al. Nutrition of the intervertebral disc: an in vivo study of solute transport. CORR 109:101-114, 1977.
34. Whalen, J.L., Parke, W.W., Mazur, J.M., Stauffer, E.S. The intrinsic vasculature of developing vertebral end plates and its nutritive significance to the intervertebral discs. Journal Pediatric Orthopaedic 5:403-410, 1985.

35. White, A.A., Panjabi, M.M. The basic kinematics of the human spine. Spine 3:12-29, 1978.
36. Yaoui, N., et al. Immunohistochemical localization of Types I, II, and III collagens in the ossified posterior longitudinal ligament of the human cervical spine. Calcif. Tissue International, 35:159-163, 1983.

Table I

Structures Causing Neck Pain

Acromioclavicular joint
Heart and coronary artery disease
Apex of lung, Pancoast's tumor, bronchogenic cancer, (C3, C4, C5 nerve roots in common)
Diaphragm muscle (C3, C4, C5 innervation)
Gallbladder
Spinal cord tumor
Temporomandibular joint
Fibrositis and fibromyositis syndromes (upper thoracic spine, proximal arm and shoulder)
Aorta
Pancreas
Disorders of any somatic or visceral structure (produces cervical nerve root irritation)
Peripheral nerves
Central nervous system (posterior fossa lesions)
Hiatus hernia (C3, C4, C5)
Gastric ulcer

Table II

Causes of Neck and Neck Related Pain Syndromes

Localized Neck Disorders
    Osteoarthritis (apophyseal joints, C1-C2-C3 levels most often)
    Rheumatoid arthritis (atlantoaxial)
    Juvenile rheumatoid arthritis
    Sternocleidomastoid tendinitis
    Acute posterior cervical strain
    Pharyngeal infections
    Cervical lymphyadenitis
    Osteomyelitis (staphylococcal, tuberculosis)
    Meningitis
    Ankylosing spondylitis
    Paget's disease
    Torticollis (cogenital, spasmodic, drug-involved, hysterical)
    Neoplasms (primary or metastatic)
    Occipital neuralgia (greater and lesser occipital nerves)
    Diffuse idiopathic skeletal hyperostosis
    Rheumatic fever (infrequently)
    Gout (infrequently)

Lesions Producing Neck and Shoulder Pain
    Postural disorders
    Rheumatoid arthritis
    Fibrositis syndromes
    Musculoligamentous injuries to neck and shoulder
    Osteoarthritis (apophyseal and Luschka)
    Cervical Spondylosis
    Intervertebral osteoarthritis
    Thoracic outlet syndromes
    Nerve injuries (serratus anterior, C3-C4 nerve root, long thoracic nerve)

Lesions Producing Predominantly Shoulder Pain
    Rotator cuff tears and tendinitis
    Calcareous tendinitis
    Subacromial bursitis
    Bicipital tendinitis
    Adhesive capsulitis
    Reflex sympathetic dystrophy

ANATOMY AND PATHOPHYSIOLOGY OF NECK PAIN

    Frozen shoulder syndromes
    Acromioclavicular secondary osteoarthritis
    Glenohumeral arthritis
    Septic arthritis
    Tumors of the shoulder

Lesions Producing Neck and Head Pain with Radiation
    Cervical spondylosis
    Rheumatoid arthritis
    Intervertebral disc protrusion
    Osteoarthritis (appophyseal and Luschka joints; intervertebral disc; osteoarthritis)
    Spinal cord tumors

    Cervical Neurovascular syndromes
        Cervical rib
        Scalene muscle
        Hyperabduction syndrome
        Rib-clavicle compression

Table III

Mean Range of Cervical Motion of the Spine (Degrees)

Level	Flexion/Extension	Lateral Flexion	Rotation
0-C1	13	8	0
C1-C2	10	0	47
C2-C3	8	10	9
C3-C4	13	11	11
C4-C5	12	11	12
C5-C6	17	8	10
C6-C7	16	7	9
C7-T1	9	4	8

White, A.A., Panjabi, M.M. *Clinical Mechanics of the Spine,* Philadelphia, J.P. Lippincott Co., 1978. Reprinted by permission.

Table IV

Physical Examination—Disc Herniation

Nerve Root	Disc Level	Symptoms	Weakness: Reflex Change
C3	C2-C3	Pain and numbness in back of neck, particularly around mastoid process and pinna of ear	No readily detectable weakness or reflex change except by EMG
C4	C3-C4	Pain and numbness in back of neck, radiating along levator scapula muscle and occasionally down anterior chest	No readily detectable weakness or reflex change except by EMG
C5	C4-C5	Pain radiating from side of neck to shoulder top, numbness over middle of body of deltoid muscle (axillary nerve distribution)	Weakness of extension of arm and shoulder, particularly above 90 degrees; atrophy of deltoid muscle; no reflex change
C6	C5-C6	Pain radiating down lateral side of arm and forearm, often into thumb and index finger; numbness of tip of thumb or on dorsum of hand over first dorsal interosseous muscle	Weakness of biceps muscle; depression of biceps reflex
C7	C6-C7	Pain radiating down middle of forearm, usually to middle of finger, although index and ring fingers may be involved	Weakness of triceps muscle; depression of triceps reflex

Table IV (Continued)
Physical Examination—Disc Herniation

Nerve Root	Disc Level	Symptoms	Weakness: Reflex Change
C8	C7-T1	Pain down medial aspect of forearm to ring and small finger; numbness can involve small finger and medial portion of ring finger but rarely extends above wrist	Weakness of triceps and small muscles of the hand; no reflex change

Figure 1

The Atlas Viewed From Above and Below

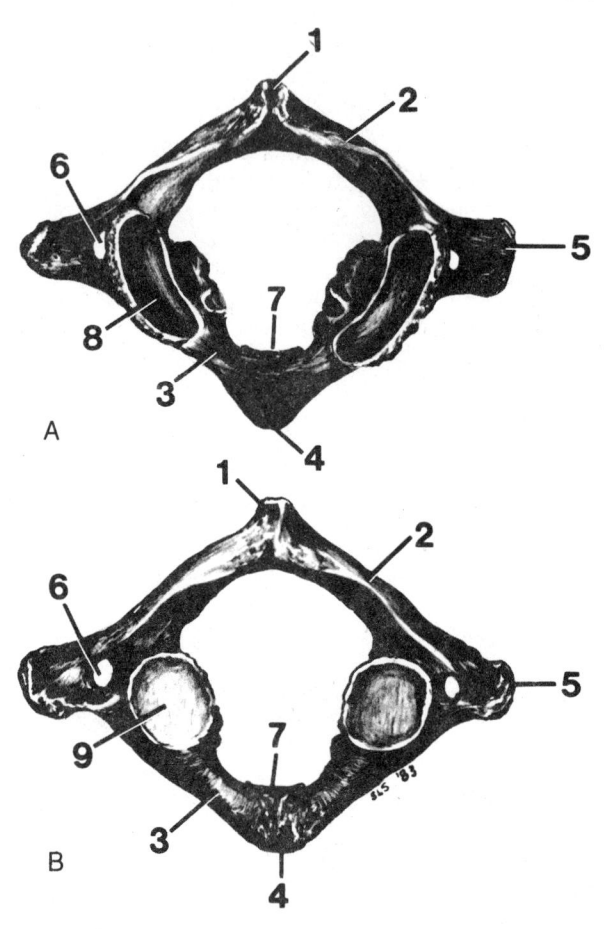

The atlas viewed from above (A) and below (B). 1, posterior tubercle; 2, posterior arch; 3, anterior arch; 4, anterior tubercle; 5, transverse process; 6, transverse foramen; 7, facet articulation for dens; 8, superior articular facet; 9, inferior articular facet.

Cruess, R.L., Rennie, W.R.J. (eds.) *Adult Orthopaedics*, Vol. 2, New York, Churchill Livingstone, Inc., 1984. Reprinted by permission.

Figure 2

The Axis

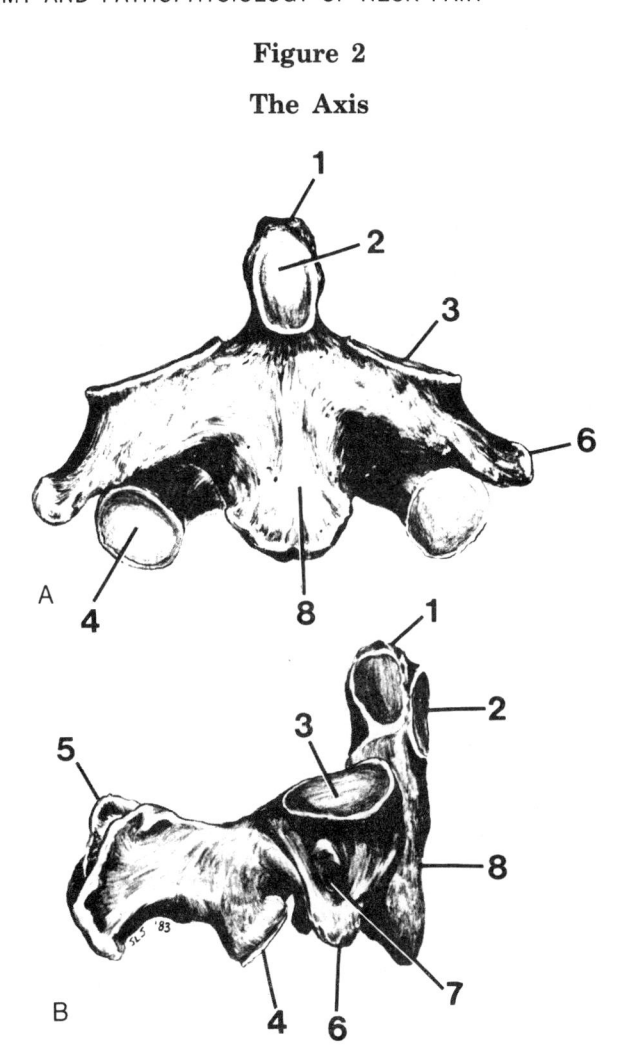

The axis. (A) Anterior view and (B) lateral views, 1, dens; 2, facet for anterior arch of atlas; 3, superior facet; 4, inferior facet; 5, spinous process; 6, transverse process; 7, transverse foramen; 8, body.

Cruess, R.L., Rennie, W.R.J. (eds.) *Adult Orthopaedics,* Vol. 2, New York, Churchill Livingstone, Inc., 1984. Reprinted by permission.

Figure 3

Typical Lower Cervical Vertebra

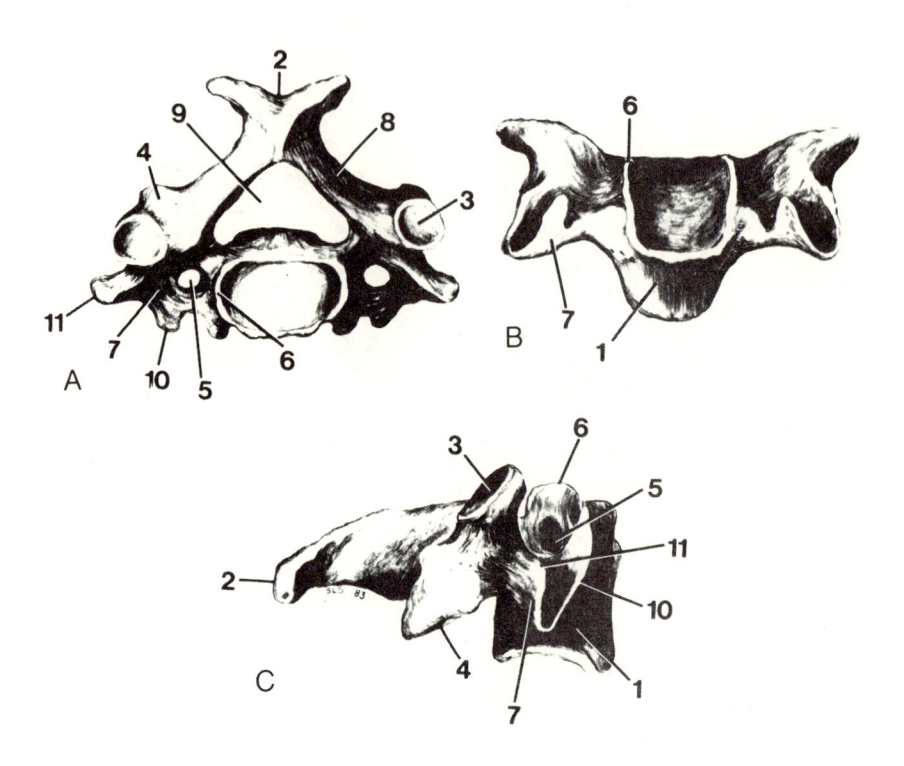

A. Superior Aspect. B. View from the front. C. Lateral view. 1, body; 2, spinous process; 3, superior facet; 4, inferior facet; 5, transverse foramen; 6, uncinate process; 7, gutter-shaped transverse process; 8, lamina; 9, vertebral canal; 10, anterior tubercle of transverse process; 11, posterior tubercle of transverse process.

Cruess, R.L., Rennie, W.R.J. (eds.) *Adult Orthopaedics,* Vol. 2, New York, Churchill Livingstone, Inc., 1984. Reprinted by permission.

Figure 4

Three Dimensional Anatomy of the Cup-Like Articulations of the Occipital-Atlantal Joints

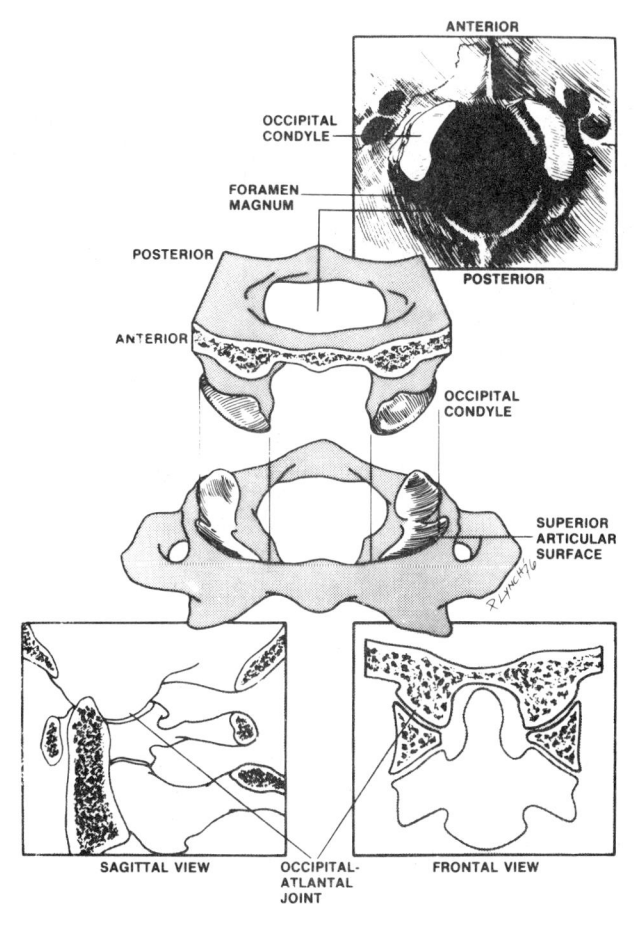

The cup is relatively more shallow in the sagittal than in the frontal plane. Consequently, the joint is probably more unstable to anteroposterior displacement or dislocation than to lateral displacement.

White, A.A., Panjabi, M.M., *Clinical Biomechanics of the Spine,* Philadelphia, J.P. Lippincott Co., 1978. Reprinted by permission.

NECK PAIN

Figure 5

The Cruciform and Tectorial Ligaments

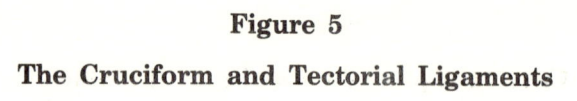

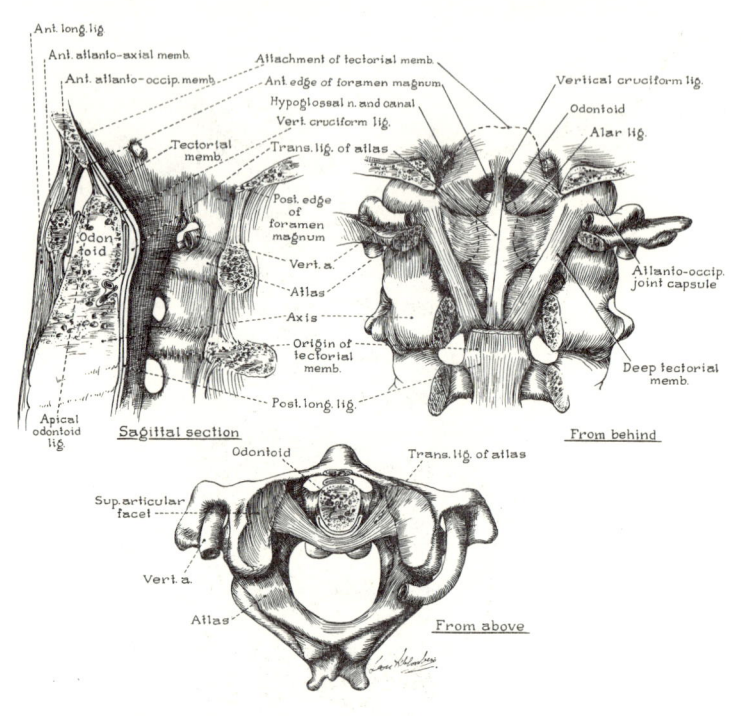

The cruciform and tectorial ligaments seen from within the spinal canal looking anteriorly, in sagittal section and from above. The cruciform ligament holds the odontoid in a sling to the anterior ring of the atlas. It is composed of a superior arm, which inserts on the basiocciput, an inferior arm, which reinforces the base of the dens, and two lateral arms, the transverse ligament. The transverse ligament inserts on the ring of the atlas and is one of the primary stabilizers of the atlantoaxial joint. This is reinforced by the tectorial and deep tectorial membranes or ligaments. The odontoid is fixed to the base of the skull through the apical odontoid and alar ligaments.

Rothman, R.H., Simeone, F.A., *The Spine,* 2d ed., Philadelphia, W.B. Saunders Co., 1982. Reprinted by permission.

ANATOMY AND PATHOPHYSIOLOGY OF NECK PAIN

Figure 6

Cervical Spine Viewed From the Side

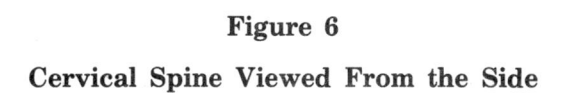

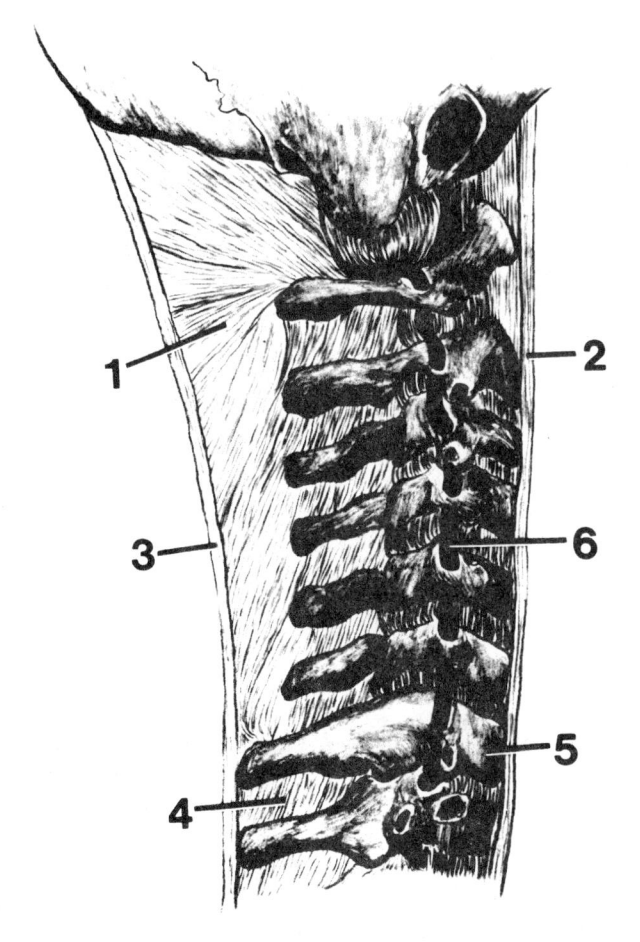

1, Ligamentum nuchae; 2, anterior longitudinal ligament; 3, supraspinatus ligament; 4, interspinous ligament; 5, body of vertebra; 6, vertebral artery.

Cruess, R.L., Rennie, W.R.J. (eds.) *Adult Orthopaedics,* Vol. 2, New York, Churchill Livingstone, Inc., 1984. Reprinted by permission.

Figure 7
Lower Cervical Spine in Neutral Position

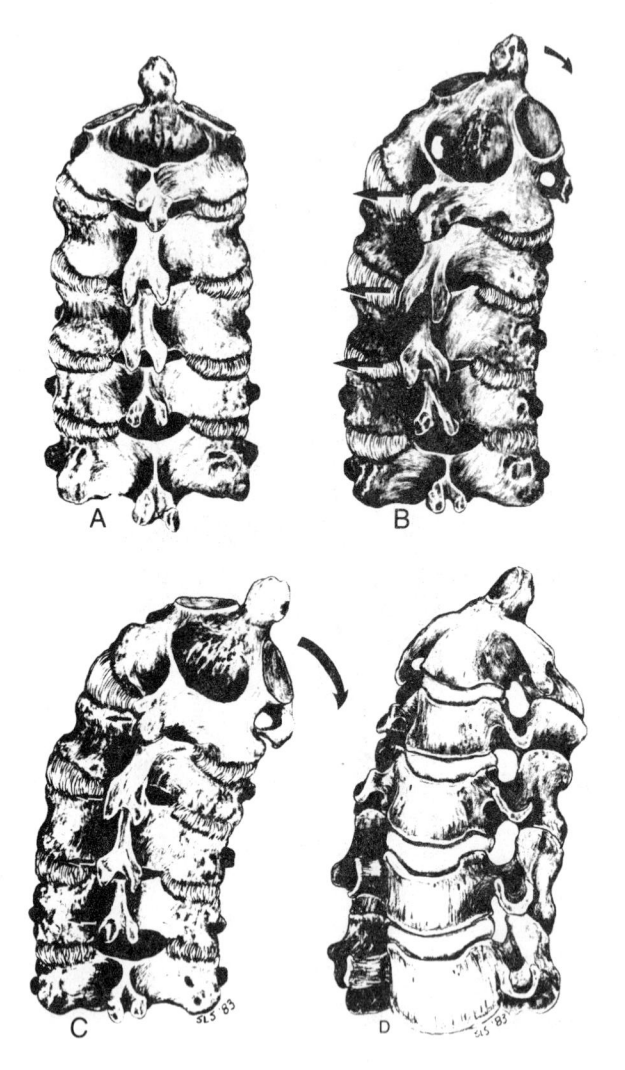

Cruess, R.L., Rennie, W.R.J. (eds.) *Adult Orthopaedics,* Vol. 2, New York, Churchill Livingstone, Inc., 1984. Reprinted by permission.

ANATOMY AND PATHOPHYSIOLOGY OF NECK PAIN

Figure 8

Vertebral Artery

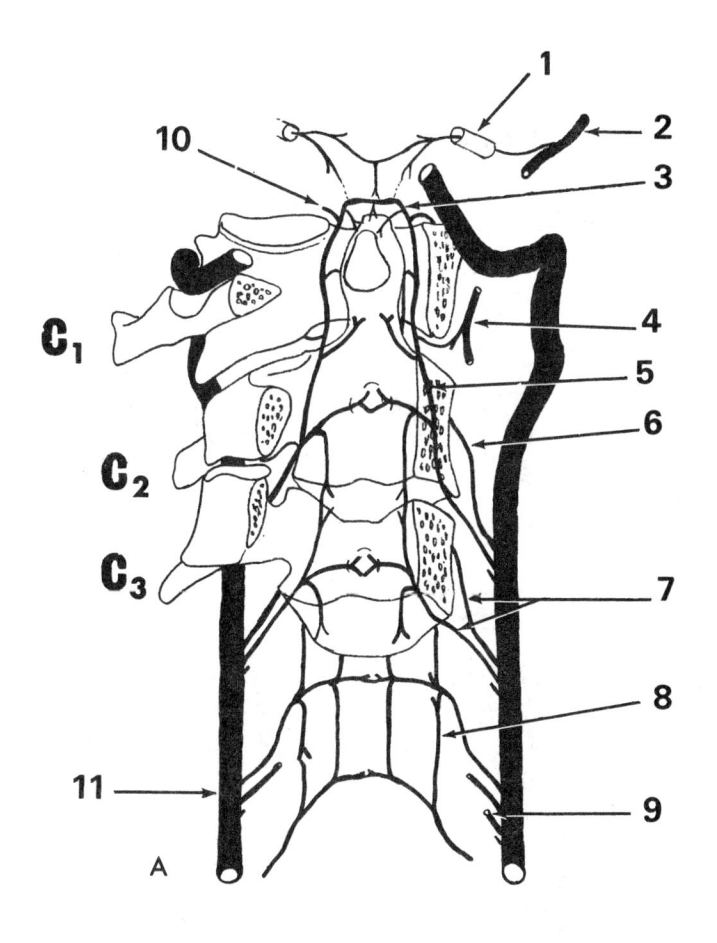

Rothman, R.H., Simeone, F.A., *The Spine,* 2d ed., Philadelphia, W.B. Saunders Co., 1982. Reprinted by permission.

Figure 9

Sinuvertebral Nerve

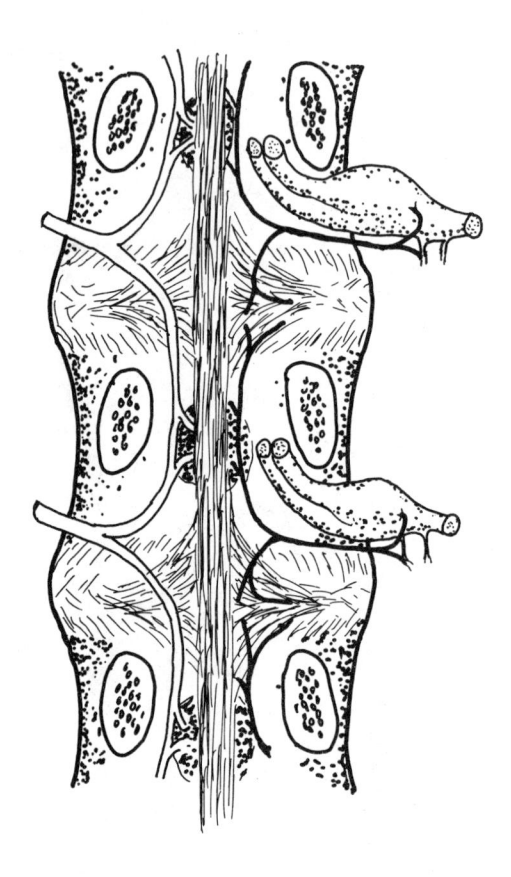

Schema of the distribution of the major channels of the branches of the spinal arteries to intravertebral elements (left) and the ramifications of the vertebral branches of the sinuvertebral nerve (right).

Rothman, R.H., Simeone, F.A., *The Spine*, 2d ed., Philadelphia, W.B. Saunders Co., 1982. Reprinted by permission.

ANATOMY AND PATHOPHYSIOLOGY OF NECK PAIN

Figure 10

Brachial Plexus and Lower Cervical Spine

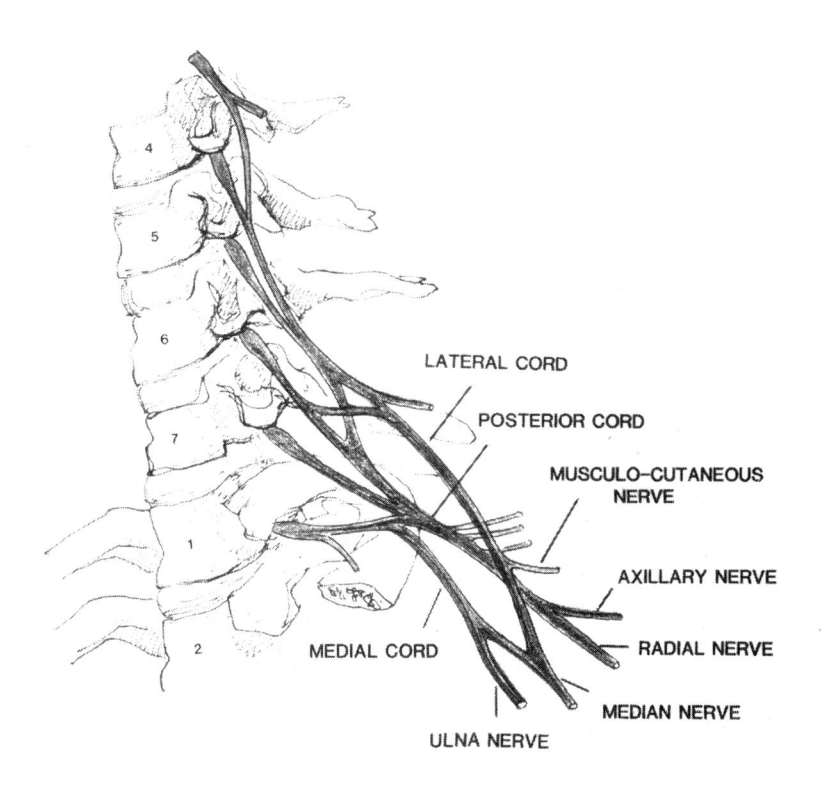

Brachial plexus and lower cervical spine. Note nerve roots, trunk, cords, and the peripheral nerves. The brachial plexus goes under the clavicle and over the first rib, accompanied by the subclavian artery and vein.

CHAPTER 3

A STANDARDIZED APPROACH TO THE DIAGNOSIS AND TREATMENT OF NECK PAIN

Sam W. Wiesel, M.D.

§ 3-1. The Algorithm.
§ 3-2. Cervical Spine Protocol.
§ 3-3. Neck Pain Predominant.
§ 3-4. Arm Pain Predominant (Brachialgia).
§ 3-5. Treatment Modalities.
§ 3-6. Immobilization.
§ 3-7. Drug Therapy.
§ 3-8. Traction.
§ 3-9. Trigger Point Injection.
§ 3-10. Manipulation.
§ 3-11. Exercises.
Bibliography.
Figure 1. Cervical Spine Algorithm.
Figure 2. Differential Diagnosis of Neck Pain.

The cervical spine is a frequent area of complaints for those physicians dealing with car accidents or industrial injuries. When a patient is initially evaluated by a physician, he complains of a symptom and does not arrive labeled with a specific diagnosis. The problem confronting the examining physician is to integrate the patient's symptoms, physical findings, and laboratory findings (including X-rays) into a logical diagnosis and then formulate a rational plan of treatment.

The primary purpose of this chapter is to present a standardized protocol for the diagnosis and treatment of patients with neck pain. This will give some insight into a physician's thought process in assessing cervical spine problems. Next, several of the more common treatment regimens such as trigger point injections and traction will be discussed, with attention given to their efficacy and current role in the treatment of neck pain.

§ 3-1. The Algorithm.

The task of the physician, when confronted with the cervical spine patient, is to integrate his complaints into an accurate diagnosis and to prescribe appropriate therapy. Achieving this goal depends on the accuracy of the physician's decision making. Although specific information is not available for every aspect of neck pain, there is a large body of data to guide us in handling these patients. Using this knowledge, which has already been presented, an algorithm for neck pain has been designed.

Webster defines an algorithm as "a set of rules for solving a particular problem in a finite number of steps." It is, in effect, an organized pattern of decision making and thought processes found useful in approaching the universe of cervical spine patients. The algorithm can be followed in sequence (Figure 1) and is also presented in table form (Figure 2), which are at the end of this chapter.

The primary objective for the physician is to return the patient to his normal function as quickly as possible. In the course of achieving this goal, he must be concerned with other circumstances which include making efficient and precise use of diagnostic studies, minimizing the use of ineffectual surgery, and making therapy available at a reasonable cost to society. The algorithm follows well-delineated rules, established from the consensus of a broad segment of qualified spine surgeons. It allows the patient to receive the most helpful diagnostic and therapeutic measures at optimal times.

§ 3-2. Cervical Spine Protocol.

The protocol (see algorithm) begins with the universe of patients who are initially evaluated for neck pain with or without arm pain. Patients with major trauma including fractures are not included. After an initial medical history and physical examination, and with the assumption that the patient's symptoms are originating from the cervical spine, the first major decision is to rule in or out the presence of a cervical myelopathy.

A cervical myelopathy is essentially the compression of the neural elements in the cervical spine (entry 9). It can lead to a progressive and profound neurologic deficit in any one case. The etiology of the compression is usually a combination of osteoarthritis and degenerative disc disease which leads to a decrease in the volume of the spinal canal. If the spinal canal becomes too small, the nerves (spinal cord) which pass through it are compromised.

The character and severity of the problem depends on the size, location and duration of the lesion. Ventrolateral lesions encroach on the nerve roots and lateral aspects of the spinal cord, producing all the manifestations accompanying nerve root compression. The chief radicular signs are weakness and loss of tone and volume of the muscles of the upper extremity, while the pressure on the spinal cord may produce pyramidal tract signs and spasticity in the lower extremities.

Midline lesions intrude on the central aspect of the anterior portion of the spinal cord. They produce no signs of nerve root compression. Both lower extremities are primarily involved and the most common problem relates initially to gait disturbances. As the disease progresses, bowel and bladder control may be affected.

In the absence of an acute central disc herniation, the natural history of a cervical myelopathy is one of very slow development over the course of many years. It should be appreciated that an automobile accident or an industrial injury does not cause a cervical myelopathy but aggravates a pre-existing condition. This is sometimes very difficult for a patient to understand when they had never experienced any symptoms until an injury. What is occurring is that the osteoarthritis and disc degeneration has been developing over time and the accident triggers the symptoms.

Once a diagnosis of a cervical myelopathy is made, surgical intervention should be considered quickly. The best results are attained in patients with one or two motor units involved and with a myelopathy of a relatively short duration. The longer pressure is applied to the neural elements, the poorer the results. A cervical myelogram should be obtained in these patients to precisely define the neural compression and an adequate surgical decompression should be performed as soon as possible to achieve the best results.

After a cervical myelopathy has been ruled out, the remaining patients, which constitute an overwhelming majority, should be started on a course of conservative management. At this stage of the patient's course a specific diagnosis, whether it be a herniated disc or neck strain, is not important because the entire group is treated in the same fashion.

The primary mode of therapy in both acute and chronic cervical spine disease is immobilization (entry 2). In the acute neck injuries, immobilization allows for healing of torn and attenuated soft tissues, whereas in chronic conditions immobilization is aimed at reduction of inflammation in the supporting soft tissues and around the nerve roots of the cervical spine.

Immobilization is best achieved by the use of a soft felt collar. It needs to be properly fitted and comfortable for the patient. Initially the collar is worn 24 hours a day. The patient must understand that during sleep the neck is totally unprotected from awkward positions and movement and that the collar is most important.

The other mainstay of the initial treatment is drug therapy. It is directed at reducing inflammation — especially in the soft tissues. There are a variety of anti-inflammatory medications available; however, there is no one drug that has proven to be significantly better than all the others. Salicylates have proven to be as effective and safe as the rest and are the least expensive. The dosage must be adequate to achieve a therapeutic blood level. The efficacy of this treatment regimen is predicated on the patient's ability to understand the disease process and the role of each therapeutic modality.

The vast majority of patients will respond to this approach in the first ten days, but a certain percentage will not heal rapidly. This group should be placed at bed rest to relieve the cervical spine's burden of supporting the weight of the head. While at bed rest, these patients should continue full-time use of the collar and anti-inflammatory medication.

At this juncture a local injection into the area of maximum tenderness should be considered. Localized tender areas in the paravertebral musculature and trapezii will be found in many individuals and are referred to as trigger points. Marked relief of symptoms often is achieved dramatically by infiltration of these trigger points with a combination of lidocaine (Xylocaine) and 1 ml. of a steroid preparation. The object of the injection is to decrease the inflammation in a specific anatomic area. The more localized the trigger point, the more effective this form of therapy.

The patient should be treated conservatively for up to six weeks. The majority of cervical spine patients will get better. In some cases the problem arises in distinguishing those patients who have a true neck problem from those individuals using their neck as an excuse to stay out of work and collect compensation or for some other cause (auto accident with subsequent litigation).

There is no one good answer to this problem. The treating physician is in a ticklish situation: on the one hand, as the patient's representative he must accept what the patient tells him (synonymous with a lawyer representing a client who may not be telling the complete truth); on the other hand, he has a responsibility to society to keep medical costs down, return people to work as quickly as possible, and not prescribe unnecessary treatments. If there are no objective findings to substantiate a patient's subjective complaints, the patient should be strongly encouraged to return to some type of work as soon as possible. In spite of this some patients will complain of continued pain and inability to work.

The best solution for the primary physician is to recommend an independent medical examination (IME). This does not destroy the patient physician relationship. If the IME concurs with the primary physician that no serious pathology exists, the primary physician, with reinforcement from the "expert" IME, can recommend that the patient return to work as quickly as possible. The sooner an IME is consulted the more effective it is.

The patients that do get better should be encouraged to gradually increase their activities and begin a program of exercises. The goal is a return to their normal lifestyles. The exercises should be directed at strengthening the paravertebral musculature, not at increasing the range of motion.

The pathway along this top portion of the algorithm is reversible. Should regression occur — with exacerbation of symptoms — the physician can resort to more stringent conservative measures. These may include additional bed rest and stronger anti-inflammatory medication. The majority of patients with neck pain will respond to therapy and return to a normal life pattern within two months of the beginning of their problem.

If the initial conservative treatment regimen fails, symptomatic patients are divided into two groups. The first is comprised of people with neck pain as a predominant complaint, with or without interscapular radiation. The second group is made up of those who complain primarily of arm pain (brachialgia).

§ 3-3. Neck Pain Predominant.

After six weeks of conservative therapy with no symptomatic relief, plain roentgenograms with lateral flexion-extension films are carefully examined for abnormalities. One group of patients will have objective evidence of instability (entry 12). In the lower cervical spine (C-3 through C-7), instability is identified by horizontal translation of one vertebra on another of more than 3.5 mm, or of an angulatory difference of adjacent vertebrae of more than eleven degrees. The majority of patients with instability will respond well to further nonoperative measures, including a through explanation of the problem and some type of bracing. In some cases, these measures will fail and a fusion of the involved spinal segments will be necessary.

Another group of patients complaining mainly of neck pain will be found to have degenerative disease on their plain X-ray films. The roentgenographic signs include loss of height of the intervertebral disc space, osteophyte formation, secondary encroachment of the intervertebral foraminae, and osteoarthritic changes in the apophyseal joint. The difficulty is not in identifying these abnormalities on the roentgenogram, but in determining their significance (entries 4, 5).

Degeneration in the cervical spine can be a normal part of the aging process. In a study of matched pairs of asymptomatic and symptomatic patients, it was concluded that large numbers of asymptomatic patients show roentgenographic evidence of advanced degenerative disease. The most significant roentgenographic finding relevant to symptomatology was found to be narrowing of the intervertebral disc space, particularly between C5-6 and C6-7. There was no difference between the two groups as far as changes at the apophyseal joints, intervertebral foraminae, or posterior articular processes.

These patients should be treated symptomatically with anti-inflammatory medication, support, and trigger point injections as required. In the quiescent stages they should be placed on isometric exercises. Finally, they should be re-examined periodically because some will develop significant pressure on the neurologic elements (myelopathy) (entry 3). As discussed, the earlier this is diagnosed the better the treatment outcome.

The majority of patients with neck pain will have normal roentgenograms. The diagnosis for this group is neck strain. At this point, with no objective findings, other pathology must be considered. These patients should undergo a bone scan and medical evaluation. The bone scan is an excellent tool, often identifying early spinal tumors or infections not seen on routine roentgenographic examinations. A thorough medical search also may reveal problems missed in the early stages of neck pain evaluation. If these diagnostic studies are positive, the patient is treated appropriately.

If the above workup is negative, the patient should have a thorough psychosocial evaluation. This is predicated on the belief that a patient's disability is related not only to his pathologic anatomy but also to his perception of pain and his stability in relationship to his sociologic environment. Drug habituation, alcoholism, depression, and other psychiatric problems frequently are seen in association with neck pain. If the evaluation reveals this type of pathology, proper measures are instituted to overcome the disability.

Should the psychosocial evaluation prove normal, the patient is considered to have chronic neck pain. One must be aware that other outside factors such as compensation and/or litigation can influence a patient's perception of his subjective pain. Patients with chronic neck pain need encouragement, patience, and education from their physicians. They need to be detoxified from narcotic drugs and placed on an exercise regimen. Many will respond to antidepressant drugs such as amitriptyline (Elavil). All of them need periodic re-evaluation to avoid missing any new problems.

§ 3-4. Arm Pain Predominant (Brachialgia).

Patients who have pain radiating into their arm may be experiencing their symptoms secondary to mechanical pressure and inflammation of the involved nerve roots. This mechanical pressure may arise from a ruptured disc or from bone secondary to degenerative changes (entry 8). Other pathologic causes of arm pain should be carefully considered. Extrinsic pressure on the vascular structures or on the peripheral nerves are the most likely imitators of brachialgia. Pathology in the chest and shoulder also should be ruled out.

A careful physical examination, including Adson's test, shoulder evaluation, and Tinel's test at the ulnar and carpal tunnels should be conducted. If there is any question about these findings, appropriate roentgenograms and an electromyogram (EMG) should be obtained. If any of these are positive for peripheral pressure on the nerves or other pathology, the appropriate therapy should be administered.

Should all these studies prove negative and the EMG is consistent, the patient is considered to have brachialgia. One must carefully re-evaluate the patient who has a neurologic deficit and/or a positive EMG; those who have either one are subjected to a myelogram. If the myelogram is positive and is consistent with the physical findings, surgical decompression should be considered at this juncture.

It has been documented repeatedly that for surgery to be effective, unequivocal evidence of nerve root compression must be found at surgery (entries 10, 11). One must have firm confirmation of mechanical root compression from the neurologic and roentgenographic data before proceeding with any surgery. The indications for surgery are the subjective complaint of arm pain and a neurologic deficit or positive EMG. If the patient does not have these, there is inadequate clinical evidence of root compression to proceed with surgery regardless of the roentgenographic findings. For individuals who have met these criteria for cervical decompression, the results will usually be satisfactory: 95% of them can expect good or excellent results.

§ 3-5. Treatment Modalities.

Most patients with neck pain will achieve relief from a conscientious program of conservative care. As the algorithm indicates all patients with either chronic or acute neck pain (except those with myelopathy) deserve an initial period of conservative therapy. There are a multitude of treatment modalities available but many of them are based on empiricism and tradition. The purpose of this section is to discuss the rationale behind the use of some of the more common therapeutic measures.

§ 3-6. Immobilization.

The cornerstone of conservative therapy is immobilization of the cervical spine (entry 9). The goal of immobilization is to rest the neck so that healing of torn and/or attenuated soft tissues in acute cervical injuries can take place. In the chronic situation, the purpose of immobilization is to reduce any inflammation.

Immobilization can best be achieved by the use of a soft cervical collar that holds the head in a neutral or slightly flexed position. It is very important that the collar is fitted properly. If the neck is held in hyperextension the patient is usually quite uncomfortable and does not derive any benefit from its use. In acute neck injuries, the collar should be worn on a full-time basis, night and day, until the acute pain subsides. This may sometimes take as long as four to six weeks and the patient should be aware of this time course from the outset of treatment so that the physician will not feel pressured to discontinue immobilization before the proper time.

Other types of devices are available to achieve immobilization such as plastic collars and metal braces. These are more burdensome to the patient than soft collars and are less effective in the relief of pain. When the rigid devices are used for a prolonged period of time, they can lead to marked soft tissue atrophy and stiffness, which are not found with the use of a soft collar.

In some instances, patients fail to attain adequate pain relief with ambulatory use of the soft collar. These people should be put to bed to relieve the cervical spine from the burden of supporting the weight of the head. While at bed rest, these patients should be instructed to continue using their collar on a full-time basis. The amount of immobilization prescribed varies for each patient: these people should not be mobilized until reasonably comfortable at which time exercises can be considered.

§ 3-7. Drug Therapy.

There are three different groups of medications that have proved helpful in the treatment of neck pain: anti-inflammatory drugs, analgesics, and muscle relaxants. They are used as an important adjunct to adequate immobilization.

Anti-inflammatory drugs are used because it is felt that inflammation in the soft tissues is a major contributor to pain production in the cervical spine. This is especially true for those patients with symptoms secondary to a herniated disc. The arm pain that these people experience is due not only to the mechanical pressure from the ruptured disc, but also to the inflammation around the involved nerve roots. If one can get rid of the inflammation, the patient's pain usually will markedly decrease.

There is a spectrum of anti-inflammatory agents available but none have been proven superior. The author's usual treatment plan is to begin the patient on adequate doses of aspirin, which is effective and inexpensive. If the patient response is not satisfactory, other anti-inflammatory agents such as Naprosyn, Motrin or Indocin are tried. Most patients will get significant relief from one of the agents presently available. It should be stressed that anti-inflammatory medications are utilized in conjunction with immobilization; they do not replace adequate rest.

Analgesic medication is also very important during the acute phase of neck pain. The goal is to keep the patient comfortable. Most patients will respond to the equivalent of 30-60 mg of codeine every four to six hours. If stronger medication is required the patient should be monitored very closely and in some instances admitted to the hospital for observation. In many cases narcotics will be abused by the patient and addiction to some degree will become a problem. The treating physician must maintain control of the patient's drug use at all times.

Injuries to the cervical spine frequently result in painful muscle spasm. A vicious cycle is established, whereby pain leads to muscle spasm, which leads to ischemia and a further increase in pain. Once the cycle is established, it tends to be self-perpetuating. An effective muscle relaxant frequently breaks this painful cycle and allows more comfort and an increased range of motion in the cervical spine. Methocarbanol or carisoprodol in adequate doses are the drugs recommended. They are safe and quite effective.

§ 3-8. Traction.

Cervical traction has been used for many years. Today opinions regarding its effectiveness range from that of it being a valuable clinical therapy (entry 6) to the conclusion that it is either ineffective and/or potentially harmful (entry 1).

There is no uniform idea as to how traction actually works and there are a number of methods of actually applying the traction. The three major ways of administering traction are mechanical, manual, and home traction. Many feel that manual traction is preferred due to the interaction between the therapist and patient and the potential specificity of individually varying the traction.

In certain situations cervical traction is contraindicated. Malignancy, cord compression, infectious disease, osteoporosis, and rheumatoid arthritis are the major entities where cervical traction should not be employed. It is also felt that when there is a herniated disc present either in the midline or laterally traction should not be considered.

The author feels that cervical traction is useful when a collar has proved ineffective in those patients with a cervical strain or a hyperextension injury. The major benefit is felt to be continued rest and a home traction device is preferred. When used in this situation, only minimal amounts of weight (4 to 6 lbs.) should be utilized and the direction of pull should be in slight flexion. As already mentioned there are other ways of applying traction, but to date there is no valid scientific evidence available that traction in and of itself is effective.

§ 3-9. Trigger Point Injection.

Many patients will complain of a very localized tender spot in the paravertebral area. In some of these cases relief of the discomfort can be achieved with the infiltration of the trigger point with a combination of Xylocaine and a steroid preparation or Xylocaine by itself. There have been no true randomized clinical trials to study the efficacy of trigger injections, but they empirically seem to work on some patients. It is interesting to note that although the pharmacologic effects of these drugs may wear off in two to three hours, the relief may last indefinitely. The effect may be entirely the result of pyschological suggestion.

Before actually injecting a patient, a history of allergy to the drugs to be used should be obtained. The more localized the trigger point, the more effective the injection tends to be. An area of diffuse tenderness does not respond very well to this approach.

§ 3-10. Manipulation.

Manipulation of the cervical spine should be approached very carefully. In the United States this is mainly performed by chiropractors although other health care professionals are involved. The goal of manipulation is to correct any malalignment of the spinal structures which is assumed to be the etiology of the patient's pain. There is no real scientific evidence that manipulation of the cervical spine is effective in the treatment of acute or chronic neck problems.

Unfortunately, there have been a number of tragic complications associated with the use of cervical manipulation (entry 7). In one clinical study the morbidity was as high as seven percent. Injuries from manipulation include joint injury, nerve damage, vascular injury, and fracture-dislocation. Although some patients do receive a good symptomatic response after cervical manipulation, it is the author's feeling that the hazards are too great to warrant its use and that manipulation at this time has no place in the treatment of cervical spine disorders.

§ 3-11. Exercises.

After a patient's acute symptoms have cleared and there is no significant pain or spasm, an exercise regimen is reasonable. The exercises should be directed at strengthening the paravertebral musculature and not at increasing the range of motion. Motion will return with the disappearance of pain.

The exercises are isometric in nature. They are performed once each day with increasing repetitions. It should be appreciated that at present there are no scientific studies which demonstrate that isometric exercises or any other type of cervical exercises will reduce the frequency and/or recurrent neck pain episodes. Empirically, they do appear to have a positive psychologic effect and give the patient an active part in his treatment program.

BIBLIOGRAPHY

1. British association of physical medicine: pain in the neck and arm: a multicentre trial of the effects of physiotherapy. Br Med J, 1966: 1:253.
2. DePalma, A.P., and Rothman, R.H. *The Intervertebral Disc.* Philadelphia, W.B. Saunders Co., 1970.

3. DePalma, A.P., et al. The natural history of severe cervical disc degeneration. Acta Orthopaedic Scand 43:392-396, 1972.
4. Friedenberg, Z.B., and Miller, W.T. Degeneration disc disease of the cervical spine. J. Bone Joint Surg, 45A:1171-1178, 1963.
5. Friedenberg, Z.B., Edeiken, J., Spencer, H.N., et al. Degenerative changes in the cervical spine. J. Bone Joint Surg, Am 41:61-70, 1959.
6. Harris, W. Cervical traction: review of the literature and treatment guidelines. Physical Therapy 1977, 57:8.
7. Livingston, M.C.P. Spinal manipulation causing injury. (A three-year study), CORR 81:82-86, 1971.
8. Rothman, R.H., and Marvel, J.P. The acute cervical disc, CORR 129:59-68, 1975.
9. Rothman, R.H., and Simeone, F. *The Spine,* 2d ed., Philadelphia, W.B. Saunders Co., 1982.
10. Saunders, R.L., and Wilson, D.H. The surgery of cervical disc disease: new perspectives. CORR 146:119-127, 1980.
11. Scoville, W.B. Types of cervical disc lesions and their surgical approaches. JAMA 196:479-481, 1966.
12. White, A.A., Panjabi, M.M., Posner, I., Edwards, W.T., and Hayes, W.C. Spinal stability: evaluation and treatment. Instr. Course Lectures, Vol. 30:457-483, 1981.

APPROACH TO DIAGNOSIS AND TREATMENT

Figure 1

Cervical Spine Algorithm

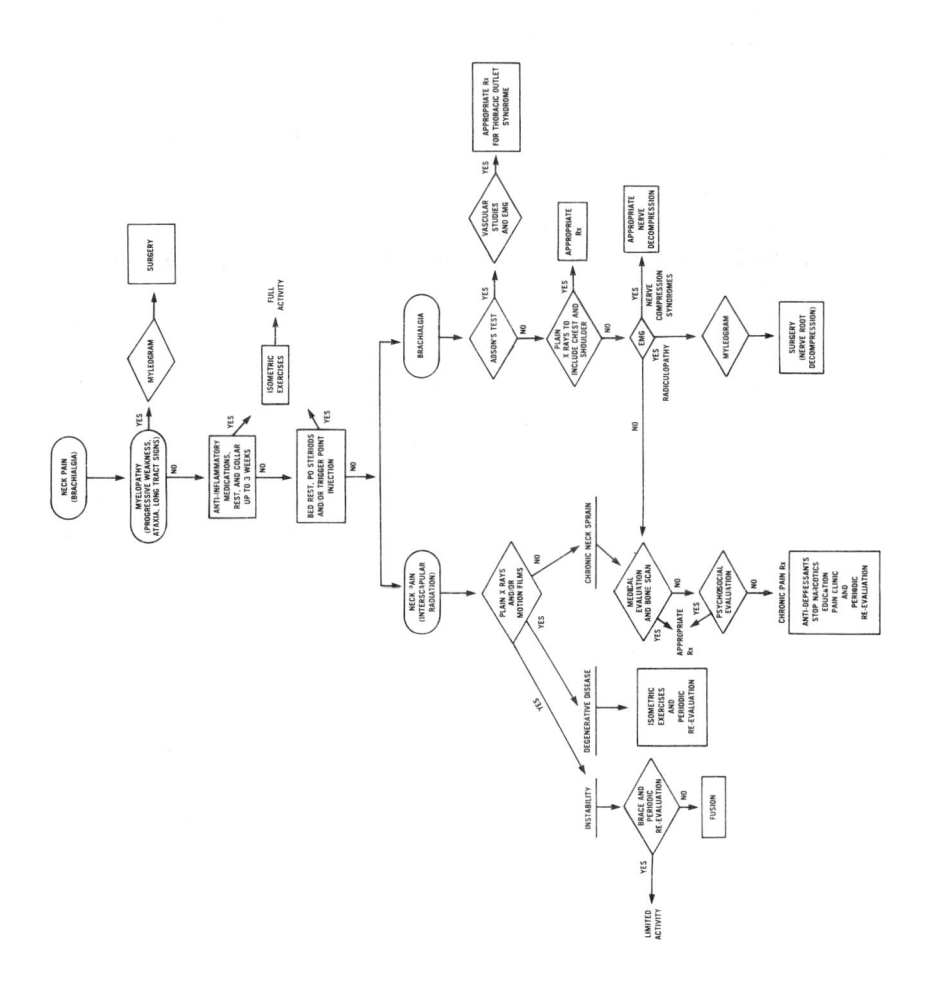

NECK PAIN

Figure 2

Differential Diagnosis of Neck Pain

EVALUATION	NECK STRAIN	HNP	INSTABILITY	DEGENERATIVE DISC DISEASE	MYELOPATHY	TUMOR	SPONDYLO-ARTHROPATHY	METABOLIC	INFECTION
PREDOMINANT PAIN (ARM vs. NECK)	NECK	ARM	NECK	NECK	NECK	NECK	NECK	NECK	NECK
CONSTITUTIONAL SYMPTOMS						+	+	+/−	+
COMPRESSION TEST		+							
NEUROLOGIC EXAM		+			+				
PLAIN X-RAYS			+/−	+	+/−	+/−	+		+/−
LATERAL MOTION X-RAYS			+						
C.A.T. SCAN		+		+	+/−	+			+
MYELOGRAM		+			+				
BONE SCAN						+	+	+/−	+
E.S.R.							+		+
Ca/P/ALK PHOS						+		+	

86

CHAPTER 4

NON-MECHANICAL CAUSES OF NECK PAIN

David G. Borenstein, M.D.

§ 4-1. Introduction.
§ 4-2. Rheumatologic Disorders of the Cervical Spine.
  § 4-2(A). Introduction.
  § 4-2(B). Rheumatoid Arthritis.
    § 4-2(B)(1). Prevalence and Etiology.
    § 4-2(B)(2). Clinical Symptoms.
    § 4-2(B)(3). Physical Findings.
    § 4-2(B)(4). Laboratory Findings.
    § 4-2(B)(5). Radiographic Findings.
    § 4-2(B)(6). Differential Diagnosis.
    § 4-2(B)(7). Treatment.
    § 4-2(B)(8). Prognosis and Course.
  Bibliography.
  § 4-2(C). Ankylosing Spondylitis.
    § 4-2(C)(1). Prevalence and Etiology.
    § 4-2(C)(2). Clinical Features.
    § 4-2(C)(3). Physical Examination.
    § 4-2(C)(4). Laboratory Findings.
    § 4-2(C)(5). Radiologic Findings.
    § 4-2(C)(6). Differential Diagnosis.
    § 4-2(C)(7). Treatment.
    § 4-2(C)(8). Course and Outcome.
  Bibliography.
  § 4-2(D). Reiter's Syndrome.
    § 4-2(D)(1). Prevalence and Etiology.
    § 4-2(D)(2). Clinical Findings.
    § 4-2(D)(3). Physical Findings.
    § 4-2(D)(4). Laboratory Findings.
    § 4-2(D)(5). Radiologic Findings.
    § 4-2(D)(6). Differential Diagnosis.
    § 4-2(D)(7). Treatment.
    § 4-2(D)(8). Course and Outcome.
  Bibliography.
  § 4-2(E). Psoriatic Arthritis.

§ 4-2(E)(1). Prevalence and Etiology.
§ 4-2(E)(2). Clinical Features.
§ 4-2(E)(3). Physical Findings.
§ 4-2(E)(4). Laboratory Findings.
§ 4-2(E)(5). Radiologic Findings.
§ 4-2(E)(6). Differential Diagnosis.
§ 4-2(E)(7). Treatment.
§ 4-2(E)(8). Course and Outcome.
Bibliography.
§ 4-2(F). Enteropathic Arthritis.
§ 4-2(F)(1). Prevalence and Etiology.
§ 4-2(F)(2). Clinical Features.
§ 4-2(F)(3). Physical Findings.
§ 4-2(F)(4). Laboratory Findings.
§ 4-2(F)(5). Radiographic Findings.
§ 4-2(F)(6). Differential Diagnosis.
§ 4-2(F)(7). Treatment.
§ 4-2(F)(8). Course and Outcome.
Bibliography.
§ 4-2(G). Diffuse Idiopathic Skeletal Hyperostosis (DISH).
§ 4-2(G)(1). Prevalence and Etiology.
§ 4-2(G)(2). Clinical Findings.
§ 4-2(G)(3). Physical Findings.
§ 4-2(G)(4). Laboratory Findings.
§ 4-2(G)(5). Radiographic Findings.
§ 4-2(G)(6). Differential Diagnosis.
§ 4-2(G)(7). Treatment.
§ 4-2(G)(8). Course and Outcome.
Bibliography.
§ 4-2(H). Polymyalgia Rheumatica.
§ 4-2(H)(1). Prevalence and Etiology.
§ 4-2(H)(2). Clinical Findings.
§ 4-2(H)(3). Physical Examination.
§ 4-2(H)(4). Laboratory Findings.
§ 4-2(H)(5). Radiologic Findings.
§ 4-2(H)(6). Differential Diagnosis.
§ 4-2(H)(7). Treatment.
§ 4-2(H)(8). Course and Etiology.
Bibliography.
§ 4-2(I). Fibrositis.
§ 4-2(I)(1). Prevalence and Etiology.

NON-MECHANICAL CAUSES OF NECK PAIN

§ 4-2(I)(2). Clinical Findings.
§ 4-2(I)(3). Physical Examination.
§ 4-2(I)(4). Laboratory Findings.
§ 4-2(I)(5). Radiographic Findings.
§ 4-2(I)(6). Differential Diagnosis.
§ 4-2(I)(7). Treatment.
§ 4-2(I)(8). Course and Outcome.
Bibliography.
Table I. Rheumatic Diseases Associated With Neck Pain.
Table II. Non-Steroidal Anti-Inflammatory Drugs.
§ 4-3. Infections of the Lumbosacral Spine.
 § 4-3(A). Introduction.
 § 4-3(B). Vertebral Osteomyelitis.
  § 4-3(B)(1). Prevalence and Etiology.
  § 4-3(B)(2). Clinical Findings.
  § 4-3(B)(3). Physical Findings.
  § 4-3(B)(4). Laboratory Findings.
  § 4-3(B)(5). Radiographic Findings.
  § 4-3(B)(6). Differential Diagnosis.
  § 4-3(B)(7). Treatment.
  § 4-3(B)(8). Course and Outcome.
 Bibliography.
 § 4-3(C). Meningitis.
  § 4-3(C)(1). Prevalence and Etiology.
  § 4-3(C)(2). Clinical Findings.
  § 4-3(C)(3). Physical Findings.
  § 4-3(C)(4). Laboratory Findings.
  § 4-3(C)(5). Radiographic Findings.
  § 4-3(C)(6). Differential Diagnosis.
  § 4-3(C)(7). Treatment.
  § 4-3(C)(8). Course and Outcome.
 Bibliography.
 § 4-3(D). Paget's Disease of Bone.
  § 4-3(D)(1). Prevalence and Etiology.
  § 4-3(D)(2). Clinical Findings.
  § 4-3(D)(3). Physical Findings.
  § 4-3(D)(4). Laboratory Findings.
  § 4-3(D)(5). Radiographic Findings.
  § 4-3(D)(6). Differential Diagnosis.
  § 4-3(D)(7). Treatment.
  § 4-3(D)(8). Course and Outcome.

Bibliography.
§ 4-4. Tumors and Infiltrative Lesions of the Cervical Spine.
  § 4-4(A). Introduction.
  § 4-4(B). Osteoblastoma.
    § 4-4(B)(1). Prevalence and Etiology.
    § 4-4(B)(2). Clinical Findings.
    § 4-4(B)(3). Physical Findings.
    § 4-4(B)(4). Laboratory Findings.
    § 4-4(B)(5). Radiographic Findings.
    § 4-4(B)(6). Differential Diagnosis.
    § 4-4(B)(7). Treatment.
    § 4-4(B)(8). Course and Outcome.
  Bibliography.
  § 4-4(C). Giant Cell Tumor.
    § 4-4(C)(1). Prevalence and Etiology.
    § 4-4(C)(2). Clinical Findings.
    § 4-4(C)(3). Physical Findings.
    § 4-4(C)(4). Laboratory Findings.
    § 4-4(C)(5). Radiographic Findings.
    § 4-4(C)(6). Differential Diagnosis.
    § 4-4(C)(7). Treatment.
    § 4-4(C)(8). Course and Outcome.
  Bibliography.
  § 4-4(D). Aneurysmal Bone Cyst.
    § 4-4(D)(1). Prevalence and Etiology.
    § 4-4(D)(2). Clinical Findings.
    § 4-4(D)(3). Physical Findings.
    § 4-4(D)(4). Laboratory Findings.
    § 4-4(D)(5). Radiographic Findings.
    § 4-4(D)(6). Differential Diagnosis.
    § 4-4(D)(7). Treatment.
    § 4-4(D)(8). Course and Outcome.
  Bibliography.
  § 4-4(E). Hemangioma.
    § 4-4(E)(1). Prevalence and Etiology.
    § 4-4(E)(2). Clinical Findings.
    § 4-4(E)(3). Physical Findings.
    § 4-4(E)(4). Laboratory Findings.
    § 4-4(E)(5). Radiographic Findings.
    § 4-4(E)(6). Differential Diagnosis.
    § 4-4(E)(7). Treatment.

NON-MECHANICAL CAUSES OF NECK PAIN

§ 4-4(E)(8). Course and Outcome.
Bibliography.
§ 4-4(F). Eosiniphilic Granduloma.
  § 4-4(F)(1). Prevalence and Etiology.
  § 4-4(F)(2). Clinical Findings.
  § 4-4(F)(3). Physical Findings.
  § 4-4(F)(4). Laboratory Findings.
  § 4-4(F)(5). Radiographic Findings.
  § 4-4(F)(6). Differential Diagnosis.
  § 4-4(F)(7). Treatment.
  § 4-4(F)(8). Course and Outcome.
Bibliography.
§ 4-4(G). Multiple Myeloma.
  § 4-4(G)(1). Prevalence and Etiology.
  § 4-4(G)(2). Clinical Findings.
  § 4-4(G)(3). Physical Findings.
  § 4-4(G)(4). Laboratory Findings.
  § 4-4(G)(5). Radiographic Findings.
  § 4-4(G)(6). Differential Diagnosis.
  § 4-4(G)(7). Treatment.
  § 4-4(G)(8). Course and Outcome.
Bibliography.
§ 4-4(H). Chordoma.
  § 4-4(H)(1). Prevalence and Etiology.
  § 4-4(H)(2). Clinical Findings.
  § 4-4(H)(3). Physical Findings.
  § 4-4(H)(4). Laboratory Findings.
  § 4-4(H)(5). Radiographic Findings.
  § 4-4(H)(6). Differential Diagnosis.
  § 4-4(H)(7). Treatment.
  § 4-4(H)(8). Course and Outcome.
Bibliography.
§ 4-4(I). Lymphomas.
  § 4-4(I)(1). Prevalence and Etiology.
  § 4-4(I)(2). Clinical Findings.
  § 4-4(I)(3). Physical Findings.
  § 4-4(I)(4). Laboratory Findings.
  § 4-4(I)(5). Radiographic Findings.
  § 4-4(I)(6). Differential Diagnosis.
  § 4-4(I)(7). Treatment.
  § 4-4(I)(8). Course and Outcome.

Bibliography.
§ 4-4(J). Skeletal Metastases.
  § 4-4(J)(1). Prevalence and Etiology.
  § 4-4(J)(2). Clinical Findings.
  § 4-4(J)(3). Physical Findings.
  § 4-4(J)(4). Laboratory Findings.
  § 4-4(J)(5). Radiographic Findings.
  § 4-4(J)(6). Differential Diagnosis.
  § 4-4(J)(7). Treatment.
  § 4-4(J)(8). Course and Outcome.
Bibliography.
§ 4-4(K). Intraspinal Neoplasm.
  § 4-4(K)(1). Prevalence and Etiology.
  § 4-4(K)(2). Clinical Features.
  § 4-4(K)(3). Physical Findings.
  § 4-4(K)(4). Laboratory Findings.
  § 4-4(K)(5). Radiographic Findings.
  § 4-4(K)(6). Differential Diagnosis.
  § 4-4(K)(7). Treatment.
  § 4-4(K)(8). Course and Outcome.
Bibliography.
§ 4-5. Endocrinologic and Metabolic Disorders of the Cervical Spine.
§ 4-6. Hematologic Disorders of the Cervical Spine.

§ 4-1. Introduction.

Neck pain is frequently associated with mechanical stresses or trauma to the cervical spine. Although occurring less frequently, systemic diseases which affect bone, cartilage, synovium, nerves, blood vessels, muscle, or connective tissue can cause damage to these same structures in the cervical spine.

The non-mechanical causes of neck pain include rheumatologic, infectious, infiltrative, endocrinologic, and hematologic. While rheumatologic, infectious, and infiltrative diseases may cause destructive changes exclusively in the cervical spine, endocrinologic and hematologic disorders cause neck disease in the setting of systemic musculoskeletal involvement. Rheumatologic disorders of the spine cause inflammation of the joints of the spine resulting in decreased motion and pain. Infections of the spine may occur in bone and are associated with localized and systemic symptoms. Infection of the meninges, meningitis, may cause severe neck pain, meningismus, and neurologic dysfunction on an acute or chronic basis. Neoplasms, both benign and malignant, may arise in the spine in association with severe, progressive pain. Neck pain, in the setting of systemic disease, is a hallmark of endocrinologic and hematologic disorders. Despite the wide range of disorders associated with cervical spine disease, the specific diagnosis of the cause of a patient's neck pain can be differentiated by the careful evaluation of the clinical history, physical examination, and laboratory data.

In most circumstances, neck pain secondary to medical causes arises totally removed from events which occur in the work place. Occasionally, however, the onset of symptoms may coincide with trauma from a work-related injury, with the worker ascribing all subsequent medical symptoms to that event. The result of this serendipitous event is a medical evaluation which concentrates on the mechanical causes of neck pain, while overlooking a potentially serious systemic illness. Alternatively, a patient may ascribe his symptoms to trauma, delaying medical evaluation, allowing the disease process to progress to his own disadvantage.

Work-related events may have a deleterious effect on the illness causing neck pain. For example, patients with ankylosing spondylitis with fusion of the cervical area have a spine which is limited in motion and more brittle. Heavy labor with twisting motion may have an adverse effect on the patient's disease because of poor body positioning which increases stress on the axial skeleton and extremities. These patients are also at risk of cervical spine fracture from minor trauma.

Limitation of work potential may also be related to the systemic illness associated with neck pain. For example, patients with enteropathic arthritis may have severe gastrointestinal symptoms causing weight loss and fatigue while being minimally limited by neck pain.

This chapter will describe those diseases associated with non-mechanical neck pain. The historical, physical, laboratory, radiographic findings, and therapy of each illness is reviewed. The course of the illnesses and its effect on work potential is described.

§ 4-2. Rheumatologic Disorders of the Cervical Spine.

§ 4-2(A). Introduction.

Rheumatologic disorders of the cervical spine are common causes of neck pain. These disorders affect the bone, joints, ligaments, tendons, and muscles which are components of the cervical spine. While muscle strain, whiplash, and osteoarthritis of the cervical spine are frequent causes of neck pain, there are a number of other inflammatory and non-inflammatory disorders associated with pain in the cervical spine. The most important rheumatic disorders which cause inflammation of the synovium and joints include rheumatoid arthritis and the seronegative spondyloarthropathies. Rheumatoid arthritis, a disease which causes chronic inflammation of the synovial lining of joints, affects the cervical spine at the attachment of the first and second cervical vertebrae and the facet joints. These changes occur in patients with diffuse disease of long duration. Patients with cervical spine involvement with rheumatoid arthritis may complain of a wide range of symptoms from mild neck pain and headaches to severe neurologic symptoms and signs including radiculopathy, paresthesias, and quadriplegia.

The seronegative spondyloarthropathies include ankylosing spondylitis, Reiter's syndrome, psoriatic arthritis, and enteropathic disease. These diseases are associated with genetic factors which predispose patients to these illnesses. Environmental factors play a role as the trigger of the inflammatory response in genetically predisposed individuals. Among the environmental triggers which have been suggested but unproven are bacterial infections and trauma. Neck pain usually occurs in a patient who has developed arthritis in the lumbosacral portion of the axial skeleton.

In rheumatoid arthritis and the spondyloarthropathies, physical examination demonstrates localized tenderness with palpation and limitation of motion in all directions of the cervical spine. Laboratory abnormalities are consistent with systemic inflammatory disease, but are non-specific except for the presence of rheumatoid factor in rheumatoid arthritis. Radiographic evaluation of the skeleton may identify characteristic changes in the cervical spine and peripheral joints which may help in the differential diagnosis of the patient with neck pain.

Non-inflammatory lesions affecting bone in the cervical spine include osteoarthritis, discussed in another portion of this book, and diffuse idiopathic skeletal hyperostosis. Muscle syndromes associated with neck pain include polymyalgia rheumatica and fibrositis.

Therapy for inflammatory and non-inflammatory disorders includes a number of modalities including patient education, physical and occupational, drug and surgical therapy. Although there are no cures for these illnesses, medical therapy can be very effective in controlling symptoms.

The prognosis and outcome of rheumatic conditions are rarely related to the extent of cervical spine disease alone. Occasionally, atlanto-axial subluxation secondary to rheumatoid arthritis may result in severe neurologic dysfunc-

§ 4-2(B)   NECK PAIN

tion which may have a deleterious effect on the patient's health. In most circumstances, the status of disease in other areas of the skeleton and the severity of constitutional symptoms (weight loss, anemia, for example) have a greater effect on work capabilities.

§ 4-2(B). Rheumatoid Arthritis.

Rheumatoid arthritis is a chronic systemic inflammatory disease which causes pain, heat, swelling, and destruction in synovial joints. The joints characteristically affected by rheumatoid arthritis are the small joints of the hands and feet, wrists, elbows, hips, knees, ankles and cervical spine. A large proportion of rheumatoid arthritis patients have cervical spine involvement manifested by neck pain, headaches, or arm numbness. Signs of cervical spine disease include decreased neck motion with stiffness, undue prominence of the spinous process of the axis (C-2), and neurologic abnormalities including sensory and motor loss, long tract signs, and rarely, paraplegia. The diagnosis of rheumatoid arthritis is made in the setting of a history of persistent joint inflammation in the appropriate distribution, and the presence of specific serum antibodies (rheumatoid factor). The extent of cervical spine involvement in rheumatoid arthritis may not correlate with patient symptoms and is detected by radiographic evaluation. Rheumatoid arthritis of the cervical spine responds to the same therapy which is effective for joint disease in other locations. However, in patients with persistent neck pain with neurologic deficits, surgical fusion of the cervical spine may be necessary to control symptoms. The disability of rheumatoid arthritis in the cervical spine is specifically related to the neurologic deficits associated with spinal cord compression. However, since patients with neck disease commonly experience severe, generalized rheumatoid arthritis, the disability these patients experience in regard to work potential is more closely related to the extent of joint destruction in all locations rather than to cervical spine disease alone.

§ 4-2(B)(1). Prevalence and Etiology.

The prevalence of rheumatoid arthritis is approximately 1% to 3% of the United States population (entry 24). Rheumatoid arthritis is found in all racial and ethnic groups. The disease affects all age groups. The male to female ratio is approximately 1:3. Symptoms of cervical spine involvement occur in 40% to 80% of patients with rheumatoid arthritis (entries 29, 9). Radiographic evidence of cervical spine involvement is found in up to 86% of patients with rheumatoid arthritis, while neurologic symptoms from cervical spine disease occur less frequently in approximately 10% of patients with radiographic changes (entries 4, 2).

The etiology of rheumatoid arthritis is probably multifactorial and mediated through the interaction of genetic (immune response genes) and environmental factors (viral infection). Clinical symptoms and signs, laboratory abnormalities, and characteristic histologic patterns in the synovium of patients with rheumatoid arthritis suggests that immunologic factors play an important role in the pathogenesis (entry 31).

In general, rheumatoid arthritis causes inflammation which is centered in the lining tissue layer of joints, the synovial membrane. This membrane lines many structures in the body associated with movement: joints, tendons, bursae, and ligaments. The inflammation associated with rheumatoid arthritis causes hypertrophy of this membrane along with the production of humoral factors which cause destruction of cartilage and bone cells. This process, if left unchecked, leads to the degradation of cartilage and bone along with disruption of the supporting structures of the joint, capsule, ligaments, tendons and bursae; a destroyed joint.

In the cervical spine, the structures lined with synovial membrane may be involved in rheumatoid arthritis. These structures include the atlantoaxial joint. This joint connects the atlas (C-1) with the axis (C-2) and is responsible for rotation of the skull on the cervical spine. Other synovial joints include the zygoapophyseal or facet, and uncovertebral.

Rheumatoid arthritis causes disease in the cervical spine by causing chronic inflammatory changes to occur in the atlanto-occipital, atlantoaxial, facet, and uncovertebral joints along with the discs, ligamentous, and bursal structures. At the level of the atlantoaxial joint, synovial inflammation of the bursae and ligaments results in laxity of the transverse ligament which holds the atlas and axis together. Normally, the distance between the bones does not exceed 2.5 to 3 mm in adults (entry 15). The relaxation of supporting ligaments results in excess motion of the axis in relation to the atlas, atlantoaxial subluxation (entry 21). Luxation of the atlantoaxial joint may occur anteriorly, posteriorly, superiorly, or laterally (entries 12, 26, 32, 7). Abnormal motion of this joint in any direction may result in compression of the cervical spinal cord which results in the development of neurologic symptoms and signs of myelopathy including paresthesias, muscle weakness, reflex changes, and incontinence (entry 19). The vertebral arteries may also be compressed during subluxation of the atlantoaxial joint by the odontoid process of the axis and the posterior arch of the atlas. Vertebral artery compression may cause tetraplegia, coma, or sudden death (entry 11).

Subluxation may occur between cervical vertebrae below the atlantoaxial joint. Common levels include the third and fourth and fourth and fifth cervical vertebrae. Inflammation in the facet joints and surrounding bursae undermine the stability of these joints resulting in excessive motion and angulation of the cervical spine (entry 8). The intervertebral discs may be invaded by growing synovial tissue resulting in disc space narrowing (entry 3).

Myelopathy may also occur in patients without atlantoaxial or cervical spine subluxation. In these patients, synovitis from the facet joints along with intervertebral disc lesions may compromise the blood supply to the spinal cord through stenosis of vertebral vessels which feed the anterior spinal artery. Ischemic myelopathy is the result (entry 11).

§ 4-2(B)(2). Clinical Symptoms.

Patients with rheumatoid arthritis develop joint pain, heat, swelling and tenderness. The joint involvement is additive and symmetrical. The joints at greatest risk of being affected by the disease process include the proximal interphalangeal, metacarpal-carpal, wrist, elbow, hip, knee, ankle, and metatarsal-phalangeal joints. Patients have joint pain and stiffness most severely in the morning. Activity improves stiffness. As a component of systemic inflammation, afternoon fatigue, anorexia and weight loss are usual complaints.

In the axial skeleton, the cervical spine is most frequently affected. Neck movement frequently precipitates or aggravates neck pain which is deep and aching in quality. Disease of the atlantoaxial joint is first felt in the upper part of the cervical spine and then radiates over the occiput into the temporal and frontal regions with more severe disease. Occipital headaches are frequently associated with active rheumatoid involvement of the cervical spine. Pain associated with rheumatoid disease in lower segments of the cervical spine is found in the lateral aspects of the neck and clavicles (C3-C4) and over the shoulders (C5-C6). Neurologic symptoms include paresthesias and numbness. The paresthesias have a burning quality which may be attributed to an entrapment neuropathy (carpal tunnel syndrome) but is sufficiently different, not to be confused with arthritic pain. Patients with sensory symptoms alone may have their problem ascribed to arthritis, delaying the diagnosis of cervical myelopathy (entry 19).

The appearance of muscular weakness, spasticity, and urinary and rectal dysfunction signifies significant compression of the spinal cord. Symptoms suggesting vertebrobasilar artery insufficiency include visual disturbances, dizziness, paresthesias of the face, ataxia and dysarthria (entries 17, 22).

In general, patients with severe, generalized rheumatoid arthritis develop neck symptoms with cervical subluxation. However, patients may develop marked subluxation with little peripheral arthritis (entry 3). Similarly, the degree of cervical subluxation may not be closely correlated with the degree of neck pain or neurologic dysfunction. This may occur because there is adequate room at the C1-C2 level (the most spacious area of the spinal column) to allow the spinal cord to slip laterally around the odontoid, escaping compression (entry 4).

§ 4-2(B)(3). Physical Findings.

Physical examination of a rheumatoid arthritis patient with cervical spine disease reveals diffuse joint inflammation characterized by heat, swelling, tenderness, and loss of motion. Examination of the cervical spine may show tenderness with palpation over the bony skeleton and limitation of all spinal movements. Inspection may show fixation of the head tilted down and to one side. This lateral tilt is caused by the asymmetrical destruction of the lateral atlantoaxial joints. The normal cervical lordosis may also be absent. With the neck flexed, the spinous process of the axis may be prominent in the midline of the neck of the patient with atlantoaxial subluxation. Palpation of the posterior pharynx during flexion may reveal abnormal separation of the anterior arch of the atlas from the body of the axis. Antero-posterior laxity may also be detected by applying pressure on the forehead while palpating the spinous process of the axis. In the patient with subluxation, the flexed head will glide backward as the subluxation is reduced. This test is not frequently utilized however for fear of causing neurologic symptoms.

Neurologic abnormalities may include loss of sensation and weakness of muscles of the upper or lower extremities. Positive Babinski signs may occur but are uncommon. Vertigo, nystagmus, dysphagia, or coma will be present in the occasional patient with vertebral artery compression. In general, neurologic abnormalities are seen in approximately 7% of patients (entry 9).

§ 4-2(B)(4). Laboratory Findings.

Abnormal laboratory findings include anemia, elevated erythrocyte sedimentation rate, and increases in serum globulins. Rheumatoid factors (antibodies directed against host antibodies) are present in 80% of patients with rheumatoid arthritis. Antinuclear antibodies are present in 30% of rheumatoid arthritis patients. Synovial fluid analysis demonstrates an inflammatory fluid characterized by poor viscosity, increased numbers of white blood cells, decreased glucose, and increased protein.

Histologic examination of the synovium from affected joints demonstrates an inflammatory, hyperplastic tissue characterized by mononuclear cell infiltration, synovial cell proliferation, fibrin deposition and fibrosis. Examination of the cervical spine apophyseal joints reveal pannus formation (synovial proliferation) associated with destruction of cartilage and subchondral bone (entry 3).

§ 4-2(B)(5). Radiographic Findings.

Characteristic radiographic changes of rheumatoid arthritis include soft tissue swelling, bony erosion without reactive sclerotic bone, joint space narrowing, and periarticular osteopenia. Radiographic examination of the cervical spine includes antero-posterior, lateral, oblique and full flexion lateral views. The latter view is necessary to show maximal atlantoaxial subluxation.

The radiographic criteria for diagnosis of cervical spine rheumatoid arthritis include the following: (1) atlantoaxial subluxation of 2.5 mm or more, (2) multiple subluxation of C2-3, C3-4, C4-5, C5-6, (3) narrow disc spaces with little or no osteophytosis, (4) erosion of vertebrae, especially vertebral plates, (5) odontoid, small, pointed, eroded, loss of cortex, (6) basilar impression, (7) apophyseal joint erosion, blunted facets, (8) osteoporosis, generalized, (9) wide space (less than 5 mm) between posterior arch of the atlas and spinous process of the axis (flexion to extension), (10) osteosclerosis, secondary, atlantoaxial-occipital area (entry 5).

Anterior subluxation is present when the distance between the odontoid and atlas is greater than 2.5 mm in women and 3.0 mm in men (entry 20). Vertical subluxation occurs when the odontoid protrudes through the foramen magnum into the posterior fossa of the skull. Any projection of the odontoid 4.5 mm or above a line which connects the posterior edge of the hard palate and the most caudal part of the occipital curve is pathognomonic for vertical subluxation (entry 14). Posterior subluxation occurs when the atlas is partially destroyed or the odontoid eroded or fractured (entry 33). Lateral subluxation is associated with atlantoaxial joint space narrowing, erosion of subchondral bone resulting in collapse of the lateral mass of the atlas (entry 13).

In addition to changes at the atlantoaxial joints, radiographic abnormalities including subaxial subluxation, facet joint narrowing and discitis may be noted (entry 18). Subaxial subluxation occurs in up to 29% of rheumatoid arthritis patients and is present when greater than a 3.5 mm subluxation of one vertebral body on another is measured on a lateral radiograph. Multiple subluxations may occur producing a "staircase" appearance on lateral radiographs (entry 29). Facet joint changes include narrowing, sclerosis and erosions of the joint. Disc destruction in the cervical spine of the rheumatoid patient is associated with disc space narrowing and is caused by extension of erosive disease from uncovertebral joints or by ongoing trauma to vertebral endplates secondary to instability.

Radiographic techniques, other than a plain X-ray, may be useful in discovering specific abnormalities in the cervical spine. Computed tomography is better than a plain radiograph in revealing soft tissue abnormalities in the spinal canal and may be able to detect the position of an eroded odontoid process which may not be seen on the open mouth view radiograph (entry 6). Patients with arachnoid space obliteration with cervical subluxation on CT scan may be at risk for progressive myelopathy (entry 27). Angiography may identify vertebrobasilar artery compression in the patient with neurologic signs of syncope, vertigo or visual changes (entry 17). Myelography is usually reserved for patients who are candidates for surgical correction of cervical spine subluxation.

§ 4-2(B)(6). Differential Diagnosis.

The diagnosis of rheumatoid arthritis is a clinical one based upon the history of the quality and duration of joint pain, distribution of joint involvement, presence of rheumatoid subcutaneous nodules and characteristic laboratory abnormalities (rheumatoid factor). In the setting of generalized, active disease, the finding of neck pain associated with multiple abnormalities including facet joint erosion

§ 4-2(B)

without sclerosis, disc space narrowing without osteophytes, multiple subluxations, are most appropriately attributed to rheumatoid arthritis. The cervical spine abnormalities of ankylosing spondylitis, psoriatic arthritis, and diffuse idiopathic skeletal hyperostosis, are associated with new bone formation or ligamentous calcification which differentiate them from rheumatoid arthritis. Occasionally, atlantoaxial subluxation may occur alone in the setting of little peripheral arthritis. In those circumstances other disease processes which may be associated with subluxation include ankylosing spondylitis, psoriatic arthritis, Reiter's syndrome, trauma or local infection (entry 28). Characteristics of these specific diseases are listed in Table I at the end of and in other portions of this chapter.

§ 4-2(B)(7). Treatment.

The treatment for control of generalized rheumatoid arthritis includes a regimen of patient education, physical therapy, non-steroidal anti-inflammatory drugs, remittive agents (gold, penicillamine, hydroxychloroquine), corticosteroids, and immunosuppressive agents (entry 16). Therapy is directed at the control of pain and stiffness, reduction of inflammation, maintenance of function, and prevention of deformity. Patients are educated about their disease so they may be an active participant in their care. They are encouraged to continue with as normal a life style as possible. Physical therapy provides temperature modalities (heat or cold) which relieve pain, exercises which maintain muscle strength, and assistive devices (canes, crutches) which promote normal function and ambulation.

Medications to control pain and inflammation are useful in the patient with rheumatoid arthritis (Table II). Aspirin is a very effective agent for rheumatoid arthritis if given in adequate doses to reach a serum concentration of 20 to 25 mg/dl. In patients who are unable to take the number of tablets necessary to reach that serum level, who are intolerant of the drug, or who have no effect, other nonsteroidal anti-inflammatory medications are useful in controlling symptoms. These agents include ibuprofen, tolmetin, fenoprofen, indomethocin, piroxicam, sulinidac and mefenamic acid.

Patients who continue with joint inflammation or who demonstrate joint damage (joint space narrowing, bony erosions or cysts) despite adequate nonsteroidal therapy are candidates for remittive therapy. Remittive agents, such as hydroxychloroquine, gold salts or penicillamine have a delayed onset of action compared to nonsteroidal drugs. However, the remittive agents are capable of slowing the progression of joint destruction and may allow for healing of damaged osseous structures.

Systemic corticosteroids are effective in controlling the inflammatory components of rheumatoid arthritis but are unable to slow the progression of disease. Corticosteroids are also associated with a wide spectrum of toxicities ranging from hypertension and diabetes to cataracts and osteonecrosis of bone. Intraarticular corticosteroid injections are used when a single joint remains active in the face of general control of the arthritic process.

Immunosuppressives are associated with severe toxicities (aplastic anemia and cancer) which limit their benefit to the severely affected patient. Only a very small proportion of patients with rheumatoid arthritis require this therapy.

Rheumatoid arthritis of the cervical spine is responsive to the same therapy which is effective in controlling generalized disease. A major therapeutic dilemma for patients with cervical subluxation is the necessity for surgical fusion of the spine to control neck pain and neurologic signs. Despite the presence of marked subluxation, many patients with cervical spine disease are asymptomatic. In a prospective study of 350 adults with rheumatoid arthritis, only 1.7% of the patients required surgical fusion for control of their disease. Most patients do well with conservative therapy which includes a cervical collar to decrease excess motion in the spine. It may also be appropriate for the patient with cervical subluxation to wear a collar in motor vehicles to prevent complications associated with whiplash injuries. Care should also be given to patients undergoing surgery so that hyperextension of the neck during intubation does not cause neurologic dysfunction. Surgical fusion of the cervical spine should be considered for patients with severe pain, gross vertebral displacement, or progressive neurologic dysfunction including weakness. These patients benefit from decompression and fusion (entry 1).

§ 4-2(B)(8). Prognosis and Course.

The course of rheumatoid arthritis cannot be predicted at time of onset. Some patients develop sustained disease which is associated with joint destruction and resistance to therapy. Patients with seropositive generalized disease, with nodules, who are older are at greater risk of developing cervical spine disease. The natural history of cervical subluxation is usually benign. In a five to fourteen-year follow-up period, 25% of patients have an increase in subluxation, 50% will remain the same, and 25% will improve (entry 30). Despite persistent subluxation, progressive neurologic sequelae are uncommon. Patients who are at greater risk of neurologic damage are those with subaxial subluxations since the spinal column diameter is narrower at lower levels.

On occasion severe neurologic dysfunction or death are associated with cervical subluxation. The first case of subluxation reported in the literature was associated with medullary compression and death (entry 10). Other cases of subluxation and sudden death have also been reported (entry 23).

Patients with rheumatoid arthritis are not disabled specifically because of cervical spine involvement. However, patients with cervical spine disease have extensive generalized involvement which usually affects their functional status and their ability to function in a job.

BIBLIOGRAPHY

1. Awerbuck, M.S., Henderson, D.R.F., Milazzo, S.C., White, R.G., and Utturkar, A.B. Longterm follow-up of posterior cervical fusion for atlanto-axial subluxation in rheumatoid arthritis. J Rheumatol, 8:423-432, 1981.
2. Bernhard, G. Extra-articular rheumatoid arthritis: clinical features and treatment overview in *Rheumatoid Arthritis,* Utsinger, P.D., Zvarfler, N.J., Ehrlich, G.E. (eds), Philadelphia, J.B. Lippincott, 1985, p 337.
3. Bland, J. Rheumatoid arthritis of the cervical spine. Bull Rheum Dis, 18:471-476, 1967.
4. Bland, J.H., Davis, P.H., London, M.G., Van Buskirk, F.W., and Duarte, C.G. Rheumatoid arthritis of cervical spine. Arch Intern Med, 112:892-898, 1963.
5. Bland, J.H., Van Buskirk, F.W., Tampas, J.P., Brown, E., and Clayton, R. A study of roentgenologic criteria for rheumatoid arthritis of the cervical spine. Am J Roentgenol, 95:949-954, 1965.
6. Braunstein, E.M., Weissman, B.N., Seltzer, S.E. Sosman, J.L., Wang, A., and Zamani, A. Computed tomography and conventional radiographs of the craniocervical region in rheumatoid arthritis: a comparison. Arthritis Rheum, 27:26-32, 1984.
7. Burry, H.C., Tweed, J.M., Robinson, R.G., and Howes, R. Lateral subluxation of the atlanto-axial joint in rheumatoid arthritis. Ann Rheum Dis, 37:525-528, 1978.
8. Bywaters, E.G.L. Rheumatoid and other diseases of the cervical interspinous bursae, and changes in the spinous process. Ann Rheum Dis, 41:360-370, 1982.
9. Colon, P.W., Isdale, I.C., and Rose, B.S. Rheumatoid arthritis of the cervical spine: an analysis of 333 cases. Ann Rheum Dis, 25:120-126, 1966.

10. Davis, Jr., F.W., and Markley, H.E. Rheumatoid arthritis with death from medullary compression. Ann Intern Med, 35:451-456, 1951.
11. Editorial: Rheumatoid atlantoaxial subluxation. Br Med J, 2:200-201, 1976.
12. Friguard, E. Posterior atlanto-axial subluxation in rheumatoid arthritis. Scand J Rheumatol, 7:65-68, 1978.
13. Halla, J.T., Fallahi, S., and Hardin, J.G. Non-reducible rotational head tilt and lateral mass collapse. Arthritis Rheum, 25:1316-1324, 1982.
14. Hinck, V.C., Hopkins, C.E., and Savara, B.S. Diagnostic criteria of basilar impression. Radiology, 76:572-584, 1981.
15. Jackson, H. Diagnosis of minimal atlanto-axial subluxation. Br J Radiol, 23:672-674, 1950.
16. Jacobs, R.P. Update on the treatment of rheumatoid arthritis. Primary Care, 6:483-503, 1979.
17. Jones, M.W., and Kaufmann, J.C.E. Vertebrobasilar artery insufficiency in rheumatoid atlantoaxial subluxation. J Neuro Neurosurg Psy, 39:122-128, 1976.
18. Komusi, T., Munro, T., and Harth, M. Radiologic review: the rheumatoid cervical spine. Semin Arthritis Rheum, 14:187-195, 1985.
19. Marks, J.S., and Sharp, J. Rheumatoid cervical myelopathy. Quart J Med, 199:307-319, 1981.
20. Martel, W. The occipito-atlanto-axial joints in rheumatoid arthritis and ankylosing spondylitis. Am J Roentgenol, 86:223-240, 1961.
21. Mathews, J.A. Atlanto-axial subluxation in rheumatoid arthritis: a five-year follow-up study. Ann Rheum Dis, 33:526-531, 1974.
22. Mayer, J.W., Messner, R.P., and Kaplan, R.J. Brain stem compression in rheumatoid arthritis, JAMA, 236:2094-2095, 1976.
23. Mikulowski, P., Wollheim, F.A., Rotmil, P., and Olsen, I. Sudden death in rheumatoid arthritis with atlanto-axial dislocation. Acta Med Scand, 198:445-451, 1975.
24. O'Sullivan, J.B., and Cathcart, E.S. The prevalence of rheumatoid arthritis: follow-up evaluation of the effect of criteria on rates in Sudbury, Massachusetts. Ann Intern Med, 76:573-577, 1972.
25. Pellicci, P.M., Ranawat, C.S., Tsairis, P., and Bryan, W.J. A prospective study of the progression of rheumatoid arthritis of the cervical spine. J Bone Joint Surg, 63A:342-350, 1981.
26. Rana, N.A., Hancock, D.O., Taylor, A.R., Hill, A.G.S. Upward translocation of the dens in rheumatoid arthritis. J Bone Joint Surg, 55B:471-477, 1973.

27. Raskin, R.J., Schnapf, D.J., Wolf, C.R., Killian, P.J., and Lawless, O.J. Computerized tomography in evaluation of atlantoaxial subluxation in rheumatoid arthritis. Arthritis Rheum, 10:33-41, 1983.
28. Resnick, D., and Niwayama, G. *Rheumatoid Arthritis in Diagnosis of Bone and Joint Disorders.* Resnick, D. and Niwayama, G. (eds), Philadelphia, W.B. Saunders, 1981, p 1000.
29. Sharp, J., Purser, D.W., and Lawrence, J.S. Rheumatoid arthritis of the cervical spine in the adult. Ann Rheum Dis, 17:303-313, 1958.
30. Smith, F.H., Benn, R.T., and Sharp, J. Natural history of rheumatoid cervical luxations. Ann Rheum Dis, 31:431-439, 1972.
31. Stastny, P. Immunogenetic factors in rheumatoid arthritis. Clin Rheum Dis, 3:315-332, 1977.
32. Swinson, D.R., Hamilton, E.B.D., Mathews, J.A., and Yates, D.A.H. Vertical subluxation of the axis in rheumatoid arthritis. Ann Rheum Dis, 31:359-363, 1972.
33. Weiner, S., Bassett, L., and Spiegel, T. Superior, posterior, and lateral displacement of C-1 in rheumatoid arthritis. Arthritis Rheum, 25:1378-1381, 1982.

§ 4-2(C). Ankylosing Spondylitis.

Ankylosing spondylitis is a chronic inflammatory arthritis which causes progressive disease in the sacroiliac and axial skeleton joints. Inflammation in these joints causes spine pain and limitation of motion. Ankylosing spondylitis occurs most commonly in men who have back pain as their initial complaint. Neck pain and limitation of cervical spine motion occurs later in the course of the illness. Ankylosing spondylitis occurs less frequently in women but is associated with more severe symptoms in the cervical spine as an initial manifestation of disease. Physical examination demonstrates decreased range of motion of the spine associated with abnormal curvature. The diagnosis of ankylosing spondylitis is made in the setting of axial skeletal arthritis, the absence of rheumatoid factor in serum (seronegative), the lack of rheumatoid nodules, and the presence of a tissue factor on host cells, HLA-B27. Ankylosing spondylitis is the prototype to which the other seronegative spondyloarthropathies are compared. Disability in ankylosing spondylitis occurs in patients with extensive axial skeletal disease and hip arthritis. Cervical spine disease alone rarely limits work capabilities of a patient.

§ 4-2(C)(1). Prevalence and Etiology.

Ankylosing spondylitis and rheumatoid arthritis have the same prevalence, approximately 1% of the Caucasian population. While once thought to be predominantly a male disease, recent studies have demonstrated a male:female ratio in the range of 3:1 (entry 3). Women have less severe back pain and milder disease which may account for their under representation in earlier studies.

The etiology of ankylosing spondylitis is unknown. Most current theories propose a pathogenesis for the illness including a genetic predisposition in a host exposed to an environmental factor. The genetic predisposition for the seronegative spondyloarthropathies involves HLA (Human Leukocyte Antigen), antigens which are cell surface markers present on all nucleated human cells. The portion of the sixth chromosome of man which determines the expression of HLA is the major histocompatibility complex (MHC) which is associated with control of the immune response of the host. In the MHC region are loci which code for the A, B, C, and D Antigens. Antibody for the A, B, and C loci, and lymphocytes for the D locus, identify specific antigens for each locus. In the seronegative spondyloarthropathies, an association between HLA-B27 and axial skeletal disease has been demonstrated. HLA-B27 is present in over 90% of Caucasian patients with ankylosing spondylitis compared to a frequency of 8% in a normal Caucasian population (entry 28). HLA-B27 occurs with a prevalence of 4% of the normal Black population but in 50% of American Blacks with ankylosing spondylitis (entry 8). Approximately 20% of individuals with HLA-B27 have evidence of spondylitis (entry 3). That leaves 80% of HLA-B27 individuals without disease suggesting that genetic factors alone will not result in disease expression. Identical twins who are HLA-B27 positive may remain normal, may both develop ankylosing spondylitis or may become discordant with one developing ankylosing spondylitis and the other a non-ankylosing spondylitis spondyloarthropathy (entry 9).

Some environmental factors which may be associated with ankylosing spondylitis are infections and trauma. Bacteria, Klebsiella, in the urinary tract or gut were thought to be associated with the initiation of the disease. However, studies which reported heightened lymphocyte sensitivity to Klebsiella antigens in spondylitic patients have not been corroborated by other investigators (entries 5, 32).

The role of trauma to the axial skeleton in initiation of the inflammatory process of ankylosing spondylitis is unproven. In one large study of patients with ankylosing spondylitis, 23% related the onset of their symptoms to a traumatic event (entry 26). However, the authors state that the injuries precipitated symptoms of a disease already established. Patients with ankylosing spondylitis who sustain injury in the form of a surgical procedure (joint replacement) are at risk of developing myositis ossificans, calcification of soft tissues surrounding a joint. It may be possible that in patients predisposed to this disease, significant tissue injury to the axial skeleton or peripheral joints can result in an inflammatory process which promotes tissue calcification and joint ankylosis (entry 23). However, the scientific data that associates the inflammation of healing with chondritis, inflammation of cartilage and osteitis, inflammation of bone, which results in ankylosis of joints and ossification of ligaments surrounding vertebrae (syndesmophytes) are not available.

§ 4-2(C)(2). Clinical Features.

The usual patient with ankylosing spondylitis is between the ages of fifteen and forty who has had low back pain for a period of months (entry 18). The mode of onset is variable with 60% of patients developing pain in the lumbosacral area. About 20% of patients have pain in peripheral joints such as hips, shoulders, knees, elbows, and ankles as their initial symptom. Iritis, inflammation of the iris, occurs in 10% while sciatica occurs in a similar number (entry 13). Rarely do patients develop ankylosis of the spine without back pain (entry 10).

Cervical spine pain is a symptom that men with ankylosing spondylitis experience when they have had the disease for a number of years. In contrast to spondylitis in men, women with the disease have cervical spine symptoms in the absence of pain in other areas of the axial skeleton, and have a higher incidence of initial and subsequent peripheral joint disease (entry 24).

Arthritis in different areas of the spine result in corresponding clinical symptoms. Patients with lumbosacral disease have low back pain and flattening of the lumbar spine. Thoracic spine involvement results in shortness of breath secondary to decreased motion at the costovertebral joints, reduced chest expansion and decreased pulmonary function. Head and neck pain associated with decreased motion in all planes is characteristic of cervical spine disease.

Other areas of the musculoskeletal system which are affected by ankylosing spondylitis include the peripheral joints and entheses, the area of attachment of tendon to bone. Peripheral joint arthritis, particularly the knees, hips, shoulders, elbows, occurs in 30% of patients within the first ten years of disease (entry 4). Enthesopathy at the plantar fascia of the calcaneus causes heel pain and spurs, while inflammation at the attachment of the Achilles tendon also causes heel pain.

Neurologic complications of ankylosing spondylitis in the cervical spine are secondary to instability or trauma. The transverse ligament is responsible for keeping the anatomic relationship of the first and second cervical vertebrae intact. The inflammation of ankylosing spondylitis causes erosion of the ligament allowing for excess motion (subluxation) of the two vertebrae. This abnormal motion, when excessive, causes impingement of the spinal cord. This abnormality is rare but may be associated with neurologic symptoms including headaches, decreased spinal mobility, and decreased strength (entries 31, 29, 15).

Minimal trauma to the cervical spine may be associated with fracture in the patient with ankylosing spondylitis of long duration. Although the disease is associated with calcification of ligaments and joints, the loss of motion causes the vertebrae to become osteopenic. Osteopenia is associated with bone with decreased bone calcium per unit volume. Osteopenic bones are weaker and are at greater risk of fracture. In addition, the bones which are ankylosed are more brittle and unable to withstand minimal trauma. The most common location for fracture is the fifth through seventh cervical vertebrae (entries 11, 17). Although patients who develop fractures may complain of nothing more than localized pain and decreased spinal motion, severe sensory and motor functional loss corresponding to the location of the lesion may develop. Patients with minimal symptoms may be treated conservatively since fractures heal with normal bone formation. Surgical decompression and fusion is reserved for the prevention of severe neurologic abnormalities such as quadraplegia. Occasionally, fractures may go unnoticed, with no healing, resulting in a pseudoarthrosis. Although more commonly seen in the thoracic and lumbar spine, pseudoarthrosis also occurs in the cervical spine (entry 20).

Ankylosing spondylitis is associated with many non-articular abnormalities. Constitutional manifestations of disease include fever, fatigue, and weight loss which occur more commonly in the minority with peripheral joint disease. Eye disease occurs in the form of iritis, inflammation of the anterior uveal tract, which is unilateral, recurrent, and rarely causes blindness. Cardiac involvement occurs in 10% of patients with durations of disease of thirty years or longer. The most serious cardiac abnormality is aortic valve insufficiency which may result in heart failure and death. Pulmonary disease is manifested by upper lobe fibrosis which decreases lung capacity and function.

§ 4-2(C)(3). Physical Examination.

Physical examination of the patient with cervical spine involvement shows decreased range of motion, tenderness on palpation and associated muscle spasm. In most circumstances, these same patients will have decreased flexion and extension of the lumbar spine as measured by the Schober's test, decreased lateral bending, and impaired chest expansion. Examination of peripheral joints may demonstrate swelling, heat, and pain with motion particularly in larger joints such as the hips, knees, shoulders, and elbows. Extra-articular disease may be discovered with careful examination of the eyes, heart, lung, and nervous system.

§ 4-2(C)(4). Laboratory Findings.

Laboratory results are nonspecific for this illness. An elevated erythrocyte sedimentation rate is abnormal in 80% of patients while a minority will develop mild anemia. The rheumatoid factor and antinuclear antibody are absent.

Histocompatibility testing for B27 is not diagnostic for ankylosing spondylitis. Although 90% of patients with ankylosing spondylitis are HLA-B27 positive, patients with Reiter's syndrome, psoriatic spondylitis, spondylitis with inflammatory bowel disease and 8% of the normal Caucasian population are also positive. Histocompatibility testing is useful to obtain data for corroborating the diagnosis of ankylosing spondylitis in the young patient with early disease, or the woman with predominantly cervical or lumbar disease (entry 14).

§ 4-2(C)(5). Radiologic Findings.

Characteristic changes of ankylosing spondylitis in the cervical spine include straightening, symmetrical marginal vertical ossification of the outer fibers of the annulus fibrosus of the disc (syndesmophytes) and apophyseal joint fusion (entry 21). Involvement of the lumbosacral spine is manifested by symmetrical subchondral bone loss of the sacroiliac joints and "squaring" of vertebral bodies. The inflammatory process may result in eventual ankylosis of the sacroiliac and apophyseal joints which progress from the sacrum to the neck (entry 16). Scintigraphic evaluation by bone scan may demonstrate increased activity over the sacroiliac joints in early disease prior to any detectable radiographic changes in the spinal joints (entry 27).

§ 4-2(C)(6). Differential Diagnosis.

The diagnosis of ankylosing spondylitis used in clinical studies of the disease is based upon the Rome clinical criteria which include bilateral sacroiliitis on radiologic examination plus low back pain for more than three months which is not relieved by rest, pain in the thoracic spine, limited motion in the lumbar spine and limited chest expansion or iritis (entry 12). Patients with neck pain with ankylosing spondylitis will have a history of back pain as well, suggesting the diagnosis.

The differential diagnosis of neck pain and radiographic abnormalities includes other spondyloarthropathies (psoriatic spondylitis), DISH, ossification of the posterior longitudinal ligament, sternoclavicular hyperostosis, and acromegaly. Characteristics of these illnesses are listed in Table I, after § 4-2(I)(8) of this chapter, or in references (entries 25, 22).

§ 4-2(C)(7). Treatment.

The goals of therapy are to control pain and stiffness, reduce inflammation, maintain function, and prevent deformity. A therapeutic program would include patient education, physical therapy, medication, and surgical measures (entry 2). Patients are taught to maintain as normal a lifestyle as possible while maintaining normal posture and mobility. For example, to maximize neck motion and maintain normal position of the neck, patients are instructed to sleep on a hard mattress with no pillows. Physical therapy has been shown to maintain or improve neck motion (entry 19). Deep breathing exercises delay ankylosis of costovertebral joints.

Medications to control pain and inflammation are useful in the patient with ankylosing spondylitis (Table II), after § 4-2(I)(8) of this chapter (entry 7). The nonsteroidal agents which may be effective at controlling symptoms include aspirin, indomethacin, phenylbutazone, ibuprofen, tolmetin, fenoprofen, piroxicam, sulindac, mefenamic acid (entries 6, 30). In one retrospective study, phenylbutazone decreased the rate of progression of axial skeletal disease (entry 1).

Drugs which are particularly effective in rheumatoid arthritis such as injectable gold and systemic corticosteroids, are not useful for control of synovitis in ankylosing spondylitis. The same could be said of antimalarials and immunosuppressives which are ineffective in controlling axial skeletal disease.

Orthopedic therapy for ankylosing spondylitis includes braces, arthroplasties, and spinal osteotomy. Heel cups are helpful for heel pain associated with plantar fasciitis while spinal bracing may prevent forward flexion. Patients with destruction of hip joints with flexion deformities or limitation of motion because of pain benefit from total joint replacements which relieve pain and increase mobility. In patients with atlantoaxial subluxation with persistent pain or severe narrowing of the spinal canal, surgical fusion of the cervical spine relieves symptoms (entry 31).

§ 4-2(C)(8). Course and Outcome.

The usual course of ankylosing spondylitis is characterized by self-limited exacerbations and remissions. The outcome is usually benign.

Most studies report that the majority of patients remain functional and employed over the course of the illness (entries 4, 33). In one study, 80% of patients continued full-time work after twenty years of disease. The prime predictor of more severe dysfunction is the presence of hip arthritis within the first ten years of disease. Patients with cervical spine disease without peripheral arthritis did not have an increased morbidity. However, patients with spinal disease with rigidity are at risk for fracture. Their work place should be designed to limit the necessity for twisting motions which would require turning the axial skeleton or heavy labor, such as lifting objects heavier than forty pounds.

BIBLIOGRAPHY

1. Boersma, J.W. Retardation of ossification of the lumbar vertebral column in ankylosing spondylitis by means of phenylbutazone. Scand J Rheumatol, 5:60-64, 1976.
2. Calin, A., and Marks, S. Management of ankylosing spondylitis. Bull Rheum Dis, 31:35-38, 1981.
3. Calin, A., and Fries, J.F. Striking prevalence of ankylosing spondylitis in "healthy" W27 positive males and females: a controlled study. N Eng J Med, 293:835-839, 1975.
4. Carette, S., Graham, D., Little, H., Rubenstein, J., and Rosen, P. The natural disease course of ankylosing spondylitis. Arthritis Rheum, 26:186-190, 1983.
5. Edmonds, J., Macauley, D., Tyndall, A., Liew, M., Alexander, K., Geczy, A., and Baskin, H. Lymphocytotoxicity of anti-Klebsiella antisera in ankylosing spondylitis and related arthropathies: patient and family studies. Arthritis Rheum, 24:1-7, 1981.
6. Fowler, P. Phenylbutazone and indomethacin. Clin Rheum Dis, 1:267-283, 1975.
7. Godfrey, R.G., Calabro, J.J., Mills, D., and Matty, B.A. A double blind crossover trial of aspirin, indomethacin, and phenylbutazone in ankylosing spondylitis. Arthritis Rheum, 15:110, 1972.
8. Good, A.E., Kawaniski, H., and Schultz, J.S. HLA-B27 in blacks with ankylosing spondylitis or Reiter's disease. N Eng J Med, 294:166-167, 1976.
9. Hochberg, M.C., Bias, W.B., and Arnett, F.C., Jr. Family studies in HLA-B27 associated arthritis. Medicine, 57:463-475, 1978.
10. Hochberg, M.C., Borenstein, D.G., and Arnett, F.C. The absence of back pain in classical ankylosing spondylitis. Johns Hopkins Med J, 143:181-183, 1978.
11. Hunter, T., and Dubo, H. Spinal fractures complicating ankylosing spondylitis. Arthritis Rheum, 26:751-759, 1983.
12. Kellgren, J.H. Diagnostic criteria for population studies. Bull Rheum Dis, 13:291-292, 1962.
13. Lehtinen, K. 76 patients with ankylosing spondylitis seen after 30 years of disease. Scand J Rheumatol, 12:5-11, 1983.
14. Levitin, P.M., Gough, W.W., and Davis, J.S., IV. HLA-B27 Antigen in women with ankylosing spondylitis. JAMA, 235:2621-2622, 1976.
15. Martel, W., and Page, J.W. Cervical vertebral erosions and subluxations in rheumatoid arthritis and ankylosing spondylitis. Arthritis Rheum, 3:546-556, 1960.

16. McEwen, C., DiTata, D., Ling, G.C., Porini, A., Good, A., and Rankin, T. Ankylosing spondylitis and spondylitis accompanying ulcerative colitis, regional enteritis, psoriasis and Reiter's disease: a comparative study. Arthritis Rheum, 14:291-318, 1971.
17. Murray, G.C., and Persellin, R.H. Cervical fracture complicating ankylosing spondylitis: a report of eight cases and review of the literature. Am J Med, 70:1033-1041, 1981.
18. Neustadt, D.H. Ankylosing spondylitis. Postgrad Med, 61:124-135, 1977.
19. O'Driscoll, S.L., Jayson, M.I.V., and Baddeley, H. Neck movements in ankylosing spondylitis and their responses to physiotherapy. Ann Rheum Dis, 37:64-66, 1978.
20. Park, W.M., Spencer, D.G., McCall, I.W., Ward, D.J., Buchanan, W.W., and Stephens, W.H. The detection of spinal pseudoarthrosis in ankylosing spondylitis. Brit J Rad, 54:467-472, 1981.
21. Resnick, D. Hyperostosis and ossification in the cervical spine. Arthritis Rheum, 27:564-569, 1984.
22. Resnick, D. Sternocostoclavicular hyperostosis. Am J Roentgenol, 135:1278-1280, 1980.
23. Resnick, D., Dwosh, I.L., Goergen, T.G., Shapiro, R.F., and D'Ambrosia, R. Clinical and radiographic "reankylosis" following hip surgery in ankylosing spondylitis. Am J Roentgenol, 126:1181-1188, 1976.
24. Resnick, D., Dwosh, I.L., Goergen, T.G., Shapiro, R.F., Utsinger, P.D., Wiesner, K.B., and Bryan, B.L. Clinical and radiographic abnormalities in ankylosing spondylitis: a comparison of men and women. Radiology, 119:293-297, 1976.
25. Resnick, D., Guerra, J., Jr., Robinson, C.A., and Vint, V.C. Association of diffuse idiopathic skeletal hyperostosis (DISH) and calcification and ossification of the posterior longitudinal ligament. Am J Roentgenol, 131:1049-1053, 1978.
26. Rosen, P.S., and Graham, D.C. Ankylosing (Strumpell-Marie) spondylitis. Arch Interamer Rheumatol, 5:158-211, 1962.
27. Russel, A.S., Lentle, B.C., and Percy, J.S. Investigation of sacroiliac disease comparative evaluation of radiological and radionuclide techniques. J Rheumatol, 2:45-51, 1975.
28. Schlosstein, L., Terasaki, P.I., Bluestone, R., and Pearson, C.M. High association of an HL antigen, W27, with ankylosing spondylitis. N Eng J Med, 288:704-706, 1973.
29. Sharp, J., and Purser, D.W. Spontaneous atlantoaxial dislocation in ankylosing spondylitis and rheumatoid arthritis. Ann Rheum Dis, 20:47-77, 1961.

30. Simon, L.S., and Mills, J.A. Nonsteroidal anti-inflammatory drugs. N Eng J Med, 302:1179-1185, 1237-1243, 1980.
31. Sorin, S., Askari, A., and Moskowitz, R.W. Atlantoaxial subluxation as a complication of early ankylosing spondylitis. Two-case reports and a review of the literature. Arthritis Rheum, 22:273-276, 1979.
32. Warren, R.E., and Brewerton, D.A. Faecal carriage of Klebsiella by patients with ankylosing spondylitis and rheumatoid arthritis. Ann Rheum Dis, 39:37-44, 1980.
33. Wilkinson, M., and Bywaters, E.G.L. Clinical features and course of ankylosing spondylitis; as seen in a follow-up of 222 hospital referred cases. Ann Rheum Dis, 17:209-228, 1958.

§ 4-2(D). Reiter's Syndrome.

Reiter's syndrome is a disease associated with the triad of urethritis, arthritis, and conjunctivitis. Commonly affected joints include those of the lower extremities and the sacroiliacs. Spondylitis occurs with Reiter's syndrome and may involve the cervical spine with little disease in other parts of the axial skeleton. The disease results from the interaction of an environmental factor, usually a specific infection, and a genetically predisposed host. Chronic disability with Reiter's syndrome is associated with unremitting disease which affects predominantly the lower extremities. Cervical spine disease alone rarely limits work potential.

§ 4-2(D)(1). Prevalence and Etiology.

The onset of Reiter's syndrome is frequently associated with a genitourinary or gastrointestinal infection. Approximately 1% of patients with non-gonococcal urethritis develop Reiter's syndrome. In patients with enteric infections secondary to Shigella, Salmonella, Campylobacter, and Yersinia, between 0.2% to 3% will develop the syndrome. The male to female ratio in venereal and enteric infection is 10:1 and 1:1, respectively.

The etiology of Reiter's syndrome is unknown. Many patients develop the clinical characteristics of the disease after dysenteric (epidemic) or venereal (endemic) infections. Antigens associated with these infecting organisms are thought to cross react with the host's immune system resulting in a systemic disease including arthritis.

Reiter's syndrome may develop in patients who have no history of enteric or venereal infection. Some of these patients associate the onset of their disease with an episode of joint trauma (entry 1). Patients may develop urethritis, conjunctivitis, or cutaneous disease after trauma to a joint (entry 4). Another possible manifestation of trauma in these patients is the presence of bony bridging or nonmarginal syndesmophytes in the spine in the absence of sacroiliitis (entries 5, 6). However, there is no scientific evidence to substantiate the role of trauma as an initiator of Reiter's syndrome.

The etiology of the spondyloarthropathies being associated with a genetic predisposition is based upon the increased prevalence of certain histocompatibility antigens. HLA-B27 is found in 60% to 80% of patients with Reiter's syndrome, particularly those with arthritis of the axial skeleton. In addition, a majority of those who are HLA-B27 negative, have B antigens which cross react with B27, including B7, BW22, B40, and BW42 (entry 2).

§ 4-2(D)(2). Clinical Findings.

The onset of Reiter's syndrome is usually acute with predominantly lower extremity oligoarthritis occurring one to three weeks after the appearance of urethritis and mild conjunctivitis. Urethritis is manifested by dysuria and urethral discharge which is more symptomatic in men. Conjunctivitis is associated with erythema and crusting of the eyelids. The inflammation is bilateral, mild, resolves spontaneously, and may not be recognized by the patient.

Arthritis is of acute onset, asymmetric in distribution, and lower extremity predominant. In many patients, arthritis may be the only recognized manifestation of disease (entry 3). The weight-bearing joints — knees, ankles, and feet — are most frequently affected.

Although pain in the axial skeleton, particularly the back, is a common symptom during the acute phase of the illness, 20% to 70% of patients develop radiographic evidence of sacroiliitis and 23% have evidence of spondylitis (entry 10). Cervical spine involvement is characterized by neck pain and stiffness and usually occurs in the setting of pain in other parts of the axial skeleton (entry 11). Neck disease is unusual in Reiter's syndrome.

Although not part of the classic triad of the disease, mucocutaneous lesions are very characteristic of Reiter's syndrome. Oral ulcers occur on the mucosa of the oropharynx, are painless and shallow, and occur in 33% of patients. Keratodermia blennorrhagica lesions are found on the heels and soles and are indistinguishable from pustular psoriasis. Keratodermia which appears on the glans penis is referred to as circinate balanitis.

Constitutional symptoms, fever, anorexia, weight loss, and fatigue, occurs in about one-third of patients. Extra-articular complications, including cardiac and neurologic disease, are late manifestations of disease and occur in few patients.

§ 4-2(D)(3). Physical Findings.

Physical examination should include all organ systems which may be involved in the disease process. Areas to be examined include the skin, eyes, oropharynx, genitalia, and musculoskeletal system. Musculoskeletal disease is predominantly lower extremity in men and upper extremity in women (entry 16). In the lower extremities, joints of the feet, ankles, and knees are affected. Percussion tenderness over the sacroiliac joints may be bilateral or unilateral dependent on the underlying joint involvement. Mobility of the entire axial skeleton may be limited in patients with extensive spondylitis. A search for evidence of enthesopathy (inflammation of tendinous attachments) is most productive over the heel or Achilles tendon.

§ 4-2(D)(4). Laboratory Findings.

Laboratory results are non-specific. Mild anemia, an elevated white blood cell and platelet count is demonstrated in a third of the patients (entry 1). The erythrocyte sedimentation rate is elevated in up to 80% of patients, but is not helpful in monitoring therapy since it may not follow the course of the illness. Rheumatoid factor and antinuclear antibodies are characteristically absent. The inflammatory synovial fluid abnormalities associated with Reiter's syndrome are nonspecific. Histocompatibility testing helps differentiate Reiter's syndrome from rheumatoid arthritis, but does not separate Reiter's syndrome from other spondyloarthropathies.

§ 4-2(D)(5). Radiologic Findings.

Although there are no pathognomonic radiologic abnormalities of Reiter's syndrome, the presence of a combination of certain features are distinctive and are helpful in confirming the diagnosis in the patient who does not manifest the complete triad (entry 14). Characteristic findings included joint destruction most severe in the feet with relative absence of osteoporosis, periosteal new bone formation contiguous to inflamed joints and at attachments of tendons, particularly to the calcaneus.

Radiographic abnormalities in the axial skeleton more closely mirror those of psoriatic arthritis than ankylosing spondylitis (entry 15). While sacroiliac involvement may be bilateral, it is usually asymmetric in the degree of sclerosis and erosions, or unilateral. Vertebral bodies are minimally squared and facet joint (apophyseal) fusion is not common.

Spondylitis in Reiter's syndrome may be indistinguishable from ankylosing spondylitis, but more commonly is unifocal or multifocal, rather than diffuse. Areas of the lumbar and cervical spine may be affected, skipping the thoracic area (entry 14). Bony hypertrophy in the axial skeleton results in vertebral hyperostoses which are markedly thickened compared to the thin syndesmophytes of ankylosing spondylitis and cause nonmarginal bridging of vertebral bodies.

Radiologic abnormalities in the cervical spine include extensive syndesmophytoses, squaring of vertebral bodies, and atlanto-axial subluxation (entries 20, 18, 12). Paravertebral ossification occurs in the cervical spine and may be noted in patients who lack radiographic signs of disease in other areas of the axial skeleton (entries 14, 21).

§ 4-2(D)(6). Differential Diagnosis.

Preliminary criteria for the diagnosis of acute Reiter's syndrome have been reported by the American Rheumatism Association (entry 22). Patients with Reiter's syndrome were distinguished from patients with other spondyloarthropathies and gonococcal arthritis by an episode of peripheral arthritis of more than one month's duration, occurring in association with urethritis and/or cervicitis. The patient with Reiter's syndrome who develops neck pain does so in the setting of established disease. The differential diagnosis includes those inflammatory and non-inflammatory arthropathies which affect the cervical spine including the other spondyloarthropathies and DISH.

§ 4-2(D)(7). Treatment.

The goals of therapy include the alleviation of pain through reduction of inflammation and the prevention of disease progression. Modalities of therapy include patient education, physical therapy, and medication. Patient education stresses that the onset of Reiter's syndrome is not necessarily related to sexual activity and that urethritis may appear without any additional exposure to infection. Physical therapy maintains muscle strength around joints affected by arthritis.

The drugs which are most effective for Reiter's syndrome are listed in Table II, after § 4-2 (I)(8) of this chapter. Indomethacin, phenylbutazone and the other newer nonsteroidal anti-inflammatory drugs are better than aspirin in controlling joint and enthesopathic manifestations of Reiter's syndrome. These drugs result in symptomatic relief for these patients. The effect of these agents on the long-term course of the disease is unknown.

Remittive therapy in the form of gold salts or immunosuppressives are reserved for those patients with progressive, destructive peripheral disease. Methotrexate is used in patients who have failed other remittive drugs and persist with active disease (entry 8). The effect of these agents on axial skeleton disease is minimal. Patients show progressive disease in the axial skeleton although peripheral joint disease may be controlled. Systemic corticosteroids are rarely used since they are less effective in Reiter's syndrome than rheumatoid arthritis in controlling symptoms. Ophthalmic or intra-articular corticosteroids are useful for iritis and persistent joint effusions, respectively.

§ 4-2(D)(8). Course and Outcome.

Reiter's syndrome has no cure and its course is unpredictable. About 30% of patients have a self-limited illness, lasting up to a year. Another 50% develop a relapsing pattern of illness with periods of complete remission. The final 20% develop chronic, unremitting disease associated with significant disability (entry 9). Painful or deformed feet or visual loss from iritis are the most frequent causes of disability. Neck disease, if it does affect job performance, occurs in patients with severe generalized disease which limits work potential. In one study, 26% of 131 patients with Reiter's syndrome had disease activity which interfered with employment (entry 9). In contrast, only 5% of 84 patients with Reiter's syndrome had permanent disability from their disease (entry 17).

Although there is evidence that patients who were HLA-B27 positive have more severe disease and greater disability, not all HLA-B27 positive Reiter's patients have poor outcomes (entries 9, 13). Patients with HLA-B27 may have more frequent chronic axial skeleton disease.

Reiter's syndrome has the potential to be a disabling illness. Early therapy with medications, physical therapy, and appropriate shoes may improve patient function. Unfortunately, even aggressive therapy is unable to prevent disease activity and progressive disability in many of Reiter's syndrome patients.

BIBLIOGRAPHY

1. Arnett, F.C., Jr. Reiter's syndrome. Johns Hopkins Med J, 150:39-44, 1982.
2. Arnett, F.C., Hochberg, M.D., and Bias, W.B. Cross-reactive HLA antigens in B27 negative Reiter's syndrome and sacroiliitis. Johns Hopkins Med J, 141:193-197, 1977.
3. Arnett, F.C., McClusky, E., Schacter, B.Z., and Lordon, R.F. Incomplete Reiter's syndrome: discriminating features and HL-A W27 in diagnosis. Ann Intern Med, 84:8-12, 1976.
4. Borenstein, D. Unpublished observation.

5. Calin, A., and Fries, J.F. Striking prevalence of ankylosing spondylitis in "healthy" W27 positive males and females: a controlled study. N Eng J Med, 293:835-839, 1975.
6. Cohen, L.M., Mittal, K.K., Schmid, F.R., Rogers, L.F., and Cohen, K.L. Increased risk for spondylitis stigmata in apparently healthy HL-A W27 men. Ann Intern Med, 84:1-7, 1976.
7. Csonka, G.W. Clinical aspects of Reiter's syndrome. Ann Rheum Dis, 385:4-8, 1979.
8. Farber, G.A., Forshner, J.G., and O'Quinn, S.E. Reiter's syndrome: treatment with methotrexate, JAMA, 200:171-173, 1967.
9. Fox, R., Calin, A., Gerber, R.C., and Gibson, D. The chronicity of symptoms and disability in Reiter's syndrome: an analysis of 131 consecutive patients. Ann Intern Med, 91:190-193, 1979.
10. Good, A.E. Involvement of the back in Reiter's syndrome: follow-up study of thirty-four cases. Ann Intern Med, 57:44-59, 1962.
11. Good, A.E. Reiter's syndrome: long-term follow-up in relation to development of ankylosing spondylitis. Ann Rheum Dis, 38:39-45, 1979.
12. Latchow, R.E., and Meyer, G.W. Reiter disease with atlanto-axial subluxation. Radiology, 126:303-304, 1978.
13. Leirisalo, M., Skylv, G., Kousa, M., Voipio-Pulkki, L., Suoranta, H., Nissila, M., Hvidman, L., Niellsen, E.D., Svejgaard, A., Tilikainen, A., and Laitinen, O. Follow-up study on patients with Reiter's disease and reactive arthritis, with special reference to HLA-B27. Arthritis Rheum, 25:249-259, 1982.
14. Martel, W. Braunstein, E.M., Borlaza, G., Good, A.E., and Griffin, P.E., Jr., Radiologic features of Reiter's disease. Radiology, 132:1-10, 1979.
15. McEwen, C., DiTata, P., Ling, G.C., Porini, A., Good, A., and Rankin, T. Ankylosing spondylitis and spondylitis accompanying ulcerative colitis, regional enteritis, psoriasis, and Reiter's disease: a comparative study. Arthritis Rheum, 14:291-318, 1971.
16. Neuwelt, C.M., Borenstein, D.G., and Jacobs, R.P. Reiter's syndrome: a male and female disease. J Rheumatol, 9:268-272, 1982.
17. Nissila, M., Isomaki, H., Kaarela, K., Kiviniemi, P., Martio, J., and Sarna, S. Prognosis of inflammatory joint diseases. Scand J Rheumatol, 12:33-38, 1983.
18. Peterson, C.C., Jr., and Silbiger, M.L. Reiter's syndrome and psoriatic arthritis: their roentgen spectra and some interesting similarities. Am J Roentgenol, 101:860-871, 1967.

19. Popert, A.J., Gill, A.J., and Laird, S.M. A prospective study of Reiter's syndrome: an interim report on the first 82 cases. Br J Vener Dis, 40:160-165, 1964.
20. Sholkoff, S.D., Glickman, M.G., and Steinbach, H.L. Roentgenology of Reiter's Syndrome. Radiology, 97:497-503, 1970.
21. Sundaram, M., and Patton, J.T. Paravertebral ossification in psoriasis and Reiter's disease. Brit J Rad, 48:628-633, 1975.
22. Willkens, R.F., Arnett, F.C., Bitter, T., Calin, A., Fisher, L., Ford, D.K., Good, A.E., and Masi, A.T. Reiter's syndrome: evaluation of preliminary criteria for definite disease. Bull Rheum Dis, 32:31-34, 1982.

§ 4-2(E). Psoriatic Arthritis.

Psoriatic arthritis is a distinct entity associated with characteristic pattern of joint damage which occurs in the setting of the skin disease, psoriasis. The characteristic patterns of psoriatic arthritis include asymmetric oligoarthritis, symmetric polyarthritis, and spondylitis. Spondylitis may occur independent of or in conjunction with peripheral arthritis. Cervical spine involvement, characterized by neck pain and stiffness occurs most commonly with joint activity in other areas of the axial skeleton. The diagnosis of psoriatic arthritis is made in the setting of specific patterns of joint involvement, skin and nail disease, and characteristic radiographic abnormalities. The arthritis is slowly progressive and is rarely associated with significant disability.

§ 4-2(E)(1). Prevalence and Etiology.

Precise data concerning the prevalence of psoriasis are not available since patients with mild disease may never come to medical attention. Estimates of the general population affected by psoriasis have ranged from 1% to 2% (entries 2, 12). Psoriatic arthritis occurs in 7% of individuals with psoriasis, and in 0.1% of the general population (entry 15). Psoriasis and psoriatic arthritis occur in equal frequency in both sexes although psoriatic spondylitis occurs more frequently in men (entry 20).

The etiology of psoriasis and psoriatic arthritis are unknown. An unspecified abnormality in the skin results in increased metabolic activity which may reside in the superficial layers (epidermis) or deeper layers (dermis). A psoriatic diathesis exists in these patients since abnormalities in protein synthesis, blood flow and metabolism are present in normal appearing skin.

A genetic predisposition for the development of psoriasis and psoriatic arthritis does exist. HLA-B13 and HLA-BW17 antigens are found with increased frequency in patients with psoriatic skin disease (entry 31). Patients with peripheral psoriatic arthritis have an increased frequency of HLA-BW38, HLA-DR4, and HLA-DR7 antigens (entry 13). Approximately 40% to 60% of patients with psoriatic spondylitis are HLA-B27 positive compared to 90% of patients with ankylosing spondylitis (entry 26).

In addition to a genetic predisposition, exposure to environmental factors are necessary to develop psoriasis and psoriatic arthritis. Trauma has been reported by a number of investigators as the initiator of arthritis or osteolysis in psoriasis (entries 8, 32). Koebner phenomenon is the reaction of the skin with swelling and erythema when stroked with an object. Trauma has been suggested as causing a "deep Koebner effect" on joints resulting in pathologic changes of psoriatic arthritis. Chronic arthritis has developed after trauma to normal joints in patients with psoriasis uncomplicated by arthritis. Other environmental factors implicated in the pathogenesis of psoriatic arthritis include infections, delayed hypersensitivity, altered vascularity, and impaired immune function.

§ 4-2(E)(2). Clinical Features.

Psoriatic arthritis has more than one clinical form (entry 25). Asymmetric oligoarthritis, affecting a few large or small joints, is the most common form of the illness, involving 70% of patients. Dactylitis, diffuse swelling of a digit, is most closely associated with this form of the disease. Symmetric polyarthritis, which affects the small joints of the hands and feet and resembles rheumatoid arthritis, occurs in 15% of patients. Classical psoriatic arthritis which involves the distal interphalangeal (DIP) joints, is associated with nail disease and occurs in 5% of psoriatic patients. Arthritis mutilans, characterized by extensive bone destruction in hands, is found in 5% of patients. Spondylitis, arthritis of the spine, with or without peripheral disease occur in 5% of patients.

In a recent report, clinical forms of psoriatic arthritis were divided into three major types — asymmetric, oligoarticular arthritis (54%); symmetric arthritis (25%); and spondyloarthritis (21%) (entry 17). DIP involvement occurs in all groups but most commonly in the asymmetric oligoarthritis group. Arthritis mulitans occurred rarely in all groups.

Patients who develop spondylitis are men who have the onset of psoriasis later in life (entry 20). Patients with psoriatic spondylitis may have cervical spine disease only although a majority of patients with spondylitis have arthritis in other parts of the axial skeleton as well. Cervical spondylitis may occur in the absence of peripheral arthritis (entry 18). Patients with spondylitis may have neck or back pain as their initial complaint although a majority have symptoms of peripheral arthritis simultaneously. Patients with psoriatic scalp disease may be more prone to cervical spine involvement (entry 30).

Psoriasis antedates the arthritis in a majority of patients. Between 10% and 20% of patients will have characteristic arthritis before the appearance of psoriatic skin lesions. Patients with severe skin involvement are more likely to develop arthritis (entry 22). Nail involvement characterized by pitting, ridging, opacification, and discoloration, occurs in 80% of patients with psoriatic arthritis, in contrast to a 30% incidence in patients with the skin disease alone.

Psoriatic arthritis differs from rheumatoid arthritis, in that the clinical appearance of an involved joint does not correlate with patient symptoms. Patients with severely affected joints, including the cervical spine, may be asymptomatic (entry 16).

§ 4-2(E)(3). Physical Findings.

Psoriatic skin lesions are characterized by erythematous, raised, circumscribed, dry scaling lesions over the elbows, knees, and scalp, and pitting of the nails. Lesions in the scalp, gluteal folds, perineum, rectum or umbilicus remain undetected unless a thorough skin examination is undertaken.

A complete musculoskeletal examination is essential in determining the extent of joint involvement. Patients may be asymptomatic in a joint although physical examination demonstrates decreased function. For example, patients may not realize decreased range of motion of the cervical spine until demonstrated on examination. Patients may describe pain with palpation over the cervical spine and may be limited in motion due to discomfort.

§ 4-2(E)(4). Laboratory Findings.

A minority of psoriatic patients have abnormalities including anemia, leukocytosis, and elevated erythrocyte sedimentation rate (entry 3). Due to an increased metabolic rate associated with protein breakdown, 20% of psoriasis patients will have hyperuricemia and are at risk of developing secondary gout. Rheumatoid factor and antinuclear antibody are absent. Synovial fluid findings are inflammatory, but nonspecific. HLA-B27 is detected in approximately 35% to 60% of patients with axial skeleton disease, but is not specific for sacroiliitis (entry 7). In one study, patients with sacroiliitis and spondylitis had 90% positively for HLA-B27 where in another study patients with spondylitis and normal sacroiliac joints had 13% positivity (entries 20, 24). Peripheral joint disease is associated with HLA-BW38 while psoriasis alone is associated with HLA-B13 and B17 (entry 14).

§ 4-2(E)(5). Radiologic Findings.

Although clinically psoriatic arthritis and rheumatoid arthritis may be confused, characteristic radiographic changes of soft tissue swelling, mineralization, erosions, and bone proliferation help differentiate the two illnesses. Psoriatic arthritis produces a symmetric fusiform soft tissue swelling around joints. Normal mineralization of bone is maintained despite the presence of erosions. Erosions may be so extensive as to cause the appearance of joint widening. The "pencil-in-cup" deformity, osteolysis of the proximal phalanx and widening of the distal phalanx, is characteristic of psoriatic arthritis. New bone formation may occur adjacent to erosions, along shafts of bones, across joints and at entheses (attachments of ligaments or tendons to bone).

Classically, DIP and PIP joints of the hands are affected in psoriatic arthritis (entries 1, 33). Similar changes may also occur in the feet. Involvement of the axial skeleton may occur with or without disease of the sacroiliac joints. Involvement of the joints, sacroiliitis, may be unilateral, asymmetric bilateral, or symmetric bilateral (entry 23).

In a radiographic study of psoriatic spondylitis, 60% of patients had cervical spine disease (entry 19). Spondylitis in this region was manifested by syndesmophytes which were asymmetric and non-marginal. Squaring of vertebral bodies occurred in 20% of patients; a smaller frequency than seen in ankylosing spondylitis. Atlantoaxial subluxation occurred in 45% of patients but none had signs of nerve compression. Facet joint fusion occurred more commonly in the cervical spine but to a lesser degree than that found with ankylosing spondylitis. Paravertebral ossification separated from the vertebral body has been reported in the cervical spine of patients with psoriatic spondylitis (entry 9). Calcification may also occur in cervical intervertebral discs in association with vertebral body fusion (entry 21). As with the other spondyloarthropathies, a bone scintiscan may demonstrate increased activity over the sacroiliac joints or axial skeleton before radiographic changes are detectable (entry 4).

§ 4-2(E)(6). Differential Diagnosis.

The diagnosis of psoriatic arthritis rests on the presence of characteristic joint disease in the setting of skin lesions. The diagnosis is more difficult in patients who present with joint disease before the appearance of skin lesions. However, the diagnosis of psoriatic arthritis can be made with confidence if characteristic radiographic changes of that disease are present.

The differential diagnosis of the neck lesions of psoriatic arthritis are limited to rheumatoid arthritis, diffuse idiopathic skeletal hyperostosis, and other spondyloarthropathies. Rheumatoid arthritis of the cervical spine causes atlantoaxial subluxation in the setting of osteoporosis and rheumatoid factor. DISH causes paravertebral ossification but without skin rash and with a normal erythrocyte sedimentation rate. Ankylosing spondylitis and inflammatory bowel disease cause symmetric disease of the axial skeleton. Gastrointestinal symptoms are common in patients with inflammatory bowel disease. The greatest difficulty arises in distinguishing Reiter's syndrome from psoriatic disease since the dermatologic findings are almost identical. The presence of conjunctivitis and urethritis is more common in Reiter's syndrome but is not exclusive.

§ 4-2(E)(7). Treatment.

The goals of therapy are the maintenance and improvement in function by the reduction of inflammation. Patient education, physical therapy, nonsteroidal anti-inflammatory drugs, and immunosuppressives are components of therapy. Although no clear cut correlation with improved skin disease and activity of arthritis can be made, non-spondylitic psoriatic arthritis may improve in patients whose skin disease responded to photochemotherapy (entry 28). Non-steroidal anti-inflammatory drugs, particularly indomethacin and phenylbutazone, are useful in controlling pain and stiffness in peripheral and axial joints. Mefenamic acid has also been suggested as useful in control of joint symptoms.

Drugs with potentially more serious side effects, including hydroxychloroquine, gold salts, corticosteroids, methotrexate, 6-mercaptopurine, and azathioprine, are reserved for patients with severe skin disease and destructive peripheral arthritis (entries 17, 10, 11). There has been no therapeutic regimen shown to stop the progression of axial disease. Therapy for psoriatic spondylitis usually includes physical therapy and non-steroidal drugs. This combination of therapies limits pain and stiffness while trying to maximize motion in the spine.

§ 4-2(E)(8). Course and Outcome.

The course of psoriatic arthritis is unpredictable although when compared to rheumatoid arthritis, patients with psoriatic disease have less pain, deformity, and long-term disability. In a ten-year longitudinal study, 97% of patients with psoriatic arthritis missed less than twelve months of work during the entire course of their disease. Over one-third lost no time from work. Over 80% of patients had clinic and radiographically stable disease over the study period. Similar findings in regard to work potential was found in another study of psoriatic arthritis (entry 27).

Patients with psoriatic spondylitis have decreased range of motion as their major limitation. Patients with documented psoriatic spondylitis should be prohibited from engaging in heavy labor. As in ankylosing spondylitis, fusion of the axial skeleton makes it more vulnerable to fracture from minimal trauma.

BIBLIOGRAPHY

1. Avila, R., Pugh, D.G., Slocumb, C.H., and Winkelman, R.K. Psoriatic arthritis: a roentgenologic study. Radiology, 75:691-701, 1960.
2. Baker, H. Epidemiological aspects of psoriasis and arthritis. Br J Dermatol, 78:249-261, 1966.
3. Baker, H., Golding, D.H., and Thompson, M. Psoriasis and arthritis. Ann Intern Med, 58:909-925, 1963.
4. Barraclough, D., Russell, A.S., and Percy, J.S. Psoriatic spondylitis: a clinical, radiological, and scintiscan survey. J Rheumatol, 4:282-287, 1977.
5. Baum, J., Hurd, E., Lewis, D., Ferguson, J.L., and Ziff, M. Treatment of psoriatic arthritis with 6-mercaptopurine. Arthritis Rheum, 16:139-147, 1973.
6. Black, R.L., O'Brien, W.M., Van Scott, E.J., Auerbach, R., Eisen, A.Z., and Bunim, J.J. Methotrexate therapy in psoriatic arthritis: double-blind study in 21 patients. JAMA, 189:743-747, 1964.

7. Brewerton, D.A., Coffrey, M., Nicholls, A., Walters, D., and James, D.C.O. HLA-B27 and arthropathies associated with ulcerative colitis and psoriasis. Lancet, 1:956-958, 1974.
8. Buckley, W.R., and Raleigh, R.L. Psoriasis with acro-osteolysis. N Eng J Med, 261:539-541, 1959.
9. Bywaters, E.G.L., and Dixon, A.S.J. Paravertebral ossification in psoriatic arthritis. Ann Rheum Dis, 24:313-331, 1965.
10. Dorwart, B.B., Gall, E.P., Schumacher, H.R., and Krauser, R.E. Chrysotherapy in psoriatic arthritis: efficacy and toxicity compared to rheumatoid arthritis. Arthritis Rheum, 21:513-515, 1978.
11. DuVivier, A., Munro, D.D., and Verbov, J. Treatment of psoriasis with azathioprine. Br Med J, 1:49-51, 1974.
12. Espinoza, L.R. *Psoriatic Arthritis: Further Epidemiologic and Genetic Considerations in Psoriatic Arthritis.* Gerber, L.H., and Espinoza, L.R. (eds), New York, Gruen and Stratton, Inc., 1985, p 9.
13. Espinoza, L.R., Vasey, F.B., Gaylord, S.W., Dietz, C., Bergan, L., Bridgeford, P., and Germain, B.F. Histocompatibility typing in the seronegative spondyloarthropathies: a survey. Semin Arthritis Rheum, 11:375-381, 1982.
14. Espinoza, L.R., Vasey, F.B., Oh, J.H., Wilkinson, R., and Osterland, C.K. Association between HLA-BW38 and peripheral psoriatic arthritis. Arthritis Rheum, 21:72-75, 1978.
15. Hellgren, L. Association between rheumatoid arthritis and psoriasis in total populations. Acta Rheum Scand, 15:316-326, 1969.
16. Jajic, I. Radiologic changes in the sacroiliac joints and spine of patients with psoriatic arthritis and psoriasis. Ann Rheum Dis 27:1-6, 1968.
17. Kammer, G.M., Soter, W.A., Gibson, D.J., and Schur, P.H. Psoriatic arthritis: a clinical, immunologic, and HLA study of 100 patients. Semin Arthritis Rheum, 9:75-97, 1979.
18. Kaplan, D., Plotz, C.M., Nathanson, L., and Frank, L. Cervical spine in psoriasis and in psoriatic arthritis. Ann Rheum Dis, 23:50-55, 1964.
19. Killebrew, K., Gold, R.H., and Sholkoff, S.D. Psoriatic spondylitis. Radiology, 108:9-16, 1973.
20. Lambert, J.R., and Wright, V. Psoriatic spondylitis: a clinical and radiological description of the spine in psoriatic arthritis. Quart J Med, 184:411-425, 1977.
21. Langelund, N., and Roaas, A. Spondylitis psoriatica. Acta Orthop Scand, 42:391-396, 1971.

22. Leczinsky, C.G. The incidence of arthropathy in a ten-year series of psoriasis cases. Acta Dermatol Vener, 28:483-487, 1948.
23. McEwen, C., DiTata, D., Lingg, C., Porini, A., Good, A., and Rankin, T. Ankylosing spondylitis and spondylitis accompanying ulcerative colitis, regional enteritis, psoriasis, and Reiter's disease: a comparative study. Arthritis Rheum, 14:291-318, 1971.
24. Metzger, A.L., Morris, R.I., Bluestone, R., and Terasaki, P.I. HLA-W27 in psoriatic arthropathy. Arthritis Rheum, 18:111-115, 1975.
25. Moll, J.M.H., and Wright, V. Psoriatic arthritis. Semin Arthritis Rheum, 3:55-78, 1973.
26. Murray, C., Mann, D.L., Gerber, L.N., Barth, W., Perlman, S., Decker, J.L., and Nigra, T.P. Histocompatibility alloantigens in psoriasis and psoriatic arthritis. J Clin Invest, 66:670-675, 1980.
27. Nissila, M., Isomaki, H., Kaarela, K., Kiviniemi, P., Martio, J., and Sarna, S. Prognosis of inflammatory joint diseases. Scand J Rheumatol, 12:33-38, 1983.
28. Perlman, S.G., Gerber, L.H., Roberts, R.M., Nigra, T.P., and Barth, W.F. Photochemotherapy and psoriatic arthritis: a prospective study. Ann Intern Med, 91:717-722, 1979.
29. Roberts, M.E.T., Wright, V., Hill, A.G.S., and Mehra, A.C. Psoriatic arthritis: follow-up study. Ann Rheum Dis, 35:206-212, 1976.
30. Vasey, F.B., and Espinoza, L.R. *Psoriatic Arthropathy in Spondyloarthropathies,* Calin, A. (ed), New York, Grune and Stratton, Inc., 1984, 169-170.
31. White, S.H., Newcomber, V.D., Micky, M.R., and Terasaki, R.I. Disturbance of HLA antigen frequency in psoriasis. N Eng J Med, 287:740-743, 1972.
32. Williams, K.A., and Scott, J.T. Influence of trauma on the development of chronic inflammatory polyarthritis. Ann Rheum Dis, 26:532-537, 1967.
33. Wright, V. Psoriatic arthritis: a comparative study of rheumatoid arthritis and arthritis associated with psoriasis. Ann Rheum Dis, 20:123-131, 1961.

§ 4-2(F). Enteropathic Arthritis.

Ulcerative colitis and Crohn's disease are inflammatory bowel diseases. Ulcerative colitis affects the colon only while Crohn's disease may involve any part of the gastrointestinal system. These diseases which are associated with abdominal cramps, fever, and weight loss cause extra-intestinal abnormalities including both a peripheral and axial skeletal form of arthritis. Peripheral arthritis is generally non-deforming and mirrors the activity of the underlying bowel disease. Patients with spondylitis may have back and neck pain as initial manifestations of disease before bowel symptoms become prominent. The course of spondylitis is independent of the activity of bowel inflammation. The diagnosis of enteropathic arthritis is made in the setting of axial skeletal arthritis in a patient with biopsy-proven inflammatory bowel disease. The work potential of patients with inflammatory bowel disease is rarely limited by spondylitis but is more significantly affected by the activity of their gastrointestinal disorder.

§ 4-2(F)(1). Prevalence and Etiology.

A patient with ulcerative colitis is most commonly a white, Jewish woman between the ages of twenty-five and forty-five years. In contrast, Crohn's disease has no racial or sexual predilection. The frequency of spondylitis is 4% of both diseases with women being half as often affected in ulcerative colitis and equally affected in Crohn's (entry 4).

The etiology of inflammatory bowel disease is unknown. The reason for the association of extraintestinal features, such as spondylitis, with bowel disease has also escaped explanation. Although no specific genetic factor has been associated with these illnesses, heredity plays a role as evidenced by the familial predilection for these diseases (entry 1).

§ 4-2(F)(2). Clinical Features.

Patients with enteropathic arthritis have changes in bowel function during the course of their illness. Patients with ulcerative colitis have an increase in bowel movements associated with bloody diarrhea. Severe disease causes fever, weight loss, and fatigue. Crohn's disease may be more indolent in onset with only mild abdominal symptoms which may go unrecognized for years.

There are two forms of arthritis associated with inflammatory bowel disease, spondylitic and peripheral. Axial skeleton involvement is similar in ulcerative colitis and Crohn's disease. Although patients may complain of lower back pain, these same individuals may describe neck pain and stiffness if questioned about these symptoms specifically (entry 12). These symptoms are most prominent in the morning and improve with activity during the day. In about 40% of patients, bowel and axial skeletal disease occur simultaneously. Bowel symptoms precede back and neck disease in 25% of patients. In the remaining percent of patients, spondylitic symptoms precede bowel disease (entry 5). Compared to ankylosing spondylitis, spondylitis associated with inflammatory bowel disease may be milder, affecting more women (entry 8). Frequently, the presence and severity of spine symptoms do not follow the course of the bowel disease.

In contrast, peripheral joint involvement does follow the activity of the bowel disease. There is a closer correlation between arthritis and ulcerative colitis than with Crohn's disease, since the latter may be associated with bowel activity which causes few symptoms. The joints most commonly affected include the knee, ankle, elbow, proximal interphalangeal, wrist or shoulder (entry 11). Patients with colonic involvement with Crohn's disease may be at greater risk of developing peripheral arthritis (entry 3). As a generalization, patients with arthritis frequently demonstrate extra-intestinal manifestations of bowel disease such as erythema nodosum, pyoderma gangrenosum and uveitis (entry 9).

§ 4-2(F)(3). Physical Findings.

Musculoskeletal examination of the patient with the spondylitic form of enteropathic arthritis may include percussion tenderness over the cervical and lumbar spine. Decreased motion is also noted with involvement of that area of the spine. A third of patients may have abnormal posture with straightening of the cervical spine. Examination for extra-intestinal disease including ulcers, erythema nodosum, pyoderma gangrenosum and uveitis is indicated. Abdominal gastrointestinal evaluation includes examination of the oropharynx, abdomen, perineum and rectum.

§ 4-2(F)(4). Laboratory Findings.

Abnormal laboratory tests include hematocrit, white blood count, platelet count, and erythrocyte sedimentation rate. Rheumatoid factor and antinuclear antibody are absent. While no specific histocompatibility typing is associated with peripheral arthritis, approximately 50% of patients with spondylitis and inflammatory bowel disease are HLA-B27 positive, while some family studies suggest that non-B27 genetic factors may play a role (entries 10, 6).

§ 4-2(F)(5). Radiographic Findings.

The radiographic features of spondylitis associated with enteropathic arthritis and ankylosing spondylitis are indistinguishable. These features include symmetric sacroiliitis, associated with widening, then fusion of the joints, "squaring" of vertebral bodies, fusion of apophyseal joints, and marginal syndesmophytes (entry 8). As mentioned, in contrast to ankylosing spondylitis, men and women have equal involvement (entry 7).

Cervical spine involvement in enteropathic arthritis occurs in the setting of disease in other parts of the axial skeleton. The disease causes radiographic abnormalities which spread from the lumbosacral to the thoracic spine and finally into the cervical area (entry 8). Approximately 35% of patients with enteropathic spondylitis longer than fifteen years have disease in the entire axial skeleton.

§ 4-2(F)(6). Differential Diagnosis.

The specific diagnosis of ulcerative colitis or Crohn's disease is based upon histologic examination of biopsies from the gastrointestinal tract. The superficial layers of the colon, including the mucosa and submucosa, are involved with inflammatory cells causing crypt abscesses and atrophy of the mucosal glands in ulcerative colitis. Transluminal granulomatous inflammation is the hallmark of Crohn's disease. The inflammatory tissue may be located at any point in the gastrointestinal tract. Radiographic studies of the gut are helpful in locating potential sites for biopsy.

The diagnosis of enteropathic spondylitis is difficult to substantiate in the patient who has no gastrointestinal symptoms. The lower frequency of HLA-B27 and female sex may help differentiate enteropathic arthritis from ankylosing spondylitis. The absence of mucocutaneous lesions, including conjunctivitis, urethritis, oral ulcers, and psoriasis, may help distinguish enteropathic arthritis from Reiter's syndrome or psoriatic arthritis.

§ 4-2(F)(7). Treatment.

Therapy for enteropathic spondylitis is similar to that of ankylosing spondylitis. This program includes patient education, physical therapy and non-steroidal anti-inflammatory drugs. The program decreases pain and stiffness and allows for maximum range of motion. Therapy which is effective for inflammatory bowel disease, including sulfasalazine, 4-6 gm. per day, corticosteroid enemas, oral corticosteroids, or colectomy, which are helpful in controlling peripheral arthritis, has little effect on the course of enteropathic spondylitis. In ulcerative colitis, colectomy should not be done with the expectation of improvement of spondylitic symptoms.

§ 4-2(F)(8). Course and Outcome.

The clinical course of enteropathic spondylitis is variable, but in contrast to ankylosing spondylitis, there is less of a tendency toward development of flexion contractions and loss of motion (entry 2). Neck disease may appear late in the course of the illness. Peripheral arthritis may accompany the axial skeleton disease and may have its onset after axial skeletal symptoms have appeared. Patients with peripheral enteropathic arthritis have non-deforming disease of short duration with little disability. Disability in enteropathic spondylitis is associated with marked decrease in mobility in patients with axial skeletal and hip disease. Patients with spinal rigidity are at risk for fracture. These patients should not perform heavy labor associated with lifting.

The ultimate outcome of these patient is dependent on the severity of their bowel disease. Cancer of the colon occurs in patients with ulcerative colitis with a severe initial attack, continuous activity of disease, and duration of ten years or longer. The mortality rate is 10% to 20% over five years with severe disease. The overall mortality rate of Crohn's disease is 5% for the first five years of disease.

BIBLIOGRAPHY

1. Almy, T.P., and Sherlock, P. Genetic aspects of ulcerative colitis and regional enteritis. Gastroenterology, 51:757-763, 1966.
2. Bowen, G.E., and Krisner, J.B. The arthritis of ulcerative colitis and regional enteritis ("intestinal arthritis"). Med Clin North Am, 49:17-32, 1965.
3. Cornes, J.S., and Stecher, M. Primary Crohn's disease of the colon and rectum. Gut, 2:189-201, 1961.
4. Dekher-Saeys, B.J., Meuwissen, S.G.M., van den Berg-Loonen, E.M., DeHaas, W.H.D., Agenant, D., and Tytgat, G.N.J. Prevalence of peripheral arthritis, sacroiliitis and ankylosing spondylitis in patients suffering from inflammatory bowel disease. Ann Rheum Dis, 37:33-35, 1978.
5. Dekhar-Saeys, B.J., Meuwissen, S.G.M., van den Berg-Loonen, E.M., DeHaas, W.H.D., Meijers, K.A.F., and Tytgat, G.N.J. Clinical characteristics and results of histocompatibility typing (HLA-B27) in 50 patients with both ankylosing spondylitis and inflammatory bowel disease. Ann Rheum Dis, 37:36-41, 1978.
6. Enlow, R.W., Bias, W.B., and Arnett, F.C. The spondylitis of inflammatory bowel disease: evidence for a non-HLA linked axial arthropathy. Arthritis Rheum, 23:1359-1365, 1980.
7. Hyla, J.F., Frank, W.A., and Davis, J.S. Lack of association of HLA-B27 with radiographic sacroiliitis in inflammatory bowel disease. J Rheumatol, 3:196-200, 1976.
8. McEwen, C., DiTata, D., Lingg, C., Porini, A., Good, A., and Rankin T. Ankylosing spondylitis and spondylitis accompanying ulcerative colitis, regional enteritis, psoriasis, and Reiter's disease: a comparative study. Arthritis Rheum, 14:291-318, 1971.
9. McEwen, C., Lingg, C., Krisner, J.B., and Spencer, J.A. Arthritis accompanying ulcerative colitis. Am J Med, 33:923-941, 1962.
10. Morris, R.I., Metzger, A.L., Bluestone, R., and Terasaki, P.I. HL-A-W27 — a useful discriminator in the arthropathies of inflammatory bowel disease. N Eng J Med, 290:1117-1119, 1974.
11. Wright, V., and Watkinson, G. The arthritis of ulcerative colitis. Br Med J, 2:670-680, 1965.
12. Zvaifler, N.J., and Martel, W. Spondylitis in chronic ulcerative colitis. Arthritis Rheum, 3:76-87, 1960.

§ 4-2(G). Diffuse Idiopathic Skeletal Hyperostosis (DISH).

Diffuse idiopathic skeletal hyperostosis is a radiographically defined illness characterized by ossification of spinal and extraspinal structures associated with the clinical symptoms of spinal stiffness and pain. Cervical spine involvement ranges from mild neck stiffness to difficulty swallowing (dysphagia). Physical findings are usually limited to decreased range of motion of affected areas of the spine. While laboratory tests are normal, radiographs of the spine demonstrate the abnormalities of paraspinous calcification of four contiguous vertebral bodies and paraarticular osteophytes. Treatment with nonsteroidal antiinflammatory drugs and exercises are effective in controlling symptoms of this illness. Rarely, patients with dysphagia may require removal of a cervical exostosis. The course of this illness is very slowly progressive and its outcome causes little morbidity or limitation of work potential.

§ 4-2(G)(1). Prevalence and Etiology.

Diffuse idiopathic skeletal hyperostosis (DISH) is a common illness found in 6% to 12% of autopsy populations (entries 5, 10). The ratio of men to women is 2:1 and Caucasians are more commonly affected than Blacks (entry 1). Most patients become symptomatic in their sixties (entry 9).

The etiology of DISH is unknown. Spinal trauma due to occupational stresses may play an etiologic role since, in at least one study, 57% of patients had occupations, construction, ranching, and roofing, which required a moderate degree of physical activity (entry 6). However, other patients in the study had the same degree of disease involvement without a history of occupational trauma. Endocrinologic abnormalities have been proposed as a possible etiology of this illness, but no consistent imbalance in growth hormone, parathormone, or glucose metabolism has been discovered (entries 9, 6).

Although one study identified an increased prevalence of HLA-B27 positivity in DISH compared to controls (34% to 8% respectively), a subsequent study found no statistically significant association of DISH with any specific genotype (entries 7, 8). DISH is not part of the spectrum of the seronegative spondyloarthropathies which includes inflammatory diseases such as ankylosing spondylitis and Reiter's syndrome.

§ 4-2(G)(2). Clinical Findings.

The predominant symptom in 80% of patients with DISH is spinal stiffness (entry 9). Stiffness is found most commonly in the thoracic spine but is also noted in the lumbar and cervical areas in patients with longer duration of disease. Duration of symptoms is not uncommonly ten to twenty years with onset in the patients' forties. Neck pain is a complaint in over 50% of patients with DISH (entry 2). Pain usually dissipates in an hour in the morning, is mild and non-radiating. Dysphagia, secondary to constriction of the esophagus by anteriorly located cervical osteophytes, occurs in 17% to 28% of patients with DISH and is their chief complaint (entries 9, 4). Dysphagia may be so severe to restrict patients' food intake to liquids only.

Extraspinal manifestations of DISH occur in 37% of patients and include symptoms of bone or joint pain. The most common areas of skeletal involvement include the shoulders, knees, elbows, and heels.

§ 4-2(G)(3). Physical Findings.

Physical examination reveals little limitation of motion of the spine in general. However, patients with cervical spine disease may have limitation of motion of the neck. A minority of patients have percussion tenderness over the spine. Patients with extraspinal disease have diminished range of motion with pain in the affected bones or joints.

§ 4-2(G)(4). Laboratory Findings.

Laboratory data is normal in patients with DISH. Abnormal parameters, when they do occur, are more closely associated with changes which occur in the elderly (elevated erythrocyte sedimentation rate, positive rheumatoid factor) than with DISH.

§ 4-2(G)(5). Radiographic Findings.

The diagnosis of DISH is a radiographic one. The three criteria for spinal involvement include flowing calcification along the anterolateral aspect of four contiguous vertebral bodies, preservation of intervertebral disc height, and absence of apophyseal joint bony ankylosis and sacroiliac joint sclerosis, erosion or fusion (entry 5). The most frequently affected area is the thoracic spine. The cervical spine has radiographic changes in about 80% of patients with DISH (entry 6).

Extraspinal radiographic changes include bony proliferation with "whiskering at tendinous and ligamentous attachments, and para-articular osteophytes" (entry 1). Common locations for these changes include the pelvis, heel, foot, patella, elbow, shoulder, and wrist.

§ 4-2(G)(6). Differential Diagnosis.

The diagnosis of DISH is based upon the presence of specific radiographic abnormalities and the absence of clinical symptoms or laboratory abnormalities associated with illnesses which cause generalized ossification. An illness which is frequently confused with DISH is ankylosing spondylitis. The presence of sacroiliac joint erosions and posterior vertebral body disease helps differentiate ankylosing spondylitis from DISH. Other illnesses which are associated with bony proliferation include other spondyloarthropathies, acromegaly, hypoparathyroidism, fluorosis, ochronosis, neuropathic arthropathy, and trauma. Specific abnormalities, such as elevated growth hormone concentration, decreased parathormone concentration, exposure to fluoride, homogentesic acid in urine, absence of sensation on neurologic examination or an injury history helps differentiate these illnesses. Rarely, DISH may occur in a patient with another disease which affects the axial skeleton, such as ankylosing spondylitis (entry 11).

§ 4-2(G)(7). Treatment.

The goals of treatment are maximizing motion while limiting musculoskeletal pain. Exercise programs are tailored to individual patients to emphasize range of motion exercises to areas of the spine with restricted motion. Nonsteroidal anti-inflammatory agents are helpful in decreasing spinal pain and stiffness. Localized areas of pain in spinal or extraspinal locations may be relieved through injections of anesthetic (lidocaine) and corticosteroid.

Patients with severe dysphagia may require surgical removal of cervical bony exostoses. These patients are restricted in their nutritional intake to liquids. Clinical evaluation of these patients must be thorough including cine-esophogram and endoscopy, since cancer of the esophagus causes dysphagia as well.

§ 4-2(G)(8). Course and Outcome.

The course of DISH is usually benign. Patients with cervical spine disease have mild limitation of motion which rarely limits their daily activities or work capacities. The illness at its worst is slowly progressive. The major difficulty for patients with cervical spine disease is dysphagia. However, this rarely is a persistent problem since surgical removal relieves symptoms.

A rare complication of DISH which may be associated with serious neurologic dysfunction is cervical spine fracture. Fracture is unusual in DISH since motion is not severely limited. However, in patients with extensive ossification, fracture is a possibility. However, as opposed to patients with ankylosing spondylitis who fracture through disc spaces, patients with DISH fracture through vertebral bodies (entry 3). With appropriate stabilization in a brace, these patients can heal their fractures with bone characteristic of the proliferative process of DISH without progression of neurologic findings and the need for surgical fusion.

BIBLIOGRAPHY

1. Forestier, J., and Lagier, R. Ankylosing hyperostosis of the spine. Clin Orthop, 74:65-83, 1971.
2. Harris, J., Carter, A.R., Glick, E.W., and Storey, G.O. Ankylosing hyperostosis: 1. Clinical and radiological features. Ann Rheum Dis, 33:210-215, 1974.
3. Houk, R.W., Hendrix, R.W., Lee, C., Lal, S., and Schmid, F.R. Cervical fracture and paraplegia complicating diffuse idiopathic skeletal hyperostosis. Arthritis Rheum, 27:472-475, 1984.
4. Meeks, L.W., and Renshaw, T.S. Vertebral osteophytosis and dysphagia: Two case reports of the syndrome recently termed ankylosing hyperostosis. J Bone Joint Surg, 55A:197-201, 1973.
5. Resnick, D., Shaul, S.R., and Robbins, J.M. Diffuse idiopathic skeletal hyperostosis (DISH): Forestier's disease with extraspinal manifestations. Radiology, 115:513-524, 1975.
6. Resnick, D., and Niwayama, G. Radiographic and pathologic features of spinal involvement in diffuse idiopathic skeletal hyperostosis (DISH). Radiology, 119:559-568, 1976.
7. Shapiro, R.F., Utsinger, P.D., Wiesner, K.B., Resnick, D., Bryan, B.L., and Castles, J.L. The association of HLA-B27 with Forestier's

disease (vertebral ankylosing hyperostosis). J Rheumatol, 3:4-8, 1976.
8. Spagnola, A.M., Bennett, P.H., and Terasaki, P.I. Vertebral ankylosing hyperostosis (Forestier's disease) and HLA antigens in Pima Indians. Arthritis Rheum, 21:467-472, 1978.
9. Utsinger, P.D., Resnick, D., and Shapiro, R. Diffuse skeletal abnormalities in Forestier's disease. Arch Intern Med, 136:763-768, 1976.
10. Vernon-Roberts, B., Pirie, C.J., and Trenwith, V. Pathology of the dorsal spine in ankylosing hyperostosis. Ann Rheum Dis, 33:281-288, 1974.
11. Williamson, P.K., and Reginato, A.J. Diffuse idiopathic skeletal hyperostosis of the cervical spine in a patient with ankylosing spondylitis. Arthritis Rheum, 27:570-573, 1984.

§ 4-2(H). Polymyalgia Rheumatica.

Polymyalgia rheumatica is a clinical syndrome characterized by severe muscle pain and stiffness in the neck, shoulders, and thighs. The usual patient is a Caucasian woman over fifty years of age. The pain is most severe in the morning and improves with activity during the day. Physical examination demonstrates muscle soreness on palpation without muscle weakness. An elevated erythrocyte sedimentation rate is the sole, consistently abnormal laboratory test. Corticosteroids in small doses are very effective in controlling symptoms, allowing patients to return to their baseline state of health without residual disability.

§ 4-2(H)(1). Prevalence and Etiology.

Polymyalgia rheumatica is not an uncommon illness occurring with an incidence of 5.4/10,000 Caucasian people over the age of fifty (entry 1). The majority of patients with polymyalgia rheumatica are over sixty years of age with increasing prevalence in older age groups (entry 12). The male to female ratio is 1:4. The etiology of this illness is unknown.

§ 4-2(H)(2). Clinical Findings.

The typical patient with polymyalgia rheumatica is a Caucasian woman, fifty years or older, who develops severe pain in the neck, shoulders, back, pelvic girdle, and thighs (entry 4). The pain is maximal in the morning and improves with activity during the day. Although these patients experience extreme pain, their affected muscles are not weak. The onset of symptoms is usually abrupt although some patients have experienced gradual onset of symptoms. Fever, weight loss, fatigue, and general malaise are frequently associated constitutional symptoms.

§ 4-2(H)(3). Physical Examination.

Physical examination demonstrates stiffness of muscles in the neck, shoulders, and upper thighs. Patients are hesitant in their motion because of pain. Muscles are not painful at rest but are with palpation. Active motion is limited while passive motion is normal. Patients frequently complain of weakness. However, careful examination will demonstrate normal strength, with no atrophy of muscle tissue. The remainder of the physical examination is usually normal except for the occasional patient with joint swelling, particularly in the sternoclavicular or wrist joints (entry 11).

§ 4-2(H)(4). Laboratory Findings.

A consistently abnormal laboratory finding is an elevated erythrocyte sedimentation rate (entry 8). Active disease may also result in a hypochromic anemia (entry 5). An isolated elevation in alkaline phosphatase, an enzyme of liver origin, is found in a third of patients (entry 9). Muscle enzymes, such as creatine kinase, are normal. Rheumatoid factor and antinuclear antibodies are present in the same proportion as found in age-matched controls.

Pathological examination of muscle biopsy specimens demonstrates no abnormalities. Non-specific inflammatory changes are noted in the occasional patient with joint swelling and polymyalgia rheumatica (entry 6).

§ 4-2(H)(5). Radiologic Findings.

Patients may have radiographic changes in the cervical spine of degenerative disc disease or osteoarthritis which are consistent with their age, but are unassociated with their polymyalgia rheumatica. Joint scans with technetium pertechnetate may demonstrate increased uptake in the shoulder joints (entry 13).

§ 4-2(H)(6). Differential Diagnosis.

Polymyalgia rheumatica is a diagnosis made after a number of other diseases with similar symptoms have been excluded since there is no pathognomonic physical finding or laboratory test for the illness. A wide range of diseases may cause muscle pain in the neck including viral infections, subacute bacterial endocarditis, malignancy, osteoarthritis, rheumatoid arthritis, polymyositis, giant cell arteritis, fibrositis, thyroid and parathyroid dysfunction. Characteristic patterns of historical, physical, and laboratory data help differentiate these illnesses, one from another. In some patients where clinical data are not absolutely characteristic, a tentative diagnosis of polymyalgia rheumatica is made and therapy is initiated. These patients are then continuously re-examined for the emergence of an illness other than polymyalgia. A diagnosis of polymyalgia rheumatica can be made with confidence only after other illnesses have been excluded, and the patient has responded to corticosteroid therapy with relief of symptoms and a normalization of the sedimentation rate.

Patients with giant cell arteritis, an inflammation of blood vessels, frequently have polymyalgia rheumatica (symptoms of neck and shoulder pain) with the addition of headaches, pain in the jaw with chewing (jaw claudication) scalp tenderness, and visual changes (entry 7). The major complication of giant cell arteritis is blindness which occurs suddenly secondary to the occlusion of the central retinal artery which supplies the retina with blood. The diagnosis of giant cell arteritis in the patients with appropriate symptoms is confirmed by the presence of giant cells in a biopsy of the temporal artery.

Polymyositis is an inflammatory muscle disease which results in muscle weakness in the proximal muscles of the neck, shoulders, and thighs. Muscle pain, with relatively little stiffness, is found in 50% of patients. Elevations of muscle enzymes, indicative of muscle fiber destruction, is found consistently in these patients. A muscle biopsy showing inflammatory changes of perivascular chronic inflammatory cell infiltrate, regenerating muscle cells, and fibrosis helps differentiate polymyositis from polymyalgia rheumatica.

§ 4-2(H)(7). Treatment.

Corticosteroids in doses of 15 mg per day are effective in controlling the symptoms of polymyalgia rheumatica (entry 2). Patients note relief of symptoms in twenty-four to forty-eight hours. The response to therapy is monitored by the return of the sedimentation rate to normal. Corticosteroid dosage is decreased slowly once the sedimentation rate is normal. Steroids are continued for at least two years, in most circumstances, since premature discontinuation may result in relapse in 30% of patients (entry 3). Nonsteroidal anti-inflammatory drugs are usually ineffective in controlling symptoms. Patients with polymyalgia rheumatica and giant cell arteritis require 60 mg or more of corticosteroids to control the disease and prevent blindness (entry 10).

§ 4-2(H)(8). Course and Etiology.

The majority of patients with polymyalgia rheumatica have a prompt response with resolution of symptoms within days of starting corticosteroids. They are able to resume their normal work activities quickly. They have no residual disability. In addition, the small amounts of corticosteroids needed to control symptoms are not usually associated with significant toxicity.

BIBLIOGRAPHY

1. Chuang, T.Y., Hunder, G.G., Ilbtrup, D.M., and Kurland, L.T. Polymyalgia rheumatica: a 10-year epidemiologic and clinical study. Ann Intern Med, 97:672-680, 1982.
2. Davison, S., and Spiera, H. Concepts and treatment in polymyalgia rheumatica. J Mt Sinai Hosp, N.Y., 35:473-478, 1968.
3. Fauchald, P., Rygvold, O., and Ystese, B. Temporal arteritis and polymyalgia rheumatica, clinical and biopsy findings. Ann Intern Med, 77:845-852, 1972.
4. Fernandez-Herliky, L. Polymyalgia rheumatica. Semin Arthritis Rheum, 1:236-245, 1971.
5. Gordon, I. Polymyalgia rheumatica: a clinical study of 21 cases. Quart J Med, 29:473-488, 1960.
6. Gordon, I., Rennie, A.M., and Branwood, A.W. Polymyalgia rheumatica: biopsy studies. Ann Rheum Dis, 23:447-455, 1964.
7. Hamilton, C.R., Shelley, W.M., and Tumulty, P.A. Giant cell arteritis including temporal arteritis and polymyalgia rheumatica. Medicine, 50:1-27, 1971.
8. Healy, L.A., Parker, F., and Wilske, K.R. Polymyalgia rheumatica and giant cell arteritis. Arthritis Rheum, 14:138-141, 1971.
9. Hunder, G.G., Sheps, S.G., Allen, G.L., and Joyce, J.W. Daily and alternate day corticosteroid regimens in treatment of giant cell arteritis: Comparison in a prospective study. Ann Intern Med, 82:613-618, 1975.

10. Hunder, G.G., and Allen, G.L. Giant cell arteritis: a review. Bull Rheum Dis, 29:980-987, 1978.
11. Miller, L.D., and Stevens, M.B. Skeletal manifestations of polymyalgia rheumatica. JAMA, 240:27-29, 1978.
12. Mowat, A.G., and Hazelman, B.L. Polymyalgia rheumatica: a clinical study with particular reference to arterial disease. J Rheumatol, 1:190-202, 1974.
13. O'Duffy, J.D., Wahner, H.W., and Hunder, G.G. Joint imaging in polymyalgia rheumatica. Mayo Clin Proc, 51:519-524, 1976.

§ 4-2(I). Fibrositis.

Fibrositis is a soft tissue, pain amplification syndrome characterized by chronic pain in discrete areas of the musculoskeletal system (trigger points) which occur in perfectionist, compulsive individuals who experience specific sleep disturbances. Pain in the cervical spine and base of the neck is a common complaint of patients with fibrositis. The pain may have a burning or aching quality which is exacerbated by excessive physical activity. Physical examination with palpation over trigger points elicits disproportionate pain locally which also radiates to other locations in neighboring musculoskeletal structures. The laboratory evaluation of fibrositis patients is normal. Therapy of fibrositis includes rest, education, physical therapy, nonsteroidal anti-inflammatory drugs, injection therapy, and agents which restore normal sleep patterns. Although not being thought of as a serious illness, fibrositis is associated with persistent pain and chronic fatigue which prevents patients from achieving their full work potential.

§ 4-2(I)(1). Prevalence and Etiology.

Although the exact number of patients with the illness is known, fibrositis is a very common condition with over ten million Americans affected (entry 8). The usual patient is a Caucasian woman in her late twenties (entry 10). The etiology of fibrositis is unknown. A number of studies suggest that abnormal sleep patterns characterized by the imposition of light stages of sleep (alpha waves on electro-encephalograms, [EEG]) on deep stages of sleep (delta rhythm) (entry 4). Further evidence for this theory is the development of fibrositic symptoms in healthy volunteers whose deep sleep was interrupted by loud noises which produced alpha rhythms on EEG. These symptoms disappeared during a night when these volunteers were not subjected to auditory stimuli (entry 5).

The role of trauma in the initiation and perpetuation of fibrositis has been suggested by Smythe (entry 7). Trauma in areas of increased sensitivity may result in perpetuation of pain long after the injury and associated pain has subsided. For example, cab drivers may develop cervical fibrositis.

Patients with increased muscle tone may be at increased risk of developing fibrositis. Fowler discovered a 50% increase, compared to controls, in electrical activity on electromyogram of patients with fibrositis (entry 2).

§ 4-2(I)(2). Clinical Findings.

Generalized aching in muscles with stiffness and fatigue are characteristic symptoms of patients with fibrositis. The aching is exacerbated by immobility and inclement weather. Stiffness may be early or late in the day in some, or continuous in others. These patients never feel rested and wake up from sleep fatigued. Neck and lumbosacral spine are common areas for symptoms of achiness. Many patients have symptoms which are of durations of twenty years or longer which have gone unrecognized.

Factors which exacerbate fibrositis include poor sleep, over activity, total inactivity, cold or humid weather. Moderate activity, warm and dry weather, and massage tend to alleviate symptoms.

§ 4-2(I)(3). Physical Examination.

Physical examination demonstrates trigger points, specific areas of the musculoskeletal system which are exquisitely tender on palpation. The area is usually less than 1 cm in diameter. When palpated, trigger points produce pain locally and in referred areas. Pressure of a surface area just outside the trigger point will not result in pain. The most commonly affected areas include the upper border of the trapezius at the base of the neck, medial part of the knees, lateral border of the elbows, posterior iliac crest and the lumbar spine. Patients with primary fibrosis usually have twelve or more discrete areas of tenderness although the number of sites may range from four to thirty-three tender points (entry 10). Except for the occasional presence of "fibrositic" nodules, which are composed of non-inflammatory fibrofatty tissue, located in neck and paraspinous muscles, the rest of the physical examination is normal.

§ 4-2(I)(4). Laboratory Findings.

Laboratory tests are normal. These include erythrocyte sedimentation rate, hematologic parameters, blood chemistries, rheumatoid factor, and antinuclear antibody.

§ 4-2(I)(5). Radiographic Findings.

Radiographic findings are normal in patients with fibrositis.

§ 4-2(I)(6). Differential Diagnosis.

There is no specific physical finding or laboratory test which is pathognomonic of fibrositis. Therefore, the diagnosis is one of exclusion and these patients require constant re-evaluation. The diagnosis of primary fibrositis is based on the presence of characteristic musculoskeletal abnormalities in the absence of any other disease process. Patients with diffuse aching and fatigue of at least three months duration, at least twelve trigger points, disturbed sleep patterns, and normal laboratory tests probably have fibrositis.

Secondary fibrositis is the same musculoskeletal syndrome occurring in the setting of an underlying disease process. Illnesses associated with secondary fibrositis include rheumatoid arthritis, osteoarthritis, spondyloarthropathies, connective tissue diseases, malignancies, hypothyroidism, hyperparathyroidism, chronic infections, and sarcoidosis (entry 1). Patients with secondary fibrositis have characteristic physical findings or laboratory abnormalities of the underlying disease process which help differentiate these individuals from those with primary fibrositis.

Fibrositis must also be differentiated from psychogenic rheumatism which is characterized by significant depression, or neurosis (entry 6). These patients have cutting or burning pain which is severe. The pain is excruciating and follows no recognizable anatomic boundaries. The patients usually deny stiffness. On examination, they have marked response to minimal pressure, jumping up from the examining table with slight pressure to the skin. The areas of tenderness do not correspond to fibrositic trigger points. The laboratory evaluation of psychogenic rheumatism patients is normal.

§ 4-2(I)(7). Treatment.

An essential part of the multifactorial therapy of fibrositis is educating the patient about his illness. Many of these patients have been labelled as malingerers or psychotic. Frequently, they are given no name for their clinical symptoms and are given a variety of analgesic medicines which are only minimally effective in controlling the pain these patients experience. Many patients are reassured by having a specific diagnosis and have relief of some of their symptoms.

Many fibrositic patients have a compulsive, perfectionist attitude towards their daily activities. Long periods of work at a computer terminal, for example, increase neck fatigue and increase symptoms. Patients are encouraged to modify their daily work routine to limit excessive fatigue (entry 10). Some patients may require a lighter duty job. Physical fitness is important for patients with fibrositis as a way to relax and stretch and strengthen muscle groups. Exercises are done for short periods of time, in a non-competitive manner.

Drug therapy, including nonsteroidal anti-inflammatory agents are useful as analgesics (entry 1). Narcotics, because of their toxicities, are not indicted for the symptoms of fibrositis. The same might also be said for systemic corticosteroids. Corticosteroids and an anesthetic agent, in combination, may be helpful when injected into trigger points for control of localized pain (entry 3). Antidepressant medications, which have central nervous system effects by normalizing sleep patterns, are useful in small doses in fibrositis. Amitriptyline in a dose of 10 to 75 mg, two hours before bedtime may allow a patient to feel rested in the morning.

Fibrositis is a chronic illness and patients with this illness will experience exacerbations. It must be impressed upon these patients that it is important to follow the recommendations for stress management, physical exercise, and rest. Compliance with this program results in a patient who requires little in the way of injection or drug therapy who has control of his/her symptoms and remains productive at work.

§ 4-2(I)(8). Course and Outcome.

Patients with fibrositis may have neck and other musculoskeletal pains which limit their work performance. Wood, in a study of English workers, reported that non-articular rheumatism, which included patients with fibrositis, accounted for 10.9% of absences from work, and corresponded to 10.5% of lost days from work (entry 9). Recognition of the disease may improve the output of a worker who was thought to be a malingerer. Although fibrositis is not as disabling as rheumatoid arthritis of the cervical spine, recognition of the illness and institution of appropriate therapy can have a beneficial effect on a worker's performance who has chronic neck pain secondary to fibrositis.

BIBLIOGRAPHY

1. Beetham, W.P., Jr. Diagnosis and management of fibrositis syndrome and psychogenic rheumatism. Med Clin North Am, 63:433-439, 1979.
2. Fowler, R.S., Jr., and Kraft, G.H. Tension perception in patients having pain associated with chronic muscle tension. Arch Phys Med Rehabil, 55:28-30, 1974.
3. Kraus, H. Trigger points. NY State J Med, 73:1310-1314, 1973.
4. Moldofsky, H., Scarisbrick, P., England, R., and Smythe, H. Musculoskeletal symptoms and non-REM sleep disturbances in patients with "fibrositis syndrome" and healthy subjects. Psychosom Med, 37:341-351, 1975.
5. Moldofsky, H., and Scarisbrick, P. Induction of neurasthenic musculoskeletal pain syndrome by elective sleep stage deprivation. Psychosom Med, 38:35-44, 1976.
6. Rotes-Queral, J. The syndromes of psychogenic rheumatism. Clin Rheum Dis, 5:797-805, 1979.
7. Smythe, H.A. Non-articular rheumatism and the fibrositis syndrome. Hollander, J.L., McCarty, D.J., Jr., eds., *Arthritis and Allied Conditions*, 8th ed., Philadelphia, Lea and Febiger, 1972, pp. 874-884.

8. The American Rheumatism Association Committee on Rheumatologic Practice: a description of rheumatology practice. Arthritis Rheum, 20:1278-1281, 1977.
9. Wood, P.H.N. Rheumatic complaints. Br Med Bull, 27:82-88, 1971.
10. Yunus, M., Masi, A.T., Calabro, J.J., Miller, K.A., and Feigenbaum, S.L. Primary fibromyalgia (fibrositis): clinical study of 50 patients with matched normal controls. Semin Arthritis Rheum, 11:151-171, 1981.

Table I
Rheumatic Diseases Associated With Neck Pain

	Rheumatoid Arthritis	Ankylosing Spondylitis	Reiter's Syndrome	Psoriatic Spondylitis
Sex	Female	Male	Male	=
Age at Onset	20 - 30	15 - 40	20 - 30	30 - 40
Presentation	Generalized Arthritis	Back Pain	Arthritis Urethritis Conjunctivitis	Back Pain
Cervical Spine	+	+/-	+/-	+
Peripheral Joints	Hands, Feet	Hip, Shoulder	Feet	Knees
Erythrocyte Sedimentation Rate	Elevated	Elevated	Elevated	Elevated
Rheumatoid Factor	+	-	-	-
HLA-B27	8%	90%	80%	60%
Course	Continuous	Continuous	Relapsing	Continuous
Therapy	Nonsteroidals, Gold, Methotrexate, Exercises	Nonsteroidals, Exercises	Nonsteroidals, Gold Methotrexate	Nonsteroidals, Gold, Methotrexate
Disability	Neurologic Dysfunction	Hip	Lower Extremity	Lower Extremity

Table I (Continued)

	Enteropathic Arthritis	Osteoarthritis of the Spine	Polymyalgia Rheumatica	Fibrositis
Sex	=	=	Female	Female
Age at Onset	15 - 45	40 - 50	60 - 70	20 - 40
Presentation	Abdominal Pain	Neck Pain	Neck Pain Thigh Pain	Neck Pain Back Pain Knee Pain Elbow Pain
Cervical Spine	+/-	+	-	-
Peripheral Joints	Knees	Hands, Knees Hips	-	-
Erythrocyte Sedimentation Rate	Elevated	Normal	Elevated	Normal
Rheumatoid Factor	-	-	-	-
HLA-B27	50%	8%	8%	8%
Course	Continuous	Relapsing	Continuous	Relapsing
Therapy	Nonsteroidals Corticosteroids Antibiotics	Nonsteroidals	Corticosteroids	Nonsteroidals Antidepressants
Disability	Hip	Neurologic Dysfunction	Muscle Pain	Muscle Pain

Table II
Non-Steroidal Anti-Inflammatory Drugs

	Brand Name	Size (mg)	Dose mg/day	Frequency/day	Loading	Major Toxicities
Salicylates						
Aspirin	Bayer	325	5300	4		GI, renal
Enteric-Coated	Ecotrin	325	5300	4		GI, renal
	Easprin	975	3900	4		GI, renal
Diflunisol	Dolobid	250, 500	500-1000	2	+	GI, renal
Phenylalkanoic Acids						
Ibuprofen	Motrin	300, 400, 600, 800	1200-2400	4		GI, renal
Fenoprofen Calcium	Nalfon	200, 300, 600	600-2400	3-4		GI, renal
Naproxen	Naprosyn	250, 375, 500	500-1000	2		GI, renal
Naproxen sodium	Anaprox	275	550-825	2		GI, renal
Indoles						
Sulindac	Clinoril	150, 200	300-400	2		GI
Tolmetin Sodium	Tolectin	200, 400	600-1600	4		GI, renal
Indomethacin	Indocin	25, 50, 75 (SR)	75-200	2-4		GI, renal, hematologic

Table II (Continued)
Non-Steroidal Anti-Inflammatory Drugs

	Brand Name	Size (mg)	Dose mg/day	Frequency/day	Loading	Major Toxicities
Anthranilic Acid						
Meclofenamate Sodium	Meclomen	50, 100	200-400	4		GI
Pyrazolone						
Phenylbutazone	Butazolidin	100	300-400	3	+	GI, renal, hematologic
Oxicam						
Piroxicam	Feldene	10, 20	10-20	1		GI, renal

§ 4-3. Infections of the Lumbosacral Spine.

§ 4-3(A). Introduction.

Infections of the cervical spine are uncommon causes of neck pain, however, physicians must include them in the differential diagnosis of patients who present with this symptom. The recognition of the infectious etiologies of neck pain is important because early recognition and appropriate therapy is important for an excellent outcome. Vertebral osteomyelitis and meningitis, when not promptly recognized, can lead to serious complications, including spinal deformity, spinal cord compression, and death.

The clinical symptoms and course of osteomyelitis and meningitis are dependent on the organism involved. Bacterial and viral infections cause acute toxic symptoms while tuberculous and fungal infections are more indolent in onset and course. The primary symptom of patients with osteomyelitis is pain which is localized over the involved anatomic structure, while with meningitis, neck pain and meningismus are the presenting symptoms. Physical examination demonstrates restriction of neck motion, muscle spasm, percussion tenderness, and neurologic dysfunction manifested by muscular weakness, sensory changes or sphincter incompetence. Laboratory evaluation is not helpful in making the diagnosis of osteomyelitis or meningitis since the abnormalities are non-specific. However, inspection of cerebrospinal fluid may help differentiate bacterial meningitis from other forms of meningeal infection. Radiographic abnormalities including vertebra body subchondral bone loss, disc space narrowing and erosions of contiguous bony structures are helpful when present, but often lag behind clinical symptoms by weeks to months.

The definitive diagnosis of osteomyelitis or meningitis requires identification of the offending organism by culturing aspirated body fluid and/or biopsied material from the lesion. Treatment consists of antimicrobial agents directed against the specific organism causing the infection, external support for the neck if spinal instability is present and surgical drainage of paraspinal abscesses if associated with spinal cord compression. With prompt diagnosis and treatment, patients with infectious causes of neck pain have resolution of their disease without residual disability. Mortality or marked morbity may be the final outcome if an infection is overlooked.

Paget's disease of bone has been included in this section on infectious etiologies of neck pain since there is increasing evidence that it is caused by a viral infection of bone. This disease, when it is associated with neck pain, is caused by abnormal bone resorption and formation in the skull and cervical spine. Treatment with agents which normalize bone growth, such as calcitonin, relieve painful symptoms and slow bone enlargement.

§ 4-3(B). Vertebral Osteomyelitis.

Vertebral osteomyelitis is an infection of the bones which comprise the axial skeleton. The organisms associated with this infection include bacteria — Staphylococcus aureus, and Escherichia coli; mycobacteria — Mycobacteria tuberculosis; and fungi — Coccidiodes immitis. In the cervical spine, vertebral osteomyelitis develops from hematogenous spread through the blood-stream from a distant location or by contiguous spread from local structures, i.e., the pharynx. The clinical symptoms and course of the infection are dependent on the infecting organism and host inflammatory response. Bacterial infections cause more acute, toxic reactions while granulomatous infections associated with tuberculous or fungal organisms cause more indolent symptoms with slowly progressive destruction of vertebrae.

The diagnosis of cervical osteomyelitis is easily missed unless the treating physician has a high index of suspicion. Presenting symptoms of neck pain and stiffness are nonspecific and patients may not develop constitutional symptoms of fever and anorexia until months into the course of their infection. Radiographic abnormalities lag behind the activity of the infection. The definitive diagnosis is confirmed by culturing the offending organism from fluid obtained from lesion aspirates or from blood cultures. Recent studies have suggested that if discovered early in the course of infection, vertebral osteomyelitis can be cured with antibiotic therapy alone. Patients with extensive destruction of bone, paravertebral abscesses which compress other organs, or neurologic dysfunction require surgical intervention. Neurologic function is maintained, the long term outlook of these patients is good. Most patients with this infection heal by fusing contiguous vertebrae resulting in a minimal decrease in motion and a resolution of clinical symptoms.

§ 4-3(B)(1). Prevalence and Etiology.

Over the past decade, 348 cases of vertebral osteomyelitis have been reported (entry 28). Vertebral osteomyelitis constitutes approximately 2% to 4% of patients with bone sepsis (entry 22). With decreasing frequency, the lumbar, thoracic and cervical spine are affected in vertebral osteomyelitis. Between 4% to 20% of patients with vertebral osteomyelitis have cervical spine involvement (entries 9, 27, 29, 20). Vertebral osteomyelitis occurs in older individuals in the fifth through seventh decade. The male to female ratio is 3:1.

Hematogenous spread through the blood stream is the most common mechanism of introduction of organisms into vertebral body bone. Vertebrae are supplied by the paravertebral venous system and nutrient arteries (entries 2,

31). The venous plexus is a network of valveless veins whose flow is modified by differential pressure. For example, greater pressure outside the vertebral column will force blood from potentially infected areas into the vertebral venous system. Blood which drains from the posterior nasopharyngeal region may drain through the pharyngovertebral veins into the epidural veins (entry 21). An alternative reason for localization of early foci of osteomyelitis in vertebral bodies in the subchondral region is nutrient arteries which supply these regions of vertebral bodies.

Vertebral osteomyelitis in the cervical spine may occur by spread from contiguous structures. Tuberculous infection may have its origin in lymph nodes in the neck (entry 16). Operations or penetrating trauma to the neck may cause an infection (entries 3, 12).

Approximately 40% of patients with vertebral osteomyelitis have an extraspinal primary source of infection. The genitourinary tract, skin and respiratory tract are common locations (entry 24). Parenteral drug abusers may develop cervical spine osteomyelitis more frequently than the general population (entries 22, 30). Patients with chronic illnesses which impair immune function such as diabetes mellitus, alcoholism, malignancy and hemoglobinopathies are at risk of developing this infection.

The location of the initial site of infection corresponds with the site of the capillary loops in the central portion of the vertebral body in the subchondral area. This results in infections which cause destruction of anterior, central and paradiscal areas of the vertebral body. Pyogenic and tuberculous involvement affects the posterior elements of the vertebral body in less than 2% of cases (entry 16).

Infections which originate in the vertebral body may remain in that one area or more commonly, extend out of the confines of the bones. Extension anteriorly, longitudinally, or posteriorly in the cervical spine will result in different clinical symptoms and signs. Anterior extension results in a retropharyngeal abscess. Longitudinal extension causes destruction in contiguous vertebral bodies and the possibility of mediastinitis. Posterior extension may cause life-threatening complications including meningitis and epidural abscess.

§ 4-3(B)(2). Clinical Findings.

The primary symptom of patients with cervical spine osteomyelitis is neck pain. The onset of symptoms may be abrupt or gradual but usually increases in intensity over weeks' time. The neck pain radiates to the occiput, shoulder, arm, or shoulder blade. Patients with an anterior abscess may present with dysphagia or dyspnea from retropharyngeal compression. Posterior extension with compression of the cord may manifest as radicular pain, muscle weakness, sensory loss or bowel or bladder dysfunction.

Tuberculous infection of the cervical spine has a different clinical picture. Most patients in the United States with tuberculous spondylitis are forty to fifty years old (entries 4, 10). Skeletal tuberculosis occurs as a result of hematogenous spread usually, from the lung during an acute infection, or as a reactivation of a quiescent focus present in bone for many years (entry 5). The organisms slowly grow causing formation of granulomatous inflammation and caseation necrosis of bone. The inflammation involves contiguous structures including the discs, paraspinous ligaments, and muscles. A "cold abscess" forms undermining the structural integrity of the spine resulting in angular deformity. At its most destructive stage, spinal cord compression may occur.

The clinical presentation of a patient with tuberculous spondylitis consists of pain over the involved vertebrae which has slowly been increasing. The onset of symptoms is gradual and the time before presentation to a physician may be three years (entry 11). Associated symptoms may include anorexia, low grade fever, and dysphagia.

Infections secondary to Actinomyces israelii, a bacterium frequently confused with fungi, and fungal organisms, Candida albicans, Coccidiodes immitis and Blastomyces dermatidis, are very rare causes of vertebral osteomyelitis in general and cervical disease in particular. The clinical course of these infections is similar to that of tuberculosis. These patients will present with an extended history of neck pain (entries 32, 26).

§ 4-3(B)(3). Physical Findings.

Physical findings include severe restriction of spinal motion, paravertebral muscle spasm, and percussion tenderness over the involved bone. Fever occurs more commonly in pyogenic than granulomatous infections. Neurologic abnormalities occur rarely, but may be associated more often with cervical spine lesions (entry 17). Neurologic lesions may include motor or sensory deficits, long tract signs or sphincter incontinence (entry 23).

§ 4-3(B)(4). Laboratory Findings.

Commonly ordered blood tests, including CBC, ESR, and serum chemistries, are normal or nonspecifically abnormal. White blood cell counts may be elevated in acute, pyogenic infection. The sedimentation rate, elevated in any inflammatory disease process, is abnormal in the majority of patients with vertebral osteomyelitis (entry 6).

The definitive diagnosis is based upon the growth of offending organisms from blood or bone. Blood cultures are positive in the bulk of patients with acute osteomyelitis, obviating the need for bone biopsy (entry 20). Bone aspiration or open biopsy is reserved for patients with appropriate histories and negative blood cultures (entry 24). Staphylococcus aureus causes 60% of vertebral osteomyelitis (entry 8). Gram negative organisms cause infection in older patients with genitourinary disorders (E. coli, proteus) or young parenteral drug abusers (pseudomons) (entries 28, 30). Cultures from peripheral sources of bacteria (skin, urinary tract, and respiratory tract) may be positive and should be obtained in patients with suspected osteomyelitis.

The skin test for delayed hypersensitivity to the tubercle bacillus (PPD) is a good screening procedure for the diagnosis of tuberculous spondylitis. Patients are PPD positive with spine involvement unless they are anergic secondary to miliary, widespread infection. The number of organisms is very low in bone, less than 50 colonies per cultures in a majority of cases (entry 18). Therefore, culture of purulent material and biopsy specimens improves the potential for making the appropriate diagnosis. Histologic examination of biopsy material for granulomatous inflammation and caseous necrosis increases the documentation of infection. Culturing biopsy material and histologic examination of same is also essential for the diagnosis of fungal osteomyelitis since a rise in antibody titers to fungal antigens or reactive skin tests are nonspecific.

§ 4-3(B)(5). Radiographic Findings.

Radiographic changes follow the onset of symptoms by six weeks. Radiographic changes occur almost exclusively in the anterior portion (body) of a vertebrae and cause subchondral bone loss, disc space destruction, erosions of end plates and contiguous vertebrae, and soft tissue swelling manifested as an increase in the retropharyngeal space. With healing, bone regeneration appears with osteosclerosis and eventual bony fusion across the disc space. Infection involving the first and second cervical vertebrae may lead to complete destruction of the odontoid process resulting in severe instability of the atlantoaxial region.

In contrast, tuberculous infection is more insidious and may cause more destructive radiographic abnormalities at the time of presentation. The tuberculous lesion causes subchondral bone loss, disc space destruction, and paraspinal abscesses, but causes much less sclerosis of bone compared to pyogenic infections.

Vertebral coccidiodomycosis differs from tuberculous spondylitis by sparing the intervertebral discs, involving anterior and posterior elements of the vertebral body and rarely causing vertebral collapse. In contrast, blastomycosis causes disc destruction and radiolucent anterior erosions secondary to anterior ligamentous extension of infection. Actinomycosis causes marked vertebral body destruction associated with soft tissue abscesses or sinuses.

Bone scan demonstrates an area of increased osteoblastic activity, which corresponds to the area of infection, at an earlier stage of disease than do plain radiographs. The scan may demonstrate the extent of the infection and may demonstrate noncontiguous areas of infection. Bone scan abnormalities are nonspecific and may also be caused by trauma with fracture, neoplasms or arthritis.

Computerized tomography may show bony changes before their appearance on plain radiographs. Soft tissue abscesses are more easily identified by this method (entry 13).

§ 4-3(B)(6). Differential Diagnosis.

The diagnosis of vertebral osteomyelitis is confirmed by the identification of the causative organism from aspirated material or biopsy. Examination of histologic specimens may increase the recognition of infection in those patients with granulomatous infections. A diagnosis of infection may be suspected on the basis of historical, physical and other laboratory findings but are too non-specific. A listing of disease processes which may cause neck pain and vertebral body destruction include metastatic tumors, multiple myeloma, aneurysmal bone cyst, giant cell tumor and hemangioma. Severe neck pain may also occur in the absence of vertebral destruction. For example, patients with acute calcific retropharyngeal tendinitis have severe pain with loss of motion of the neck which may be confused with acute infection (entry 25).

§ 4-3(B)(7). Treatment.

Bed rest, immobilization with bracing, and antibiotics are components of basic therapy for cervical osteomyelitis. A short period of rest associated with institution of drug therapy is helpful in controlling symptoms of pain and muscle spasm. External bracing will allow ambulation during treatment when vertebral destructive changes are mild. The choice of antibiotic therapy is decided by the organism causing the infection and its sensitivity to specific agents. Penicillin or semi-synthetic penicillin (Nafcillin, Methicillin) are effective against gram positive bacteria such as Staphylococcus, while aminoglycosides are more effective against gram negative bacteria including E. coli. Patients are treated with parenteral antibiotics for four to six weeks followed by oral antibiotics for an additional six-month period. Prolonged antibiotic therapy reduces the possibility of recurrences of the infection.

Tuberculous spondylitis has been treated with surgical fusion in the past, but is no longer required as an initial mode of therapy in most patients. An initial course of isoniazid, ethambutol, rifampin or streptomycin for two to three months followed by an additional sixteen months on two drugs has been successful in eradicating the infections (entry 19).

Fungal osteomyelitis requires parenteral amphotericin B therapy at a dose that the patient can tolerate without developing renal dysfunction. A total dose of 2.5 gm is adequate as an initial course of therapy. External bracing is useful to decrease symptoms during the course of drug therapy.

A more controversial component of therapy is surgical intervention in cervical osteomyelitis. Surgical intervention is clearly indicated to obtain appropriate material to make the diagnosis of infection. Other indications for surgery include advanced destruction of multiple vertebrae, instability of the spine, relief of neurologic compression, removal of avascular bone, drainage of abscesses, and continued constitutional symptoms (fever) despite drug therapy (entries 9, 1). Anterior fusion of the affected cervical vertebrae and drainage of abscesses help decompress areas of nerve impingement and add stability to the spine (entry 14). Posterior laminectomy is not usually done because of an increased risk of destabilizing the spine (entry 15). In tuberculous spondylitis, anterior fusion is indicated if neurologic signs do not improve after four to six weeks of maximum medical therapy (entry 11).

§ 4-3(B)(8). Course and Outcome.

Decrease in patient's pain and fever, and a return of the sedimentation rate to normal are hallmarks of improvement in vertebral osteomyelitis. With early diagnosis and prompt institution of appropriate therapy, this infection causes minimal disability. However, when the diagnosis is delayed and the infection spreads to involve the spinal cord by compression (epidural abscess) or direct extension (meningitis) potentially life threatening complications may occur. Surgical intervention is indicated to relieve spinal cord compression. Immediate surgical decompression is indicated for quadraplegia or paraplegia since a better chance of full recovery occurs when patients have had neurologic deficits for a month or less (entry 6).

BIBLIOGRAPHY

1. Bartal, A.D., Schiffer, J., Heilbronn, Y.D., and Yakel, M. Anterior interbody fusion for cervical osteomyelitis. J Neurol Neurosurg Psychiatry, 35:133-136, 1972.
2. Batson, O.V. The function of the vertebral veins and their role in the spread of metastases. Ann Surg, 112:138-149, 1940.
3. Biller, H.F., Ogura, J.H., Rontal, M., and Ehrlich, C. Cervical osteomyelitis complicating pharyngeal resection. Arch Otolaryngol, 94:165-168, 1971.
4. Brashear, H.R., Jr., and Rendleman, D.A. Potts' paraplegia. South Med J, 71:1379-1382, 1978.
5. Chapman, M., Murray, R.O., and Stoker, D.J. Tuberculosis of the bones and joints. Semin Roentgenol, 14:266-282, 1979.
6. Collert, S. Osteomyelitis of the spine. Acta Orthop Scand, 48:283-290, 1977.
7. Dalinka, M.K., and Greendyke, W.H. The spinal manifestations of coccidioidomycosis. J Canad Assoc Rad, 22:93-99, 1971.
8. Digby, J.M., and Kersley, J.B. Pyogenic non-tuberculous spinal infection: an analysis of thirty cases. J Bone Joint Surg, 61B:47-55, 1979.
9. Forsythe, M., and Rothman, R.H. New concepts in the diagnosis and treatment of infections of the cervical spine. Orthop Clin North Am, 9:1039-1051, 1978.
10. Friedman, B. Chemotherapy of tuberculosis of the spine. J Bone Joint Surg, 48A:451-474, 1966.
11. Gorse, G.J., Pais, M.J., Kusske, J.A., and Cesario, T.C. Tuberculous spondylitis: a report of six cases and a review of the literature. Medicine, 62:178-193, 1983.
12. Hagadorn, B., Smith, H.W., and Rosnagle, S. Cervical spine osteomyelitis secondary to a foreign body in the hypopharynx. Arch Otolaryngol, 95:578-580, 1972.
13. Kattapuram, S.V., Phillips, W.C., and Boyd, R. C.T. in pyogenic osteomyelitis of the spine. Am J Roentgenol, 140:1199-1201, 1983.
14. Kemp, H.B.S., Jackson, J.W., Jeremiah, J.D., and Cook, J. Anterior fusion of the spine for infective lesions in adults. J Bone Joint Surg, 55B:715-734, 1973.

15. Kemp, H.B.S., Jackson, J.W., and Shaw, N.C. Laminectomy in paraplegia due to infective spondylosis. Br J Surg, 61:66-72, 1974.
16. Key, J.A. The pathology of tuberculosis of the spine. J Bone Joint Surg, 22:799-806, 1940.
17. Ling, C.M. Pyogenic osteomyelitis of the spine. Orthop Rev, 4:23-32, 1975.
18. Medical Research Council Working Party on Tuberculosis of the Spine, Fourth Report. A controlled trial of anterior spinal fusion and debridement in the surgical management of tuberculosis of the spine in patients on standard chemotherapy. Br J Surg, 61:853-866, 1974.
19. Medical Research Council Working Party on tuberculosis of the Spine, Third Report. A controlled trial of debridement and ambulatory treatment in the management of tuberculosis of the spine in patients on standard chemotherapy. J Trop Med Hyg, 77:72-92, 1974.
20. Musher, D.M., Thorsteinsson, S.B., Minuth, J.N., and Luchi, R.J. Vertebral osteomyelitis: still a diagnostic pitfall. Arch Intern Med, 136:105-110, 1976.
21. Parke, W.W., Rothman, R.H., and Brown, M.D. The pharyngovertebral veins: an anatomical rationale for Grisels' syndrome. J Bone Joint Surg, 66A:568-574, 1984.
22. Ray, M.J., and Bassett, R.L. Pyogenic vertebral osteomyelitis. Orthopedics, 8:540-513, 1985.
23. Rimalovski, A.B., and Aronson, S.M. Abscess of medulla oblongata associated with osteomyelitis of odontoid process. Case report. J Neurosurg, 29:97-101, 1968.
24. Ross, P.M., and Fleming, J.L. Vertebral body osteomyelitis: spectrum and natural history: a retrospective analysis of 37 cases. Clin Orthop, 118:190-198, 1976.
25. Sarkozi, J., and Fam, A.G. Acute calcific retropharyngeal tendinitis: an unusual cause of neck pain. Arthritis Rheum, 27:708-710, 1984.
26. Sarosi, G.A., and Davies, S.F. Blastomycosis. Am Rev Resp Dis, 120:911-938, 1979.
27. Stone, D.B., and Bonfiglio, M. Pyogenic vertebral osteomyelitis: a diagnostic pitfall for the internist. Arch Intern Med, 112:491-500, 1963.
28. Waldvogel, F.A., and Vasey, H. Osteomyelitis: the past decade. N Eng J Med, 303:360-370, 1980.
29. Wedge, J.H., Oryschak, A.F., Robertson, D.E., and Kirkaldy-Willis, W.H. Atypical manifestations of spinal infections. Clin Orthop, 123:156-163, 1977.

30. Wiesseman, G.J., Wood, V.E., and Kroll, L.L. Pseudomonas vertebral osteomyelitis in heroin addicts: report of five cases. J Bone Joint Surg, 55A:1416-1424, 1973.
31. Wiley, A.M., and Trueta, J. The vascular anatomy of the spine and its relationship to pyogenic vertebral osteomyelitis. J Bone Joint Surg, 41B:796-809, 1959.
32. Young, W.B. Actinomycosis with involvement of the vertebral column: case report and review of the literature. Clin Radiol, 11:175-182, 1960.

§ 4-3(C). Meningitis.

Meningitis is an infection of the lining of the central nervous system, the meninges. Meningitis may be caused by bacteria — Streptococcus pneumoniae, Neisseria meningitidis; viruses — coxsackie, echo; mycobacteria — Mycobacteria tuberculosis; fungi — Coccidiodes immitis, Cryptoccoccus neoformans and protozoa — Toxoplasma gondii. Meningitis usually develops from hematogenous spread through the bloodstream from a distant, infected location or by contiguous spread from local structures, i.e., mastoid bone. The clinical symptoms and course of the infection, like in vertebral osteomyelitis, are dependent on the infecting organism and host inflammatory response. Bacterial and viral infections are associated with acute onset of a febrile illness. A more indolent course associated with gradual changes in mentation is characteristic of tuberculous, fungal and protozoal infections.

The diagnosis of bacterial or viral meningitis in the patient with acute symptoms is made without difficulty because of the high index of suspicion of the physician. The diagnosis of chronic meningitis is more difficult since symptoms and signs develop more gradually. The definitive diagnosis of meningitis is confirmed by culturing the offending organism from cerebrospinal fluid obtained by lumbar puncture. The cornerstone of therapy for meningitis is antibiotics which are selected by their ability to kill the infecting organisms and their diffusing capacity across the meninges. When diagnosed expeditiously and treated aggressively meningitis can be cured with no residual neurologic deficit. The outcome of the illness can be more serious, with severe neurologic impairment or death, if there is a delay in the diagnosis of the disease.

§ 4-3(C)(1). Prevalence and Etiology.

The prevalence of meningitis is unknown. This is due in part to the wide range of organisms associated with this infection.

The meninges are most frequently infected by hematogenous spread of organisms through the bloodstream. Organisms may also gain access to the meninges by direct spread from infected areas such as sinuses or the upper respiratory tract. A much rarer occurrence is meningitis associated with a neurosurgical procedure or lumbar puncture.

Certain characteristics of patients may predispose individuals to infection with specific organisms. Factors which may play a role include the patient's age, immunologic status, trauma, and exposure to a carrier of an organism (N. meningitidis). Adult meningitis is most frequently caused by Streptococcus pneumoniae and Neisseria meningitidis. Meningitis in children is caused by different organisms including Escherichia coli and Haemophilus influenzae.

§ 4-3(C)(2). Clinical Findings.

The primary symptoms of patients with meningitis includes head and neck pain along with neck stiffness (meningismus). Patients with bacterial meningitis usually have associated fever. Changes in mental status ranging from mild confusion to frank coma occurs in a majority of patients. The onset of symptoms is usually acute and develops over twenty-four to thirty-six hours. In a minority of patients, the progression of symptoms may be spread over a three to five-day period. The course of symptoms is from headache and neck stiffness to confusion, obtundation, and coma (entry 7).

Of the 4,000 cases of aseptic (nonbacterial) meningitis which occur each year in the United States, 25% have a defined etiology (entry 5). Of these, echovirus and coxsackieviruses are enteroviruses and cause outbreaks of meningitis during the summer. After the virus enters the body through the gastrointestinal or respiratory tract, the virus enters the meninges after a generalized viremia through the bloodstream. The incubation period for growth of the virus may range from a few days to several weeks. The patient develops fever, sore throat, and myalgias which is followed by frontal headache, photophobia, neck pain, neck stiffness and fever.

Tuberculous meningitis, while once a disease of children, occurs more commonly in the elderly (entry 4). Mycobacterium tuberculosis enters the body through the respiratory tract and grows in regional lymph nodes. Hematogenous seeding of the meninges may occur at that time. The infection may remain dormant for an extended period of time only to become activated at a time of diminished host resistance to infection. The organisms grow in the meninges which elicits an intense inflammatory reaction which is most prominent at the base of the brain. The inflammation in this location may result in inflammatory tissue which compresses cranial nerve blood vessel inflammation resulting in vessel thrombosis and infarction of tissue supplied by that vessel, or a blockage of the free flow of cerebrospinal fluid around the brain leading to increased intracranial pressure and hydrocephalus. Once the infection has started, the clinical manifestations of the infection progress over a two to three-week period. Patients develop headache, neck pain, neck stiffness, fever, altercations in mental status, seizures, coma and death.

Fungal infection with Coccidioides immitis or Cryptococcus neoformans cause similar symptoms as those of tuberculous meningitis (entry 2). Approximately 30% of patients with extrapulmonary C. immitis infection develop meningitis. The base of the brain is affected by a granulomatous inflammatory response which blocks the flow of cerebrospinal fluid resulting in hydrocephalus and cranial nerve palsies. The onset of these symptoms are gradual. Headache is the most prominent symptom of patients with fungal meningitis. Meningisms and fever are less prominent symptoms.

Cryptococcal meningitis is a very important and potentially life threatening form of this infection (entry 1). The onset of disease is usually gradual with intermittent episodes of persistent headache and fever. As the infection progresses over months, patients complain increasingly of impaired mentation, irritability, dizziness, weakness, and changes in vision. A stiff painful neck is a frequent symptom but may be absent. If left untreated both coccidioidal and cryptococcal meningitis may result in increasing neurologic deficits, coma, and death.

A more unusual form of meningitis is caused by the protozoan, Toxoplasma gondii. CNA toxoplasmosis occurs most commonly in the immunosuppressed host who has a lymphoreticular malignancy, has taken immunosuppressive drugs, or has a viral infection which impairs cellular immune function (acquired immunodeficiency syndrome) (entry 8). Patients with CNS toxoplasmosis may present with an acute or subacute course including headache, stiff neck, and seizures. If brain tissue is also infected (encephalitis), the patient may develop focal neurologic deficits which progress to cause changes in mentation and coma.

§ 4-3(C)(3). Physical Findings.

The patient with meningitis may manifest abnormalities in a number of organ systems during the physical examination. Patients with meningitis of any cause are frequently febrile. Patients with meningeal irritation develop reflex contraction of the neck muscles (nucal rigidity), Kernig's sign (pain in the hamstrings with knee extension in the supine position), and Brudzinski's sign (involuntary flexion of the hips with neck flexion). A maculopetechial or purpuric rash may be present in the patient with meningococcal meningitis or other bacterial infections. Echovirus may cause a maculopapular rash which appears on the face before other parts of the body are affected. Fundoscopic examination may demonstrate papilledema (swelling of the head of the optic nerve) which is secondary to increased intracranial pressure. Infection of the middle ear, otitis media, a possible local source of infection, would be noted on examination of the ear. Chest examination may be positive for decreased breath sounds indicative of a pneumonic process secondary to bacteria (S. pneumoniae), mycobacteria (M. tuberculosis) or fungi (C. immitis). Murmurs on cardiac examination suggest endocarditis which may be the source of the primary infection. The spectrum of neurologic abnormalities is wide. Loss of mental function in the form of memory loss, inability to perform calculations occur with all forms of meningitis. Abnormalities of cranial nerves (eye, facial, and tongue movements) occur most commonly in patients with granulomatous meningitis which affects the base of the brain.

§ 4-3(C)(4). Laboratory Findings.

Nonspecific findings such as elevation in peripheral white blood cells, and erythrocyte sedimentation rate are not helpful in making a diagnosis of meningitis, but are useful in following the response of patients to therapy.

The diagnosis of meningitis is made by the examination of cerebrospinal fluid. This fluid is obtained by lumbar puncture. In most circumstances, a lumbar puncture can be completed without complication. Contraindications for this procedure are signs of increased intracranial pressure or skin infection overlying the needle entry point. Lumbar puncture in the face of increased intracranial pressure may cause the brain to be pressed against the base of the skull causing acute compression of the brain stem which controls autonomic functions of the lungs and heart. Patients who "cone" develop cardiopulmonary arrest. Attempting an injection through an area of cellulitis may result in innoculating organisms into the central nervous system causing meningitis or vertebral osteomyelitis.

The definitive diagnosis of meningitis is based upon the growth of the offending organism from CSF or blood. Unfortunately, cultures take time to become positive, leaving the diagnosis of meningitis to be based upon other characteristic changes in CSF. Bacterial meningitis causes WBC counts greater than 1000 cells/mm (entry 4), a predominance of polymorphonuclear leukocytes (PMN), a decreased glucose which is less than 50% of the serum level, an elevated protein of greater than 100 mg/dl and positive Gram stain smear of organisms from a spun specimen (entry 3). Viral meningitis causes less of a leukocytosis (less than 500 WBC), predominantly lymphocytic in character with a normal glucose, and a slightly elevated protein.

Tuberculous and fungal meningitis causes a CSF WBC of less than 500, and a predominance of lymphocytes. Tuberculous meningitis causes a marked reduction in glucose and marked increase in protein. Organisms are rarely seen on smear. Fungal meningitis is associated with a slight reduction of glucose, moderate increase in protein, and in the case of cryptococcus, the presence of organisms by india ink examination. In toxoplasmosis, CSF examination may be normal or demonstrate mild WBC elevation with lymphocytes.

§ 4-3(C)(5). Radiographic Findings.

Radiographic examination is not useful in the diagnosis or management of uncomplicated meningitis (entry 9). Computed tomography in meningitis may detect widening of the subarachnoid space. Radiographic techniques are most useful in the patient with meningitis who has an associated abnormality such as a parameningeal focus of infection, or brain abscess. CT scan can localize the space-occupying lesion in the patient with focal cerebral signs who does not respond to usual therapy.

§ 4-3(C)(6). Differential Diagnosis.

The diagnosis of meningitis is based upon the results of cultures of cerebrospinal fluid. The clinical course, cerebrospinal fluid abnormalities along with the culture results help differentiate the various forms of meningitis (pyogenic versus granulomatous versus protozoan). Parameningeal infection such as epidural abscess, subdural empyema, or brain abscess may cause meningeal symptoms and neurologic signs. Radiographic evaluation should differentiate these entities from meningitis alone.

§ 4-3(C)(7). Treatment.

The treatment for bacterial meningitis is intravenous or intrathecal antibiotic which is bactericidal for the infecting organism. A problem obtaining and maintaining adequate concentrations of antibiotic in cerebrospinal fluid is the blood-brain barrier. The blood-brain barrier excludes proteins and antibiotics from the brain. When inflamed, the integrity of the blood-brain barrier is lost, allowing the ingress of antibiotics. Antibiotics are administered intravenously, in high, divided doses, every few hours. Penicillin (entry 8), nafcillin, ampicillin and chloramphericol are antibiotics used in gram positive infections. Gram-negative meningitis requires aminoglycoside (gentamicin) therapy. Aminoglycosides do not cross the blood-brain barrier and require intrathecal administration (lumbar puncture, ventricular pump).

The therapy for aseptic meningitis is symptomatic. There is no effective anti-viral therapy which shortens the course of the infection. Recovery begins within days and is usually complete in a few weeks.

Tuberculous meningitis requires three drug therapies including isoniazid, rifampin, and ethambutol. This therapy must be continued for twelve to eighteen months. Patients with hydrocephalus, or cranial nerve dysfunction secondary to tuberculous meningitis may benefit from a course of corticosteroids (entry 6).

Patients with fungal meningitis require amphotericin B therapy. Cryptococcal meningitis may be cured with intravenous therapy which is given in increments of 20 to 30 mg per day until a total of 2 to 3 gm. In coccidiodal meningitis, amphotericin B therapy given by an intravenous route does not reach adequate levels in cerebrospinal fluid. Intrathecal administration is necessary for control of the infection.

CNS toxoplasmosis requires prolonged therapy with pyrimethamine and sulfonamides. In adults 25 mg of pyrimethamine is given daily along with 4, 1 gram doses of sulfadiazine each day. Therapy must be continued for a minimum of six weeks.

§ 4-3(C)(8). Course and Outcome.

The course and outcome of meningitis depends on the agent which causes the infection and the immunologic status of the patients. Patients who have a compromised immune system are at risk of developing tuberculous or fungal meningitis and have a poorer prognosis than those individuals who have an episode of aseptic, viral meningitis. Patients with bacterial meningitis will have a full recovery if the diagnosis is made expeditiously and appropriate therapy is given. Antibiotic therapy is given for two weeks with the response to therapy monitored by the return of CSF abnormalities to normal. Patients with parameningeal foci of infection may not improve until the focus is drained.

Tuberculous meningitis is associated with a 20% mortality even in patients who receive drug therapy. The improvement with therapy may be slow, with survivors continuing with neurologic dysfunction.

Patients with fungal meningitis may have relapses of their disease despite receiving long courses of amphotericin B therapy. Patients who have a poor clinical outcome with cryptococcal meningitis have an underlying lymphoreticular malignancy, continued abnormal CSF white cells, or cryptococci on smear (entry 1).

CNS toxoplasmosis is uniformly fatal unless aggressively treated. In patient with AIDS, other immunocompromised state, may have a poor outcome despite maximum therapy.

BIBLIOGRAPHY

1. Diamond, R.D., and Bennett, J.E. Prognostic factors in cryptococcal meningitis: a study in 111 cases. Ann Intern Med, 80: 176-181, 1974.
2. Ellner, J.J., and Bennett, J.E. Chronic meningitis. Medicine, 55:341-369, 1976.
3. Geisler, P.J., Nelson, K.E., Levin, S., Reddi, K.J., and Moses, V.K. Community-acquired purulent meningitis: a review of 1,316 cases during the antibiotic era, 1954-1976. Rev Infect Dis, 2:725-745, 1980.

4. Hinman, A.R. Tuberculous meningitis at Cleveland Metropolitan General Hospital 1959 to 1963. Am Rev Respir Dis, 95:670-673, 1967.
5. Meyer, H.M., Johnson, R.T., Crawford, I.P., Dascomb, H.E., and Rogers, N.G. Central nervous system syndromes of "viral" etiology: a study of 713 cases. AM J Med, 29:334-347, 1960.
6. O'Toole, R.D., Thorton, G.F., Mukherjee, M.K., and Nath, R.L. Dexamethasone in tuberculous meningitis: relationship of cerebrospinal fluid effects to therapeutic efficacy. Ann Intern Med, 70:39-48, 1969.
7. Schleck, W.F., III, Ward, J.I., Band, J.D., Hightower, A., Fraser, D.W., and Broome, C.V. Bacterial meningitis in the United States, 1978 through 1981. JAMA, 253:1749-1754, 1985.
8. Townsend, J.J., Wolinsky, J.S., Baunger, J.R., and Johnson, P.C. Acquired toxoplasmosis: a neglected cause of treatable nervous system disease. Arch Neurol, 32:335-343, 1975.
9. Weisberg, L.A. Computed tomography in the diagnosis of intracranial disease. Ann Intern Med, 91:87-105, 1979.

§ 4-3(D). Paget's Disease of Bone.

Paget's disease of bone is characterized by localized areas of bone resorption which subsequently result in the formation of disorganized and irregular new bone. In the past, Paget's disease was considered a metabolic bone disease. Newer data suggest that this illness is an infectious disease caused by a virus. Cervical spine involvement is relatively uncommon compared to other locations in the bony skeleton. Patients with neck pain associated with Paget's disease develop this symptom secondary to flattening of the base of the skull around the cervical spine (platybasia) or vertebral body involvement with compression fracture or secondary osteoarthritis. Most patients with Paget's disease are asymptomatic and have no disability. More severe involvement is associated with a number of complications including bone pain, skeletal deformity, pathologic fractures, hypercalcemia, deafness, sarcomatous malignant transformation and high output cardiac failure. The diagnosis of Paget's disease is made by characteristic clinical, laboratory, and radiographic findings and rarely requires histologic confirmation. Calcitonin, diphosphonates, and mithramycin are drugs which are effective in suppressing disease activity and slowing bone growth. While cervical spine involvement with Paget's disease is usually benign, this disease may cause severe neurologic dysfunction if bone growth results in spinal cord or nerve root impingement.

§ 4-3(D)(1). Prevalence and Etiology.

Paget's disease is a common disorder found most commonly in people from Western and Eastern Europe and their descendants who have migrated to Australia, South Africa, and portions of South America. In the United States the prevalence of the disease ranges from 1% to 4% dependent on the geographic origin of the population (entry 1). Paget's disease is rare in Blacks in Africa, but is diagnosed in Blacks in the United States (entry 16). Most patients are adults over the age of forty with a male predominance at a 3:2 ratio to women.

The etiology of Paget's disease continues to be investigated. The primary abnormality resides in osteoclasts, cells which resorb bone. In the diseased state, these cells have increased numbers and sizes of nuclei. In response to the increased number and metabolic state of these abnormal osteoclasts, bone resorption is increased which results in an inadequate production of new bone from osteoblasts with limited metabolic capacity. New pagetic bone is less compact, more vascular and weaker than new bone (entry 6).

Paget's disease may be a slow virus infection of bone. The characteristics of slow virus infection, long latent period, single organ disease and lack of inflammatory response, match closely with those of Paget's disease. The nuclei of pagetic cells resemble those of cells infected with

§ 4-3(D)   NECK PAIN

paramyxoviruses (entry 15). Ultrastructural and immunohistologic studies have discovered structures which may be of viral origin. However, the infectious agent has not been cultured from cultured pagetic cells and the specific virus has not been identified. Therefore, a conclusion concerning the role of viruses as the etiologic agent of Paget's disease cannot be made at this time.

§ 4-3(D)(2). Clinical Findings.

The usual patient with Paget's disease is asymptomatic (entry 4). The diagnosis is suggested by an unexplained elevation of serum alkaline phosphatase on routine blood chemistries or the presence of an area of bony change on radiographs. When patients become symptomatic, rheumatic syndromes are frequently the source of their complaints (entry 2). These syndromes include bone deformity, pathologic fracture, and secondary osteoarthritis. The most commonly affected bones include the pelvis, femur, spine, skull, and tibia. In the axial skeleton, the lumbar, thoracic, and cervical spine are affected with decreasing frequency (entry 7). Approximately 6% of patients with spine involvement with Paget's disease have cervical involvement.

The pain of Paget's disease involving the axial skeleton may be of bone, joint or nerve origin. Vertebral bodies may fracture, facet joints may develop secondary osteoarthritis due to deformity, and neural elements may become compressed by new growth (entry 8). Patients with neck pain secondary to Paget's disease have disease in other locations in the skeleton. Rarely, the cervical spine may be the sole area of involvement and may be associated with neurologic abnormalities, including sensory loss, muscle weakness, and urinary or rectal incontinence (entry 11). Patients may also be asymptomatic with radiographic evidence of disease (entry 10).

Patients with skull disease may also have symptoms of neck pain. The skull may become soft and enlarged and settle around the opening of the skull, the foramen magnum. This basilar invagination or platybasia causes occipital headaches, and neck pain associated with decreased motion. Pressure from the odontoid process of the second cervical vertebrae on the spinal cord at the level of the medulla or upper cervical spine may cause changes in mental status secondary to a block in cerebrospinal fluid flow or ataxia, muscle weakness or respiratory distress (entries 16, 14).

Other symptoms of axial skeleton involvement is back pain which occurred in 37% of 290 Paget's patients (entry 2). Cauda equina symptom with saddle anesthesia, motor weakness and incontinence is a rare consequence of lumbar involvement. Spinal cord compression occurs most commonly in the thoracic spine where vertebral width is the most narrowed (entries 13, 18).

Other complications of Paget's disease include hyperuricemia with gout, hypercalcemia in the immobilized patient, and high output cardiac failure due to the increased blood flow to bones. Malignant degeneration develops in patients with polyostotic Paget's disease but is a rare occurrence. Less than 1% of Paget's disease patients develop osteosarcoma or fibrosarcoma (entry 20).

§ 4-3(D)(3). Physical Findings.

Patients with asymptomatic Paget's disease may have an entirely normal physical examination. Patients with significant neck involvement may have pain with palpation over the affected bone. Rapid bone metabolism and the temperature over bones may be elevated from increased blood flow. Range of motion of the cervical spine may also be limited.

Patients with neck involvement frequently have other areas of pagetic involvement. New bone formation along with bone weakening will result in dorsal kyphosis, lateral bowing of the femur and anterior bowing of the tibia with associated abnormal gait. Increased skull circumference and delated scalp veins are associated with pagetic involvement of the skull. Bone growth which results in nerve compression may cause cranial nerve, sensory, motor or cerebellar dysfunction on neurologic examination.

§ 4-3(D)(4). Laboratory Findings.

An elevated alkaline phosphatase, which corresponds to the extent of new bone, or osteoblastic activity, is the most characteristic abnormal test in Paget's disease. The test is indicative of the activity of bone disease, its progression and response to therapy. The twenty-four-hour total urinary hydroxyproline which is an amino acid released from the collagen of bone as it is remodeled also indicates activity of bone turnover, but is too difficult to obtain on a regular basis.

Elevation in serum calcium occurs in the pagetic patients if they are immobilized. Immobilization allows for the increased resorption of bone which outstrips new bone formation. Elevated calcium in a normally active patient may be a sign of coexistent primary hyperparthyroidism, or metastatic tumor. Serum uric acid concentration may be increased in men with extensive disease.

§ 4-3(D)(5). Radiographic Findings.

Radiographic abnormalities correspond to the osteolytic, mixed and sclerotic phase of the disease. In the spine, mixed or sclerotic radiographic changes are most common. The mixed phase combines areas of osseous demineralization with bone sclerosis. The bone increases in size with thickened and widely spaced trabeculae, cortical thickening, and areas of increased and reduced density. This patchy involvement is referred to as a "cotton wool" appearance. The sclerotic phase of disease appears as a homogeneous increase in bone density.

Increased cortical thickening at the inferior and superior vertebral borders results in a "picture frame" appearance of individual vertebral bodies (entry 17). Homogeneously, sclerotic "ivory" vertebra is secondary to marked osteoblastic activity. Metastatic disease may have a similar appearance but does not expand bone while Paget's disease frequently causes bone enlargement. Osteoarthritis and compression fractures, less commonly, may also be seen in the cervical spine.

Bone scans and radiographs demonstrate identical areas of involvement in 65% of Paget's patients. In most of the remaining patients, bone scan demonstrates increased osteoblastic activity in radiographically normal appearing bone. In the remaining cases, radiographs show abnormalities in bone in which osteoblastic activity has ceased (entry 19).

§ 4-3(D)(6). Differential Diagnosis.

The diagnosis of Paget's disease is confirmed by history, physical examination, chemical, radiographic, and bone scan abnormalities. Histologic confirmation is rarely necessary. Bone biopsy may be required in the rapidly growing pagetic lesion which may have undergone malignant transformation.

Diseases which cause sclerosis of bone must be included in the differential diagnosis. Illnesses to be considered include metastatic tumor, lymphoma, myelofibrosis, fluorosis, mastocytosis, renal osteodystrophy, fibrous dysplasia, tuberous sclerosis, axial osteomalacia, and fibrogenesis imperfecta ossium. Careful review of physical examination, chemical and radiologic data help differentiate Paget's disease of bone from these other diseases.

§ 4-3(D)(7). Treatment.

Therapy is not required for patients who are asymptomatic with Paget's disease. Disabling bone pain, bone fractures, vertebral compression, protrusio acetabuli, deafness, high output congestive heart failure and neurologic dysfunction secondary to bone compression are indications for therapy.

Although there is no cure for the illness, medical therapy is effective in controlling symptoms and dampening excessive bone metabolism. Calcitonin, a polypeptide hormone from the parafollicular cells of the thyroid gland, slows osteoclastic bone resorption. Decreases in bone pain and a reduction in serum alkaline phosphatase occurs with calcitonin injections of 50 to 100 units three or more times per week (entry 5). However, antibodies directed against calcitonin may develop in patients over time which decreases its beneficial effects.

The ability of osteoclasts to resorb bone is decreased by diphosphonates, which are structural analogues of pyrophosphate. Diphosphonates are given at a dose of 5 mg/kg/day for six months of the year. The drug may be given over six consecutive months for twelve months until the response to therapy is re-evaluated. Therapy with diphosphonates over a long period of time is limited since mineralization of normal bone may be adversely affected and may increase the tendency of Paget's patients to develop pathologic fractures (entry 3).

Mithramycin is an antibiotic which inhibits protein synthesis. Patients with metastatic tumor to bone with hypercalcemia have had normalization of their serum calcium through the cytotoxic effect of mithramycin on osteoclasts. The utility of this drug is limited by its toxicity (entry 12).

Therefore, this drug is used in patients who require rapid and extensive control of their Paget's disease, such as those with progressive neurologic compression syndromes.

The efficacy of drug therapy is measured by the disappearance of symptoms, decrease in serum alkaline phosphatase, and in the decrease in uptake of the affected bones on bone scan. Most patients have a good response with a single drug. Patients who require a combination of agents usually have persistent neurologic dysfunction which is resistant to usual therapy (entry 9).

§ 4-3(D)(8). Course and Outcome.

The course and outcome of Paget's disease is usually benign. Most patients have asymptomatic disease which causes no dysfunction. Patients with Paget's neck disease usually have polyostolic involvement. Disability in patients with polyostolic disease would occur more commonly because of secondary osteoarthritis in the lower extremities or pathologic fractures in weight-bearing bones. Decreased work potential may occur in patients with neck involvement with Paget's disease secondary to nerve impingement or osteoarthritis. Decompression procedures or non-steroidal anti-inflammatory drugs can be effective in controlling these complications respectively. Malignant transformation of Paget's disease is associated with a very poor prognosis but is a very rare occurrence.

BIBLIOGRAPHY

1. Altman, R.D. Paget's disease of bone (osteitis deformans). Bull Rheum Dis, 34:1-8, 1984.
2. Altman, R.D., and Collins, B. Musculoskeletal manifestations of Paget's disease of bone. Arthritis Rheum, 23:1121-1127, 1980.

3. Canfield, R., Rosner, W., Skinner, J., McWhorter, J., Resnick, K., Feldman, F., Kammerman, S., Ryan, K., Kunigonis, M., and Bohne, W. Diphosphonate therapy of Paget's disease of bone. J Clin Endocrinol Metab, 44:96-106, 1977.
4. Collins, D.H. Paget's disease of bone. Incidence and subclinical forms. Lancet, 2:51-57, 1956.
5. DeRose, J., Singer, F.R. Avramides, A., Flores, A., Dziadiw, R., Baker, R.K., and Wallach, S. Response of Paget's disease to porcine and salmon calcitonins. Effects of long-term treatment. Am J Med, 56:858-866, 1974.
6. Deuxchaines, C.N. de, and Krane, S.M. Paget's disease of bone: clinical and metabolic observations. Medicine, 43:233-266, 1964.
7. Dickson, D.D., Camp, J.D., and Ghormley, R.K. Osteitis deformans: Paget's disease of bone. Radiology, 44:449-470, 1945.
8. Franck, W.A., Bress, N.M., Singer, F.R., and Krane, S.M. Rheumatic manifestations of Paget's disease of bone. Am J Med, 56:592-603, 1974.
9. Hosking, D.J., Bijvoet, O.L.M., van Aken, J., and Will, E.J. Paget's bone disease treated with diphosphonate and calcitonin. Lancet, 1:615-617, 1976.
10. Janetos, G.P. Paget's disease in the cervical spine. Am J Roent, 97:655-657, 1966.
11. Ramamurthi, K.B., and Visvantethan, G.S. Paget's disease of the axis causing quadriplegia. J Neurosurg, 14:580-583, 1957.
12. Ryan, W., Schwartz, T.B., and Perlia, C.P. Effects of mithramycin on Paget's disease of bone. Ann Intern Med, 70:549-557, 1969.
13. Schmidek, H.H. Neurologic and neurosurgical sequelae of Paget's disease of bone. Clin Orthop, 127:70-77, 1977.
14. Simons, R.M. Paget's disease in the head and neck. Gerontology, 26:155-159, 1980.
15. Singer, F.R., and Mills, B.G. Evidence for viral etiology of Paget's disease of bone. Clin Orthop, 178:245-251, 1983.
16. Siris, E.S., Jacobs, T.P., and Canfield, R.E. Paget's disease of bone. Bull NY Acad Med, 56:285-304, 1980.
17. Steinbech, H.L. Some roentgen features of Paget's disease. Am J Roentgenol, 86:950-964, 1961.
18. Turner, J.W.A. The spinal complications of Paget's disease (Osteitis deformans). Brain, 63:321-349, 1940.
19. Waxman, A.D., Ducker, S., McKee, D., Siemsen, J.K., and Singer, F.R. Evaluation of 99mTc diphosphonate kinetics and bone scans in patients with Paget's disease before and after calcitonin treatment. Radiology, 125:761-764, 1977.

20. Wick, M.R., Siegal, G.P., Unni, K.K., McLeod, R.A., and Greditzer, H.G., III Sarcomas of bone complicating osteitis deformans (Paget's disease). Fifty years' experience. Am J Surg Path, 5:47-59, 1981.

§ 4-4. Tumors and Infiltrative Lesions of the Cervical Spine.

§ 4-4(A). Introduction.

Tumors and infiltrative lesions of the cervical spine are rare causes of neck pain compared to mechanical injuries; however, these diseases are associated with the greatest dysfunction and mortality of all causes of neck pain. A physician's differential diagnosis must include neoplastic disorders since the best outcome from these lesions occurs with early recognition and therapy. Neck pain is usually the initial complaint and is frequently attributed to a minor traumatic event. Only as the pain persists and increases in intensity does it become clear that the trauma was an incidental event unassociated with the underlying disease process.

A history of pain which increases with recumbency is a hallmark for tumors of the spine. Neurologic symptoms of sensory changes and muscle weakness may occur in the arms or legs or both. Physical examination demonstrates localized tenderness, loss of cervical spine motion, and neurologic lesions which correspond to the level of spinal cord or spinal nerve compression. Laboratory evaluation yields data which are not useful in most circumstances. In contrast, radiographic evaluation is very useful in identifying characteristic changes in the bony and soft tissue areas of the spine which help identify the location and type of neoplastic lesion. The definitive diagnosis of a tumor must be derived from histologic examination of biopsy material obtained from the lesion. Complete surgical excision of accessible lesions is the treatment of choice for both benign and malignant neoplasms. In many circumstances this is not possible and then partial resection, radiotherapy or chemotherapy may be helpful in slowing growth of the lesion and the neurologic dysfunction caused by nerve compression. In general, patients with malignant tumors have a poorer prognosis than those with benign tumors.

§ 4-4(B). Osteoblastoma.

Osteoblastoma is a benign neoplasm of bone which manifests a predilection for the vertebral column. Localized pain is a cardinal symptom in all patients which may be associated with muscle spasm, spinal curvature, and spinal cord compression. The diagnosis of osteoblastoma is confirmed by the findings of uniform osteoblasts with areas of intercellular osteoid on biopsy. Surgical excision is the treatment of choice for osteoblastomas and is curative in the vast majority of cases.

§ 4-4(B)(1). Prevalence and Etiology.

Osteoblastoma comprises 0.5 to 1.0% of biopsied bone tumors (entries 1, 2). The peak incidence occurs in patients 10 to 20 years old. Nearly 90% of patients diagnosed with osteoblastoma are younger than 30 years old (entry 3). The male to female ratio is 2:1. The etiology of the osteoblastoma is unknown.

§ 4-4(B)(2). Clinical Findings.

In contrast to most other neoplasms of bone, osteoblastoma has a predilection for the axial skeleton. Between 30% to 40% of osteoblastomas occur in the spine (entry 5). Localized bone pain of insidious onset is the most frequent presenting symptom. Seventy percent of patients have symptoms for less than a year. Pain associated with the lesion is moderately severe and is not associated with increased severity during any portion of the day. Osteoblastoma located in the cervical spine may be associated with muscle spasm and associated spinal curvature. Spinal cord compression is associated with pain which may radiate into the arms and legs (radicular) with associated neurologic deficits (entries 5, 10).

§ 4-4(B)(3). Physical Findings.

Physical examination may demonstrate local tenderness on palpation with mild swelling over the spine. Neurologic examination may demonstrate motor or sensory abnormalities with osteoblastomas which have caused spinal cord compression.

§ 4-4(B)(4). Laboratory Findings.

Laboratory findings are normal in osteoblastoma. On gross pathologic examination, the tumor is hemorrhagic, and friable due to its vascularity and varying amounts of osteoid. The lesion ranges in size from 2 to 10 cm in length and is well circumscribed. Histologic features include osteoblasts with normal maturation interspersed with large amounts of osteoid material and the absence of cartilage cells. The histologic features of osteoblastoma vary with the maturity of the lesion. Early lesions are associated with proliferating connective tissue, numerous blood vessels and giant cells, and slight osteoid formation. Later lesions contain considerable ossification (entry 1).

§ 4-4(B)(5). Radiographic Findings.

Radiographic findings of osteoblastoma are variable and non-specific. The most common location for an osteoblastoma in a vertebra is posterior in the pedicles, laminae, transverse and spinous processes (entry 6). The anterior component of a vertebra, the body, is rarely the primary location of this tumor. Osteoblastomas are expansile and may grow rapidly as measured by serial radiographic studies. Most lesions are 4 to 6 cm in size with some as large as 10 cm. Characteristically, the lesion is well outlined and is delineated by a thin rim of reactive bone. Osteoblastomas are primarily radiolucent with increased radiopaque bone in adjacent osseous tissue (entry 9). Faint, stippled densities may be present intralesionally. Small lesions in the pedicle or lamina may be missed on plain radiographs. A bone scan or tomography are helpful in localizing the exact site of an osteoblastoma when it is difficult to visualize on plain radiographs.

§ 4-4(B)(6). Differential Diagnosis.

The diagnosis of osteoblastoma is confirmed by the histologic examination of biopsied specimens. Osteosarcoma, a malignant tumor of bone, at presentation, may have similar clinical and radiographic findings with that of osteoblastoma. The histologic findings of osteosarcoma; cellular pleomorphism, bizarre nuclei, chondroid tissue, and necrotic areas, help differentiate it from those of osteoblastoma (entry 7). Malignant osteoblastoma, a locally aggressive tumor which differs from osteosarcoma, has been reported (entry 8). However, controversy remains in regard to its classification as an osteoblastoma (entry 1). Osteoid osteoma is invariably smaller than an osteoblastoma, located in long bone, has a central lucent nidus surrounded by thick reactive bone, is particularly painful at night and is usually self-limited in growth. These features help differentiate it from osteoblastoma (entry 3). Other entities which must be differentiated from osteoblastoma include giant cell tumor and aneurysmal bone cysts.

§ 4-4(B)(7). Treatment.

The ideal treatment of osteoblastoma is local excision of the entire lesion. Spinal osteoblastomas may be inaccessible for complete excision. Partial removal of accessible lesions may be associated with cessation of growth and relief of symptoms (entry 5). Radiotherapy should be limited to lesions that are inaccessible to surgical removal or demonstrate continued growth.

§ 4-4(B)(8). Course and Outcome.

Osteoblastoma has a benign course. Complete cure with no recurrence is possible with complete surgical removal of the lesion. A majority of patients will also have a cure of their tumor with partial curettage. Between 5% to 10% patients with osteoblastoma will have recurrences after partial excision. Malignant transformation is a rare occurrence and may occur more frequently in irradiated tumors (entry 4).

BIBLIOGRAPHY

1. Dahlin, D.C. *Bone Tumors: General Aspects and Data on 6,221 Cases.* Springfield, Charles C. Thomas, 1978, pp 86-98.
2. Huvos, A.G. *Bone Tumors: Diagnosis, Treatment and Prognosis.* Philadelphia, W.B. Saunders, 1979, pp 33-46.
3. Jackson, R.P., Reckling, F.W., Mantz, F.A. Osteoid osteoma and osteoblastoma: similar histologic lesions with different natural histories. Clin Orthop, 128:303-313, 1977.
4. Jackson, R.P. Recurrent osteoblastoma: a review. Clin Orthrop, 131:229-233, 1978.
5. Marsh, B.W., Bonfiglio, M., Brady, L.P., and Enneking, W.F. Benign osteoblastoma: range of manifestations. J Bone Joint Surg, 57A:1-9, 1975.
6. McLeod, R.A., Dahlin, D.C., and Beabout, J.W. The spectrum of osteoblastoma. Am J Roentgenol, 126:321-335, 1976.
7. Mirra, J.M.: *Bone Tumors: Diagnosis and Treatment.* Philadelphia, J.B. Lippincott Co., 1980, pp 108-122.
8. Schajowicz, F., and Lemos, C. Malignant osteoblastoma. J Bone Joint Surg, 58B:202-211, 1976.

9. Tonai, M., Campbell, C.J., Ahn, G.H., Schiller, A.L., Mankin, H.J. Osteoblastoma: classification and report of 16 patients. Clin Orthop, 167:222-235, 1982.
10. Wiss, D.A., Naimark, A. Osteoblastoma. Orthopedics, 6:1174-1182, 1983.

§ 4-4(C). Giant Cell Tumor.

Giant cell tumor is a common, locally aggressive tumor of non-osseous cell origin. The clinical symptoms of patients with this tumor is local pain and swelling. Neurologic symptoms and signs, including paresthesias and muscle weakness, are present with nerve root or spinal cord compression. Diagnosis is confirmed by the histologic appearance of uniformly dispersed multinucleated giant cells throughout the tumor tissue. Treatment, in the form of en bloc excision, may prevent the continued growth or recurrence of the tumor. Vertebral giant cell tumors may be controlled with partial resection alone. However, these patients are at risk of a recurrence of the tumor and additional neurologic damage.

§ 4-4(C)(1). Prevalence and Etiology.

Giant cell tumors comprise 5% of biopsied primary bone tumors (entry 9). The peak incidence of the tumor is the third decade with 85% being diagnosed after the age of 20 (entry 2). Giant cell tumors of the vertebrae predominate in women with a ratio of 3:1 (entry 3). Malignant giant cell tumors predominate in men in a ratio of 3:1 (entry 4). The etiology is not known. The tumor arises from non-bone-forming fibrous connective tissue in bones and factors which make it inherently invasive are unknown.

§ 4-4(C)(2). Clinical Findings.

Twenty-nine percent of patients with giant cell tumor of the axial skeleton above the sacrum have involvement of the cervical spine (entry 3). The most frequent presenting symptom of giant cell tumor is local pain over the site of the lesion. Subsequently, lancinating or burning pain appears associated with sensory loss, and muscle weakness. These symptoms are indicative of nerve root impingement by the tumor (entry 8).

§ 4-4(C)(3). Physical Findings.

Physical examination may demonstrate tenderness on palpation along with localized swelling if the tumor is in a superficial location. Stiffness of the neck may be present. Pain may be exacerbated by motion of the cervical spine (entry 1). Neurologic findings may show sensory, motor or reflex abnormalities dependent on the level of nerve root compression.

§ 4-4(C)(4). Laboratory Findings.

Laboratory results are normal in patients with benign giant cell tumors. The need to differentiate this tumor from hyperparathyroidism, Paget's disease, and malignant giant cell tumor require evaluation of serum calcium, phosphorus and alkaline phosphatase tests. Patients with malignant giant cell tumors are likely to develop anemia and elevated erythrocyte sedimentation rate.

The presence of multinucleated giant cells is characteristic of the histologic appearance of the tumor but is too nonspecific to establish the diagnosis (entry 5). The typical histologic picture includes giant cells separated by stromal cells. Aneurysmal dilatation of blood vessels may be present. The presence of collagenous scarring or increased numbers of stromal cells suggests malignant degeneration of the giant cell tumor or an osteosarcoma.

§ 4-4(C)(5). Radiographic Findings.

The radiographic findings of giant cell tumor are characteristic but not pathognomonic. The lesion is usually radiolucent due to rapid lytic destruction with little or no internal reparative bone formation. The lesion is expansile with irregular thinning of the cortical margin. There is scant periosteal new bone formation and no surrounding bony sclerosis. Giant cell tumors in the axial skeleton may present as ill-defined lytic areas in vertebrae (entry 6). In a vertebra, the body, pedicle, and arch are the most likely locations for the tumor. Partial collapse of a vertebral body may be noted. Myelography may be indicated to demonstrate the extent of spinal cord or nerve root compression in patients with neurologic dysfunction.

§ 4-4(C)(6). Differential Diagnosis.

Since the pathologic appearance of giant cell tumor may be mimicked by a number of other lesions, the diagnosis of this entity can only be made after a thorough review of all clinical, laboratory, radiographic, and pathologic data. Hyperparathyroidism, a disease associated with hyperactivity of the parathyroid glands which results in hypercalcemia and bone resorption, is associated with brown tumors of bone. The histology of this tumor contains giant and stromal cells in a similar pattern of that of giant cell tumor. Elevation in serum calcium, phosphorus, and parathormone concentrations are pathognomonic of hyperparathyroidism. Nonossifying fibromas have greater degrees of collagen production and contain foamy macrophages in addition to giant cells. The presence of frank anaplastic cells and rarity of osteosarcoma in the axial skeleton help differentiate it from giant cell tumor. Other diseases which may be confused with giant cell tumor include chondroblastoma, fibrosarcoma, osteoblastoma, and aneurysmal bone cyst.

§ 4-4(C)(7). Treatment.

Surgery is the preferred mode of treatment for giant cell tumor. En bloc resection results in control of the tumor in 70 to 90% of patients (entries 5, 10). The recurrence rate with partial curettage is 50% within five years (entry 7). Radiation therapy, which is rarely curative, is reserved for lesions which are inaccessible for surgical removal (entries 3, 4).

The ideal treatment for giant cell tumors of the spine associated with neurologic symptoms is complete removal of accessible lesions (entries 1, 11). Incomplete removal of the tumor is usually the rule due to the location and size of the lesion. In those circumstances partial removal with subsequent radiation therapy is considered. Decompression of the spinal cord is necessary once neurologic symptoms appear since a delay of greater than three months is associated with irreversible nerve damage (entry 8).

§ 4-4(C)(8). Course and Outcome.

Giant cell tumor of bone is a locally aggressive benign tumor which has a high local recurrence rate. Larsson suggests that giant cell tumors of the spine have a better prognosis than those located in the appendicular skeleton (entry 8). About one-third of patients are cured when treated the first time. In some circumstances up to five courses of therapy are needed to successfully cure the disease (entry 4). Most recurrences develop within four years after initial therapy. Malignant transformation of giant cell tumor occurs within an overall average of seven years (entry 5). Patients who have had surgery or radiotherapy are at risk of developing malignant transformation. Patients with giant cell tumor must be continually examined for recurrence and malignant transformation.

BIBLIOGRAPHY

1. Chow, S.P., Leong, J.C.Y., Yau, A.L.M.C. Osteoclastoma of the axis: report of a case. J Bone Joint Surg, 59A:550-551, 1977.
2. Dahlin, D.C. *Bone Tumors: General Aspects and Data on 6,221 Cases.* Springfield, Charles C. Thomas, 1978, pp 99-115.
3. Dahlin, D.C. Giant cell tumor of vertebrae above the sacrum: a review of 31 cases. Cancer, 39:1350-1356, 1977.
4. Hutter, R.V.P., Worcester, J.W., Jr., Francis, K.C., Foote, F.W., Jr., and Stewart, F.W. Benign and malignant giant cell tumors of bone: a clinicopathological analysis of the natural history of the disease. Cancer, 15:653-690, 1962.
5. Huvos, A.G. *Bone Tumors: Diagnosis, Treatment and Prognosis.* Philadelphia, W.B. Saunders, 1979, pp 265-291.
6. Jacobs, P. The diagnosis of osteoclastoma (giant-cell tumor): a radiological and pathological correlation. Br J Radiol, 45:121-136, 1972.
7. Johnson, E.W., Jr. and Dahlin, D.C. Treatment of giant cell tumor of bone. J Bone Joint Surg, 41A:895-904, 1959.
8. Larsson, S.E., Lorentzon, R., Bouquist, L. Giant cell tumors of the spine and sacrum causing neurological symptoms. Clin Orthop, 111: 201-211, 1975.
9. Mirra, J.M. *Bone Tumors: Diagnosis and Treatment.* Philadelphia, J.B. Lippincott Co., 1980, pp 332-362.
10. Parrish, F. Treatment of bone tumors by total excision and replacement with massive autologous and homologous grafts. J Bone Joint Surg, 48A:968-990, 1966.
11. Stevens, W.W., and Weaver, E.W. Giant cell tumors and aneurysmal bone cysts of the spine: report of 4 cases. South Med J, 63:218-221, 1970.

§ 4-4(D). Aneurysmal Bone Cyst.

Aneurysmal bone cyst is a benign neoplasm characterized by an expansile, cystic vascular lesion of bone. Localized pain associated with swelling is the most common symptom. Radiographically, the lesion appears as an osteolytic lesion that causes marked expansion of bone surrounded by a thin layer of calcification. The diagnosis is suggested by the characteristic radiographic findings and the close scrutiny of histopathologic specimens for cystic cavities composed of vascular channels filled with benign granulation tissue and giant cells. The treatment of choice is en bloc resection of the tumor since partial removal is associated with local recurrence.

§ 4-4(D)(1). Prevalence and Etiology.

Aneurysmal bone cyst is uncommon, comprising about 1% of primary bone tumors (entry 11). The vast majority of young adults who develop this tumor are under 30 years of age and are more frequently female (entry 6).

The etiology of aneurysmal bone cyst remains uncertain although trauma may play a role in its initiation since injuries may induce the formation of arteriovenous malformations. These malformations consist of abnormal vascular channels and several reports have suggested that trauma which initiated an AVM, may have led to the development of a cyst (entries 1, 8).

In two-thirds of cases, the lesion arises de novo in otherwise normal bone. In the remaining one-third of the cases, a cyst is superimposed upon another pathological process such as osteosarcoma, chondrosarcoma, osteoblastoma, chondroblastoma, chondromyxoid fibroma, fibrous dysplasia or nonossifying fibroma (entry 3).

§ 4-4(D)(2). Clinical Findings.

Pain and swelling are the most common symptoms associated with aneurysmal bone cyst. The duration of symptoms at the time of diagnosis ranges from weeks to a few years. Approximately 15% to 25% of aneurysmal bone cysts affect the spine (entries 5, 10). In a review of 92 cases, 22% of aneurysmal bone cysts were located in the cervical spine with a per vertebra number of 2.8 (entry 9). Neurologic symptoms and signs, ranging from sensory changes to paraplegia, may occur if the expansion of the lesion results in nerve root or spinal cord compression (entries 8, 7, 9).

§ 4-4(D)(3). Physical Findings.

Physical examination usually demonstrates tenderness with palpation over the site. The overlying skin may be erythematous and warm if the cyst is close to the surface. This finding is secondary to increased blood flow to the area. A mass may be detected in 23% of patients. In aneurysmal bone cyst of the spine, 47% of patients may develop neurologic signs. In patients with cervical lesions, the neurologic signs may include lower motor neuron abnormalities in upper or lower extremities along with paresthesias (entry 9).

§ 4-4(D)(4). Laboratory Findings.

Laboratory tests are normal in this benign lesion of bone. The pathologic findings of a cyst resected en bloc shows an eccentric expansile lesion of bone covered by a thin shell of bone. Microscopically the lesion is characterized by cavities of varying sizes, numerous giant cells, fibrous and granulation tissue (entry 2).

§ 4-4(D)(5). Radiographic Findings.

Aneurysmal bone cysts in the spine affect the posterior components of vertebrae. The areas affected are the spinous and transverse processes, lamina and pedicle. The bodies of vertebrae are affected in 40% of cases and may progress to destruction of an entire vertebral body (entry 12). The characteristic radiographic findings are that of an osteolytic, expanding lesion with a thinned cortex containing fine trabeculation of bone. While plain radiographs are usually adequate in delineating the extent of this benign tumor, CAT scan and magnetic resonance imaging may better define the location of tumor and the extent of invasion of surrounding soft tissues (entry 14).

§ 4-4(D)(6). Differential Diagnosis.

The characteristic radiographic appearance of aneurysmal bone cyst helps differentiate it from other benign and malignant lesions. Other entities to be considered include eosinophilic granuloma, hemangioma, osteoblastoma, fibrous dysplasia, and secondary malignancy. Occasionally, the diagnosis of primary versus secondary aneurysmal bone cyst cannot be confirmed without histologic evaluation of the lesion. Open biopsy of the lesion is preferred to needle biopsy since the latter procedure may be associated with neurologic deterioration secondary to bleeding (entry 9).

§ 4-4(D)(7). Treatment.

The treatment of choice for aneurysmal bone cyst is en bloc resection if the lesion is accessible. Incomplete removal with curettage may be associated with recurrences in the range of 50% (entry 11). Lesions which are too large or involve a vertebral body may be treated with radiotherapy (entry 13). However, the risk of radiation induced sarcoma must be considered (entry 6). Cryosurgery, freezing of the lesion, has been used to ablate the tumor and may prevent recurrence (entries 2, 4).

§ 4-4(D)(8). Course and Outcome.

Aneurysmal bone cyst is a benign lesion but may cause neurologic dysfunction secondary to its expansile nature. Early diagnosis and therapy help limit disability. Recurrences, if they do occur, appear within one to twelve months after initial treatment and are usually responsive to further partial or total excision with or without curettage.

BIBLIOGRAPHY

1. Barnes, R. Aneurysmal bone cyst. J Bone Joint Surg, 38B:301-311, 1956.
2. Biesecker, J.L., Marcove, R.C., Huvos, A.C., and Mike, V. Aneurysmal bone cyst: a clinicopathologic study of 66 cases. Cancer, 26:615-625, 1970.
3. Bonakdarpur, A., Levy, W., Aegerter, E. Primary and secondary aneurysmal bone cyst: a radiologic study of 75 cases. Radiology, 126:75-83, 1978.
4. Clough, J.R., and Price, C.H.G. Aneurysmal bone cyst: pathogenesis and long term results of treatment. Clin Orthop, 97:52-63, 1973.
5. Dabska, M., and Buraczewski, J. Aneurysmal bone cyst: pathology, clinical course and radiologic appearance. Cancer, 23:371-389, 1969.
6. Dahlin, D.C. *Bone Tumors: General Aspects and Data on 6,221 Cases.* Springfield, Charles C. Thomas, 1978, pp 370-375.
7. Dahlin, D.C. and McLeod, R.A. Aneurysmal bone cyst and other non-neoplastic conditions. Skeletal Radiol, 8:243-250, 1982.
8. Donaldson, W.F. Aneurysmal bone cyst. J Bone Joint Surg, 44A:25-40, 1962.
9. Hay, M.C., Patterson, D., and Taylor, T.K.F. Aneurysmal bone cyst of the spine. J Bone Joint Surg, 60B:406-411, 1978.
10. Lichtenstein, L. Aneurysmal bone cyst: observations on fifty cases. J Bone Joint Surg, 39A:873-882, 1957.
11. Mirra, J. *Bone Tumors: Diagnosis and Treatment,* Philadelphia, J.B. Lippincott Co., 1980, pp 478-492.
12. Schachar, N.S. and Edwards, G.E.: Vertebra plana (Calve's disease) due to aneurysmal bone cyst. J Bone Joint Surg, 56B:586, 1974.
13. Slowick, F.A., Campbell, C.J., and Kettelkamp, D.B. Aneurysmal bone cyst. J Bone Joint Surg, 50A:1142-1151, 1968.
14. Zimmer, W.D., Berquist, T.H., Sim, F.H., Wold, L.E., Pritchard, D.J., Shives, T.C., McLeod, R.A. Magnetic resonance imaging of aneurysmal bone cyst. Mayo Clin Proc, 59:633-636, 1984.

§ 4-4(E). Hemangioma.

Hemangiomas are benign vascular lesions composed of cavernous, capillary, or venous blood vessels which affect bone or soft tissues. Up to 10% of autopsied spines contain hemangiomas. In most circumstances, they are asymptomatic. In symptomatic hemangiomas, patients experience localized pain and muscle spasm. Cervical location of hemangioma is unusual compared to the thoracic or lumbar areas, but these lesions may be associated with serious neurologic abnormalities including compression of nerve roots or spinal cord. The diagnosis of hemangioma is suggested by the characteristic vertical striations of vertebral bodies on radiographic evaluation. Most hemangiomas require no therapy. Radiotherapy may decrease symptoms in those patients who experience pain with hemangioma. Laminectomy is reserved for those patients with neurologic deficits who require decompression of the spinal cord.

§ 4-4(E)(1). Prevalence and Etiology.

Hemangiomas are less than 1% of clinically symptomatic primary bone tumors (entry 9). Asymptomatic vertebral hemangiomas are more common, occurring in 10% to 12% of autopsies (entries 6, 11). Hemangiomas are detected in older patients; in one series most commonly in the fifth decade (entry 1). Hemangiomas occur slightly more commonly in women.

The etiology of hemangiomas remains unknown. They may be either congenital or neoplastic in origin (entry 2).

§ 4-4(E)(2). Clinical Findings.

A cervical location for a hemangioma is less common than other areas of the axial skeleton (entry 7). Most hemangiomas are asymptomatic and are discovered serendipitously on a radiograph. When symptomatic, hemangiomas produce pain and tenderness over the involved vertebrae. The pain is vague and nondescript and gradually becomes constant and throbbing in quality. Hemangiomas associated with spinal cord compression in the cervical area may be associated with radicular pain, paresthesias, motor weakness, loss of reflexes and urinary incontinence (entries 10, 3).

§ 4-4(E)(3). Physical Findings.

Physical examination may demonstrate tenderness with palpation over the affected vertebral body. Limitation of motion is noted if muscle spasm is severe. Neurologic abnormalities will correspond to the level of cord compression when present.

§ 4-4(E)(4). Laboratory Findings.

Solitary vertebral hemangiomas are not associated with any abnormal results. Pathologic examination demonstrates a brownish-red, well-delineated lesion arising in the periosteum or marrow space in a vertebral body. Microscopically, the lesions contain thickened osseous trabeculae associated with an increased number and size of capillary, cavernous or venous vessels (entry 2).

§ 4-4(E)(5). Radiographic Findings.

Vertebral hemangiomas affect the body of a vertebra most often although extension into the laminae, pedicles, transverse or spinous processes may also occur (entry 12). Characteristic plain radiographic changes of a vertebral hemangioma are diffuse, prominent vertical striations, with a lace of horizontal striations, associated with a vertebral body configuration which is unchanged. Rarely, expansion or enlargement of a vertebra may occur (entry 7). Paravertebral soft tissue extension may occur with or without a demonstrable hemangioma on plain radiographs. Spinal angiography may confirm the diagnosis, demonstrate the extent of the lesion, both intraosseously and extraosseously, and determine the location of the arterial blood supply of the lesion. Myelography is helpful at determining compression of the spinal cord which may be caused by expansion of an involved vertebral body, extradural tumor extension, compression fracture, or extradural hematoma.

§ 4-4(E)(6). Differential Diagnosis.

The diagnosis of a vertebral hemangioma is suggested by the characteristic radiographic findings in a solitary vertebral body. These lesions are not biopsied because of the potential serious complication of hemorrhage. The diagnosis of hemangioma is more difficult to make when portions of a vertebra other than the body are affected. Bone resorption of a pedicle with compression fracture is more common with metastatic tumor. Course trabeculation of the periphery of an expanding vertebral body is more characteristic of Paget's disease. Bone erosion with a paravertebral mass may suggest spinal tuberculosis. Abnormal laboratory tests (elevated ESR, serum alkaline phosphatase, cultures) should differentiate these processes from hemangioma.

§ 4-4(E)(7). Treatment.

The treatment of choice for asymptomatic hemangiomas is observation. The pain of symptomatic hemangiomas is responsive to radiation therapy although the appearance of the lesion remains unchanged. Surgical intervention followed by irradiation may yield good results but may be associated with excessive morbidity and mortality due to excessive bleeding (entry 5). Therefore, laminectomy should be reserved for those patients with neurologic deficits who require decompression of the spinal cord (entry 4).

§ 4-4(E)(8). Course and Outcome.

Vertebral hemangiomas are usually asymptomatic and require no therapy. Symptoms associated with hemangioma suggest expansion of the lesion and require therapy. The major complication of hemangioma is neural compression from an expanding lesion. Appropriate diagnosis and timely therapy may prevent this potentially disabling complication of this vascular neoplasm.

BIBLIOGRAPHY

1. Dahlin, D.C. *Bone Tumors: General Aspects and Data on 6,221 Cases.* Springfield, Charles C. Thomas, 1978, pp 137-148.
2. Huvos, A.G. *Bone Tumors: Diagnosis, Treatment, and Prognosis.* Philadelphia, W.B. Saunders, 1979, pp 345-351.
3. Krieger, A.J. Hemangioma of fifth cervical vertebra with intermittent spinal cord dysfunction. South Med J, 70:1008-1010, 1977.
4. Lozman, J., and Holmblad, J. Cavernous hemangioma associated with scoliosis and a localized consumptive coagulopathy: a case report. J Bone Joint Surg, 58A:1021-1024, 1976.
5. Manning, J.H. Symptomatic hemangioma of the spine. Radiology, 56:58-65, 1951.
6. Marcial-Rojas, R.A. Primary hemangiopericytoma of bone: review of the literature and report of the first case with metastasis. Cancer, 13:308-311, 1960.
7. McAllister, V.L., Kendell, B.F., and Bull, J.W.D. Symptomatic vertebral hemangiomas. Brain, 98:71-80, 1975.
8. Melot, C.J., Brihaye, J., Jeanmart, L., and Gompel, C. Les hemangiomes due rachis cervical. Acta radiol (Diag), 5:1067-1078, 1966.
9. Mirra, J. *Bone Tumors: Diagnosis and Treatment.* Philadelphia, J.B. Lippincott Co., 1980, pp 492-498.
10. Robbins, L.R., Fountain, E.N. Hemangioma of cervical vertebras with spinal cord compression. N Eng J Med, 258:685-687, 1958.
11. Schmorl, G., and Junghanns, H. *The Human Spine in Health and Disease,* 2d ed., New York, Grune and Stratton, 1971, p 325.
12. Sherman, R.S., and Wilner, D. The roentgen diagnosis of hemangioma of bone. Am J Roentgenol, 86:1146-1159, 1961.

§ 4-4(F). Eosinophilic Granuloma.

Eosinophilic granuloma is a benign variant of the histiocytoses which include Hand-Schuller-Christian disease and Letterer-Siwe disease. The disease is caused by the infiltration of bone by eosinophils, histiocytes, and mononuclear phagocytic cells. Eosinophilic granuloma usually occurs as a solitary lesion when it affects the spine. The lesion usually presents with pain, with swelling occurring less commonly. The radiographic findings of eosinophilic granuloma may range from an osteolytic oval area without reactive sclerosis to complete collapse of a vertebral body, vertebra plana. The diagnosis is established by the presence of eosinophils and histiocytes in biopsy specimens. The treatment of choice is total removal or partial curettage for inaccessible lesions.

§ 4-4(F)(1). Prevalence and Etiology.

Eosinophilic granuloma is a rare lesion occurring in less than 1% of biopsied primary infiltrative lesions of bone (entry 5). Approximately 10% of eosinophilic granulomas occur in patients 20 years or older. It occurs in a 2:1 ratio of men to women and is more frequent in Caucasians than Blacks (entry 1). The etiology of this illness is unknown.

§ 4-4(F)(2). Clinical Findings.

Pain is the most common symptom associated with eosinophilic granuloma. The pain is localized, aching, and constant in quality. Swelling may be present if the area of involvement is close to the skin. Patients are otherwise systemically well and have few complaints other than the localized problem. Cervical vertebrae are affected less often than those in the lower thoracic or upper lumbar segments.

§ 4-4(F)(3). Physical Findings.

A palpable mass may be present over the affected bone but it is neither tender nor associated with redness or heat. Neurologic signs may be present if vertebral body collapse results in nerve impingement.

§ 4-4(F)(4). Laboratory Findings.

Eosinophilic granuloma is associated with peripheral eosinophilia in 6% to 10% of patients (entry 5). There is also an elevated erythrocyte sedimentation rate.

The characteristic histologic picture is one of bone infiltrated with focal collections of large, swollen histiocytes surrounded by numerous eosinophilic polymorphonuclear leukocytes. The histiocytes take the form of giant cells after they have ingested necrotic tissue and convert it into cytoplasmic lipids (cholesterol). The presence of lipid in histiocytes is a secondary phenomenon and is not of pathogenetic importance.

Eosinophilic granuloma is a mimicer of benign and malignant bone diseases. The pleomorphic appearance of the histiocytes may superficially resemble malignant cells of Hodgkin's disease, or giant cell tumor.

§ 4-4(F)(5). Radiographic Findings.

Eosinophilic granuloma of the spine usually affects the vertebral body, although the posterior elements may also be affected (entry 3). The features of early lesions are those of a destructive radiolucent oval area of bone lysis without peripheral sclerosis. Progressive destruction in a vertebral body is termed vertebra plana. Eosinophilic granuloma is probably the most common cause of vertebra plana in children and adults. Vertebra plana is associated with collapse of a vertebral body which results in a wafer-like appearance of the vertebra without involvement of the intervertebral disc (entry 7). Rarely, eosinophilic granuloma can produce expansile lesions with extensive destruction of multiple vertebrae and paraspinal extension (entry 2).

§ 4-4(F)(6). Differential Diagnosis.

Close inspection of a biopsy specimen helps prevent confusing eosinophilic granuloma with a number of benign and malignant disease processes. Included in the differential diagnosis are osteomyelitis, osteoblastoma, aneurysmal bone cyst, non-ossifying fibromas, sarcoidosis, giant cell tumor, Hodgkin's disease and osteosarcoma.

§ 4-4(F)(7). Treatment.

The treatment of choice is curettage, with or without packing of the lesion with bone chips if the lesion is large. Occasionally, lesions may recede spontaneously or after biopsy (entry 4). Low dosage radiation therapy may be considered for inaccessible lesions in the spine which may lead to pathologic fractures (entry 5). Other authors believe that damaged segments may reconstitute themselves spontaneously so that radiation therapy is not indicated (entry 6).

§ 4-4(F)(8). Course and Outcome.

Eosinophilic granuloma is a benign lesion with a good prognosis. Lesions heal spontaneously or with therapy within twelve months. Patients who have a solitary lesion for six months or longer rarely develop additional lesions. Patients who develop the generalized form of histiocytosis X are more often younger patients than adults.

BIBLIOGRAPHY

1. Cheyne, C. Histiocytosis X. J Bone Joint Surg, 53B:366-382, 1971.
2. Ferris, R.A., Pettrone, F.A., McKelvie, A.M., Twigg, H.L., and Chun, B.K. Eosinophilic granuloma of the spine: an unusual radiographic presentation. Clin Orthop, 99:57-63, 1974.
3. Kaye, J.J. and Freiberger, R.H. Eosinophilic granuloma of the spine without vertebra plana: a report of two unusual cases. Radiology, 92:1188-1191, 1969.
4. Mankin, H.J. Histiocytosis of bone and of the soft tissue. Orthopaedic Rev, 12:149-153, 1983.
5. Mirra, J.M. *Bone Tumors: Diagnosis and Treatment.* Philadelphia, J.B. Lippincott Co., 1980, pp 376-382.
6. Nesbit, M.E., Kieffer, S., D'Angio, G.J. Reconstitution of vertebral height in histiocytosis X: a long-term follow-up. J Bone Joint Surg, 51A:1360-1368, 1969.
7. Ochsner, S.F. Eosinophilic granuloma of bone. Experience with 20 cases. Am J Roentgenol, 97:719-726, 1966.

§ 4-4(G). Multiple Myeloma.

Multiple myeloma is a malignant tumor of plasma cells. Plasma cells are located in bone marrow and are responsible for production of immunoglobulins and antibodies. The proliferation of these cells is associated with bone pain, pathological fractures and hypercalcemia. In the axial skeleton, the cervical spine is affected less commonly than the lumbar or thoracic areas. In addition to bone pain, patients with myeloma or solitary plasmacytoma, a localized form of myeloma, can have neurologic symptoms secondary to vertebral body compression fractures or extradural extension of tumor associated with compression of neural elements. The diagnosis of multiple myeloma is suggested by the presence of monoclonal immunoglobulins on electrophoresis, and the presence of abnormal plasma cells on histologic examination of bone marrow. Patients with clinically active multiple myeloma usually require chemotherapy for control of their disease. Patients with vertebral lesions may require radiotherapy and/or decompressive laminectomy for control of neurologic symptoms. Although patients may have an initial response to therapy, less than 50% of patients survive five years.

§ 4-4(G)(1). Prevalence and Etiology.

Multiple myeloma is the most common primary malignancy of bone in adults accounting for 27% of biopsied bone tumors in one series (entry 17) and 47% in another (entry 9). The incidence is three cases per 100,000 people in the United States (entry 14) and the usual patient age range is 50 to 70 (entry 16). Men have an increased incidence of both multiple myeloma and plasmacytoma.

The etiology of multiple myeloma is unknown. Although patients not infrequently will describe an episode of minimal trauma as the initiating factor in the onset of their pain, trauma is not a factor in the etiology of multiple myeloma (entry 16).

§ 4-4(G)(2). Clinical Findings.

Compared to other sites in the axial skeleton, the cervical spine is an uncommon location for multiple myeloma. In a review of spinal cord involvement in myeloma, 17% of myeloma patients had symptomatic cervical spine involvement compared to 69% for the thoracic spine (entry 6). Bone pain is the most common initial symptom in 75% of patients (entry 14). The pain is mild, aching, and intermittent at the onset, aggravated by weight-bearing and relieved by bed rest. Patients with cervical spine involvement may present with neck pain. Approximately 20% of myeloma patients have spinal compression which may be associated with minimal trauma (entry 6). Six percent may actually develop cord compression secondary to pathologic fractures. Bone pain may be present in areas of the skeleton without noticeable fractures. Pain may be secondary to bone marrow expansion or to microfractures (entry 5).

As a consequence of widespread bone destruction, abnormal immunoglobulin production and infiltration of bone marrow, patients with multiple myeloma develop a broad range of clinical symptoms. Hypercalcemia, due to bone destruction, is associated with bone weakness, easy fatiguability, anorexia, nausea, vomiting, mental status changes including coma, and kidney stones. Increased abnormal immunoglobulin concentrations cause progressive renal insufficiency, increased susceptibility to infection, and amyloidosis. Infiltration of bone marrow with malignant cells causes anemia, bleeding secondary to a deficiency of platelets, thrombocytopenia, and generalized weakness.

§ 4-4(G)(3). Physical Findings.

The physical examination may be unremarkable in the early stages of the disease. Bone tenderness, fever with infection, pallor and petechiae become more prominent findings with advancing disease. Neurologic examination may reveal abnormalities related to nerve compression or to metabolic effects of myeloma (entries 10, 21).

§ 4-4(G)(4). Laboratory Findings.

Laboratory examination may reveal abnormalities including normochromic, normocytic anemia, elevated leukocyte count, thrombocytopenia, or positive Coomb's test and an elevated erythrocyte sedimentation rate. Abnormal serum chemistries include hypercalcemia, hyperuricemia, and elevated creatinine.

Serum alkaline phosphatase is normal in most patients with myeloma. Characteristic serum protein abnormalities occur in the vast majority of patients with myeloma. The total serum protein concentrations are increased secondary to an increase in the globulin fraction. The increase in globulins is due to the presence of abnormal immunoglobulins of the G, A, D, E or M classes. Immunoglobulins are composed of light and heavy chains. The light and heavy chains of an antibody combine to form a site which is directed against a specific antigen. In multiple myeloma, instead of having a multitude of antibodies, one single antibody composed of a light and heavy chain, an M-protein, is produced to the exclusion of others. The balance between light and heavy chains may also be disturbed with excess light chain production resulting in Bence-Jones protein in the urine or excess heavy chain production resulting in heavy chain disease. Serum protein electrophoresis demonstrates the elevation in globulin levels, while quantitative immunoglobulin determination detects the class of immunoglobulins which is present in increased concentration. Urine protein electrophoresis will detect the presence of Bence-Jones proteinuria. Other tests associated with abnormal immunoglobulins include increased serum viscosity which results in the blockage of blood vessels and a positive rheumatoid factor (entry 16).

Gross pathologic examination of myelomatous involvement of bone reveals soft, gray friable tissue causing expansion of the affected bone associated with extraosseous extension into adjacent structures. Microscopic examination of multiple myeloma reveals dense packing of tumor cells with sparse stroma and fibrous tissue. Plasma cells are increased in number to levels of greater than 30% of bone marrow cells. Plasma cells may be classified into three histologic grades, well differentiated, moderately differentiated, and poorly differentiated (entry 2). The well differentiated plasma cells resemble normal cells. Anaplastic myeloma cells mimic undifferentiated carcinomas or small cell sarcomas.

§ 4-4(G)(5). Radiographic Findings.

The characteristic radiographic finding of "punched-out" areas of bone destruction with no surrounding zone of reactive bone is a result of the replacement of osseous structures with masses of plasma cells. Diffuse osteolysis with no reactive sclerosis resembles osteoporosis and is particularly prominent in the spine (entry 3). In individual vertebrae, the bodies are affected while the posterior elements are spared. This is in contrast with metastatic lesions which involve both vertebral bodies and pedicles (entry 15). Pathologic fractures of vertebral bodies are a usual consequence of vertebral body osteolysis. Paravertebral extension of tumor may be perceived as soft tissue swelling near the spine (entry 6).

Solitary plasmacytomas, a localized collection of plasma cells without systemic complications, have variable radiographic features. The lesion may cause an expansile lesion of a vertebral body or localized osteolysis without expansion. An involved vertebral body may fracture and disappear completely or the lesion may extend across the intervertebral disc to affect an adjacent vertebra, simulating the appearance of an infection (entry 22). Osteosclerotic lesions of vertebral bodies are associated with generalized myeloma and plasmacytoma but occur less commonly than osteolytic lesions (entry 19).

Bone scan, which is helpful detecting metastatic bone lesions, is not as useful as plain radiographs in detecting myelomatous osseous involvement since plasma cells cause little osteoblastic activity (entries 23, 24). Computed tomography is able to detect abnormalities in bone before 30% of bone calcium is lost, making it more sensitive than plain radiographs in detecting myeloma in a vertebral body (entry 13).

§ 4-4(G)(6). Differential Diagnosis.

The diagnosis of multiple myeloma is based upon the clinical history associated with plasma cell growth (bone pain, hypercalcemia) and characteristic laboratory abnormalities including monoclonal antibodies (M and Bence-Jones protein) and collections of plasma cells in a bone marrow biopsy. The diagnosis of myeloma must be considered in the patient with generalized osteoporosis since some myelomas produce no detectable myeloma protein (entry 1). Other diseases which must be considered in the differential diagnosis of myeloma include metastatic tumor, osteoporosis, chronic infections, and hyperparathyroidism.

§ 4-4(G)(7). Treatment.

Generalized, symptomatic multiple myeloma usually requires chemotherapy with prednisone and melphalan (entry 8). Approximately 70% of patients respond to therapy and have a reduction in bone pain and destruction, decreased concentration of abnormal proteins and a normalization of hematocrit, urea nitrogen, creatinine and calcium. Melphalan chemotherapy may cause bone healing, although this is not associated with any greater survival (entry 20). More aggressive disease may respond to the M-2 drug program, combining vincristine, melphalan, cyclophosphamide, prednisone, and BCNU (entry 4). In patients with neural compression secondary to vertebral collapse or extraosseous extension, decompressing laminectomy and/or local radiotherapy, dependent on the general condition of the patient, are indicated (entries 6, 11). Decompression and radiotherapy are also indicated for the solitary plasmacytoma of the spinal column.

§ 4-4(G)(8). Course and Outcome.

The usual course of multiple myeloma is one of gradual progression despite therapy. The survival rates are not encouraging with 90% succumbing in three years in one study (entry 17). Dahlin reported a 10% five-year survival (entry 9). Patients with anemia, spinal cord involvement, and renal failure have a poorer prognosis. In regard to cervical spine myelomas, there are reports which suggest a worse prognosis while others find no increased risk (entries 6, 7). Patients with D and E myeloma have poorer prognoses than those A myeloma patients (entries 12, 18). Patients with "true" solitary plasmacytomas who do not disseminate have a better prognosis than those with generalized disease (entry 22).

BIBLIOGRAPHY

1. Arend, W.P. and Adamson, J.W. Nonsecretary myeloma: immunofluorescent demonstration of paraprotein within bone marrow plasma cells. Cancer, 33:721-728, 1974.
2. Bayrd, E.D. The bone marrow on sternal aspiration in multiple myeloma. Blood, 3:987-1018, 1948.
3. Carson, C.P., Ackerman, L.V., and Maltby, J.D. Plasma cell myeloma: a clinical, pathologic, and roentgenologic review of 90 cases. Am J Clin Pathol, 25:849-888, 1955.
4. Case, D.C., Jr., Lee, B.J. III, and Clarkson, B.D. Improved survival times in multiple myeloma treated with melphalan, prednisone, cyclophosphamide, vincristine and BCNU — M-2 protocol. Am J Med, 63:897-903, 1977.
5. Charkes, N.D., Durant, J., and Barry, W.E. Bone pain in multiple myeloma: Studies with radioactive 87m SR. Arch Intern Med, 130:53-58, 1972.
6. Clarke, E. Spinal cord involvement in multiple myelomatosis. Brain, 79:332-348, 1956.
7. Cohen, D.M., Svien, H.J., and Dahlin, D.C. Long-term survival of patients with myeloma of the vertebral column. JAMA, 187:914-917, 1964.

8. Costa, G., Engle, R.L., Jr., Schilling, A., Carbone, P., Kochwa, S., Nachman, R.L., and Glidewell, O. Melphalan and prednisone — an effective combination for the treatment of multiple myeloma. Am J Med, 54:589-599, 1973.
9. Dahlin, D.C. *Bone Tumors: General Aspects and Data on 6,221 Cases.* Springfield, Charles C. Thomas, 1978, pp 159-172.
10. Davison, C., and Balser, B.H. Myeloma and its neural complications. Arch Surg, 35:913-936, 1937.
11. Gilbert, R.W., Kim, J.H., and Posner, J.B. Epidural spinal cord compression from metastatic tumor: diagnosis and treatment. Ann Neurol, 3:40-51, 1978.
12. Gompels, B.M., Votaw, M.L., and Martel, W. Correlation of radiological manifestations of multiple myeloma with immunoglobulin abnormalities and prognosis. Radiology, 104:509-514, 1972.
13. Helms, C.A. and Genant, H.K. Computed tomography in the early detection of skeletal involvement with multiple myeloma. JAMA, 248:2886-2887, 1982.
14. Huvos, A.G. *Bone Tumors: Diagnosis, Treatment and Prognosis,* Philadelphia, W.B. Saunders, 1979, pp 413-431.
15. Jacobsen, H.G., Poppel, M.H., Shapiro, J.H. and Grossberger, S. The vertebral pedicle sign: a roentgen finding to differentiate metastatic carcinoma from multiple myeloma. Am J Roentgenol, 80:817-821, 1958.
16. Kyle, R.A. Multiple myeloma: review of 869 cases. Mayo Clin Proc, 50:29-40, 1965.
17. Mirra, J.M. *Bone Tumors: Diagnosis and Treatment,* Philadelphia, J.B. Lippincott Co., 1980, pp 398-406.
18. Pruzanski, W., and Rother, I. IgD plasma cell neoplasia: clinical manifestations and characteristic features. Can Med Assoc J, 102:1061-1065, 1970.
19. Roberts, M., Rinaudo, P.A., Villinskas, J., and Owens, G. Solitary sclerosing plasma cell myeloma of the spine: case report. J Neurosurg, 40:125-129, 1974.
20. Rodriguez, L.H., Finkelstein, J.B., Shullenberger, C.C., Alexanian, R. Bone healing in multiple myeloma with melphalan chemotherapy. Annal Intern Med, 76:551-556, 1972.
21. Silverstein, A. and Doniger, D.E. Neurologic complications of myelomatosis. Arch Neurol, 9:534-544, 1963.
22. Valderrama, J.A.F. and Bullough, P.C. Solitary myeloma of the spine. J Bone Joint Surg, 50B:82-90, 1968.

23. Wahner, H.W., Kyle, R.A., and Beabout, J.W. Scintigraphic evaluation of the skeleton in multiple myeloma. Mayo Clin Proc, 55:739-746, 1980.
24. Woolfenden, J.M., Pitt, M.J., Durie, B.G.M., and Moon, T.E. Comparison of bone scintography and radiography in multiple myeloma. Radiology, 134:723-728, 1980.

§ 4-4(H). Chordoma.

Chordoma is a neoplasm that develops from the remnants of an embryonic structure, the notochord. The spinal cord is a condensation of mesoderm around the notochord. Chordomas are found only in the axial skeleton. The lesion may present with localized pain, a slowly growing mass, or neurologic dysfunction. The radiographic findings of chordoma include lytic bone destruction with calcific foci associated with a soft tissue mass. The definitive diagnosis is established by the presence of physaliphorous cells, cells of notochordal origin, which contain a large, clear area of cytoplasm with an eccentric, flattened nucleous in biopsy specimens. The treatment of choice is en bloc excision for accessible lesions.

§ 4-4(H)(1). Prevalence and Etiology.

Chordomas are rare accounting for a range of 1% to 4% of primary bone tumors (entries 3, 1, 6). The tumor usually becomes evident in patients between the ages of 30 to 70. The ratio of men to women with cervical or cranial chordomas is 1:1 as compared to 3:1 with tumors in the sacral region.

The etiology of the factors which initiates the regrowth of notochordal vestigial cells in the spine is unknown. Up to 15% of patients with chordomas of the sacral spine give a prior history of trauma (entries 3, 8). However, the evidence for the subsequent development of this tumor after trauma is conjectural.

§ 4-4(H)(2). Clinical Findings.

Approximately 35% of chordomas are located at the base of the skull (spheno-occipital area), with an additional 10% in the cervical spine area (entry 1). The symptoms of chordomas are closely related to the location and extent of the tumor. Headache, which may be present for years, is the initial and most frequent symptom of cranial chordomas and is present in over 80% of cases (entry 3). The dull and constant pain is localized to the posterior skull or neck. Neurologic, or endocrinologic dysfunction, stridor and dysphagia are associated with chordomas located in the spheno-occipital, hypophyseal, nasopharyngeal and cervical areas respectively (entries 6, 5, 7). The duration of symptoms for a majority of patients with cervical chordomas is less than one year.

§ 4-4(H)(3). Physical Findings.

Physical findings may include pain with palpation over the affected area. A soft tissue mass may be located in the retropharyngeal or paracervical areas. Neurologic findings may include abnormalities of the upper or lower extremities. Loss of sensation and motor strength, hyper-reflexia, and bilateral Babinski response have been reported with cervical lesions (entry 7).

§ 4-4(H)(4). Laboratory Findings.

Laboratory findings are unremarkable early in the course of this tumor. Elevations in cerebrospinal protein occur with tumor invasion of the spinal canal (entry 4).

Pathologically, chordoma is a soft, lobulated, gelatinous tumor. In the vertebral column, its origin is the vertebral body and it spreads along the posterior longitudinal ligament or through the intervertebral disc. On histologic examination, chordomas contain cells with large clear areas of cytoplasm, with eccentric, flattened nucleii (physaliphorous cells). These cells form columns interspersed with thick fibrous tissue. Chordomas may be confused with adenocarcinoma because of the large amounts of mucin both tumors produce.

§ 4-4(H)(5). Radiographic Findings.

Characteristic radiographic findings of vertebral chordomas are asymmetric destruction of a single vertebra with an adjacent soft tissue mass. Occasionally, multiple adjoining vertebrae may be affected (entry 9). Initially, vertebral chordoma causes destruction of vertebral bone sparing the intervertebral disc. Subsequently, the disc space narrows along with erosion of the opposing vertebral end plate (entry 7).

Intracranial chordomas cause destruction of the sella turcica and adjacent area of the sphenoid bone. Progression of the tumor results in osteolysis of the base of the skull in the midline. Chordomas in the nasopharyngeal area are associated with soft tissue swelling in the cervical area.

For complete evaluation of the epidural extension of tumor into the spinal canal, myelography is routinely utilized even in the absence of neurologic signs or symptoms. Computerized axial tomography is very useful at demonstrating the soft tissue extension of these tumors (entry 8). Carotid and vertebral angiograms prove beneficial in determining the extent of intracranial tumor.

§ 4-4(H)(6). Differential Diagnosis.

The diagnosis of chordoma is confirmed by the careful examination of a needle biopsy specimen. Other lesions which must be differentiated from chordoma include liposarcoma, chondrosarcoma, and metastatic adenocarcinoma.

§ 4-4(H)(7). Treatment.

Complete surgical removal of the tumor mass is the treatment of choice but is rarely achieved because of the location and extent of the tumor at the time of diagnosis. Vertebral chordomas are treated by decompression laminectomy, with excision of accessible tumor located in bone, soft tissues and the extradural space. Inaccessible tumors may have their growth slowed by radiotherapy. Radiotherapy is useful for intracranial as well as vertebral chordomas (entries 4, 2). Chemotherapy is usually ineffective.

§ 4-4(H)(8). Course and Outcome.

Chordomas are slowly growing tumors which metastasize in 10% of patients late in the course of their illness (entry 10). The five-year survival for vertebral chordomas is 50%, which was unaffected by the presence or absence of metastases (entry 8). Patients who receive surgical excision coupled with radiation did as well as those who received radiation alone. Chordoma has a wide spectrum of behavior from indolent to rapidly destructive. The location, pathological characteristics, and invasiveness of the tumor will decide the eventual prognosis of a patient.

BIBLIOGRAPHY

1. Dahlin, D.C. *Bone Tumors: General Aspects and Data on 6,221 Cases.* Springfield, Charles C. Thomas, 1978, pp 329-343.
2. Dahlin, D.C. and MacCarty, C.S. Chordoma: a study of fifty-nine cases. Cancer, 5:1170-1178, 1952.
3. Huvos, A.G. *Bone Tumors: Diagnosis, Treatment and Prognosis.* Philadelphia, W.B. Saunders, 1979, pp 373-391.
4. Kamrin, R.P., Potanos, J.N., and Pool, J.L. An evaluation of the diagnosis and treatment of chordoma. J Neurol Neurosurg Psychiat, 27:157-165, 1964.

5. Kragenbuhl, H., and Yasargil, M.G. Cranial chordomas. Prog Neurol Surg, 6:380-434, 1975.
6. Mirra, J.M. *Bone Tumors: Diagnosis and Treatment,* Philadelphia, J.B. Lippincott Co., 1980, pp 243-256.
7. Pinto, R.S., Lin, J.P., Firooznia, H., and Le Fleur, R.S. The osseous and angiographic manifestations of vertebral chordomas. Neuroradiology, 9:231-241, 1975.
8. Sundaresan, N., Galicich, J.H., Chu, F.C.H., and Huvos, A.C. Spinal chordomas. J Neurosurg, 50:312-319, 1979.
9. Utne, J.R., and Pugh, D.G. The roentgenologic aspects of chordoma. Am J Roentgenol, 74:593-608, 1955.
10. Wang, C.C. and James, A.E., Jr. Chordoma: brief review of the literature and report of a case with widespread metastases. Cancer, 22:162-167, 1968.

§ 4-4(I). Lymphomas.

Lymphomas are malignant diseases of lymphoreticular origin. Most commonly they arise in lymph nodes, rarely primarily in bone and are classified into two major groups: Hodgkin's and non-Hodgkin's lymphoma. In disseminated disease, 30% of patients will have cervical spine involvement. The initial and major symptom associated with lymphomatous involvement of bone is local pain. Axial skeleton involvement may result in compression of neural elements and production of neurologic symptoms. Diagnosis of lymphoma is determined by the histologic examination of biopsy material obtained from a lesion. Chemotherapy for generalized disease and radiotherapy for local disease may improve the prognosis of the patient with lymphoma.

§ 4-4(I)(1). Prevalence and Etiology.

The incidence of Hodgkin's and non-Hodgkin's (lymphosarcoma, reticulum cell sarcoma) lymphomas is approximately between 40 to 60 cases per million per year. Primary Hodgkin's and non-Hodgkin's disease of bone unassociated with lymph node involvement are rare tumors occurring in between 1% to 5% of biopsied tumors (entries 8, 7). In patients with primary disease in lymph nodes and secondary dissemination to bone, up to 50% are affected with 30% having involvement of the cervical spine (entry 8). A majority of patients who develop lymphomas are between 20 and 70 and the male to female ratio is approximately 3:2 (entry 2). The etiology of malignant lymphomas is unknown.

§ 4-4(I)(2). Clinical Findings.

Pain and localized swelling are the cardinal features of lymphoma of bone. Pain is of variable intensity but becomes persistent. An increase of pain with recumbency is not an uncommon symptom. The duration of pain before diagnosis is measured in months most commonly. Patients may feel relatively well despite extensive damage to bone (entry 5). Occasionally bone lesions may have pain increased with alcohol consumption or may be painless (entries 1, 9). Neurologic symptoms of weakness or sensory changes develop with lymphomas with contiguous involvement of the spinal canal.

§ 4-4(I)(3). Physical Findings.

A mass in the region of the tumor associated with tenderness on palpation is a common finding. Patients with axial skeleton disease may demonstrate neurologic deficits.

§ 4-4(I)(4). Laboratory Findings.

Primary lymphoma of bone is unassociated with laboratory abnormalities. The appearance of anemia, elevated sedimentation rate and increased serum chemistries suggest extension of tumor beyond the bone or that the bone lesion was part of disseminated disease which went unrecognized.

Gross pathologic examination of osseous lymphoma reveals soft tissue extension of the tumor with indistinct margins. The microscopic findings of Hodgkin's disease includes typical Reed-Steinberg cells, atypical mononuclear cells and an inflammatory component composed of lymphocytes, plasma cells and scattered eosinophils. The reactive histiocytes and eosinophils look superficially like eosinophic granuloma. Non-Hodgkin's lymphomas may exhibit marked histologic variation (entry 10). These lesions lack Reed-Steinberg cells and demonstrate different combinations of abnormal lymphocytes and supporting cells.

§ 4-4(I)(5). Radiographic Findings.

The radiographic appearance of lymphomas is quite variable and does not allow for a specific diagnosis. The bone changes in Hodgkin's disease may include lytic (75%), sclerotic (15%), mixed (5%), or periosteal lesions (5%) (entry 6). In vertebrae, the body is affected to a much greater degree than the posterior elements (pedicle, lamina, spinous process). Occasionally, fibrous replacement of marrow elements produces osteoblastic activity which results in an "ivory" vertebra (entry 3). Non-Hodgkin's lymphoma of bone has similar features characterized by lytic and blastic areas, with cortical destruction and little reactive new bone.

§ 4-4(I)(6). Differential Diagnosis.

The definitive diagnosis of lymphoma is based upon the careful examination of biopsy material. However, the diagnosis of a specific lymphoma is a difficult one to make because of the pleomorphic forms of the disease. The differential diagnosis includes metastatic carcinoma, particularly breast or prostate with osteoblastic lesions, Paget's disease, eosinophilic granuloma, and chronic osteomyelitis.

§ 4-4(I)(7). Treatment.

The treatment of lymphomas is based upon the extent of the illness. All patients must be staged before treatment is initiated. Once the stage of disease is known, the patient should receive appropriate therapy for that degree of involvement. Treatment may include radiation therapy and/or chemotherapy (entry 4).

§ 4-4(I)(8). Course and Outcome.

The therapy for lymphoma has become more effective in the control of the disease and patients have the potential for cure if the disease is not too extensive. Patients with primary lesions have a better survival than disseminated disease (entry 2). In one study, 34% of primary lymphoma of bone patients were alive at ten years.

BIBLIOGRAPHY

1. Conn, H.O. Alcohol-induced pain as a manifestation of Hodgkin's disease. Arch Intern Med, 100:241-247, 1957.
2. Dahlin, D.C. *Bone Tumors: General Aspects and Data on 6,221 Cases.* Springfield, Charles C. Thomas, 1978, pp 173-189.
3. Dennis, J.M. The solitary dense vertebral body. Radiology, 77:618-621, 1961.
4. DeVita, V.T., Jr., Serpick, A.A., and Carbone, P.O. Combination chemotherapy in the treatment of advanced Hodgkin's disease. Ann Intern Med, 73:881-895, 1970.
5. Francis, K.C., Higinbotham, N.L., and Coley, B.L. Primary reticulum cell sarcoma of bone: report of 44 cases. Surg Gynecol Obstet, 99:142-146, 1954.
6. Granger, W., and Whitaker, R. Hodgkin's disease in bone, with special reference to periosteal reaction. Br J Radiol, 40:939-948, 1967.
7. Huvos, A.G. *Bone Tumors: Diagnosis, Treatment and Prognosis.* Philadelphia, W.B. Saunders, 1979, pp 392-402.
8. Mirra, J.M. *Bone Tumors: Diagnosis and Treatment.* Philadelphia, J.B. Lippincott Co., 1980, pp 406-418.

9. Perttala, Y., and Kijanen, I. Roentgenologic bone lesions in lymphogranulomatosis maligna: analysis of 453 cases. Ann Chir Gynecol, Fenn, 54:414-424, 1965.
10. Reimer, R.R., Chabner, B.A., Young, R.C., Reddich, R., and Johnson, R.E. Lymphoma presenting in bone: results of histopathology staging, and therapy. Annal Intern Med, 87:50-55, 1977.

§ 4-4(J). Skeletal Metastases.

A principal characteristic of malignant neoplastic lesions is the growth of tumor cells distant from and noncontiguous to the primary lesion. These distant lesions are referred to as metastases and are frequently found in the skeletal system. In the skeletal system, the axial skeleton is most commonly affected by metastatic tumor. The cervical spine is the third most common site for metastases in the axial skeleton after the lumbar and thoracic areas. Skeletal lesions result from dissemination of tumor cells through the bloodstream and their deposition in the vascular channels of bones. Certain tumors such as breast, lung, kidney, and prostate have a predilection for causing skeletal metastases.

The symptoms and signs of metastatic disease are similar to those of other bone tumors affecting the spine. Radiographic findings associated with metastases include lytic, blastic or mixed bony changes. The diagnosis of metastatic disease requires a biopsy which may only be able to categorize the lesion into general groups (carcinoma or sarcoma). Although the specific types or primary location of the tumor may not be found, the skeletal symptoms associated with these lesions are responsive to surgical decompression or radiation therapy.

§ 4-4(J)(1). Prevalence and Etiology.

The skeleton is one of the commonest sites of distant metastases but the true incidence is not known since, even in autopsy studies, it is difficult to examine the entire vertebral column (entry 8). Metastatic lesions in the skeleton are much more common than primary bone tumors with an overall ratio of 25:1 (entries 7, 13). Tumors which have a predilection to metastasize to the cervical spine include breast, lung, prostate, kidney and melanoma (entry 9). Of patients with axial skeletal metastases, between 10% to 15% will have cervical spine involvement (entry 1). Of tumors causing skeletal metastases and cord compression, breast carcinoma is most common in women, and lung carcinoma in men (entry 15).

The propensity of bone and the axial skeleton, in particular, to be the site of metastases may be explained in part by the presence of Batson's plexus around the vertebral column and bone marrow inside bone. Batson's plexus is a network of veins located in the epidural space between the bony spinal column and the dura mater covering the spinal cord, and it is connected to the major veins which return blood to the heart, the inferior and superior vena cava. This plexus of veins is unique in that there are no valves to control blood flow and any increased pressure in the vena caval system results in increased flow into Batson's plexus. Metastatic cells from primary lesions in the head and neck and upper trunk may enter the venous and sinusoidal system of the cervical vertebrae that are connected to Batson's plexus (entry 2). The red bone marrow, located inside of vertebral bodies, have a rich sinusoidal system. Sinusoidal vessels are usually under low hemodynamic pressure, allowing for pooling of blood. This stagnant flow may encourage tumor growth.

§ 4-4(J)(2). Clinical Findings.

Pain is the most frequent and, usually, initial manifestation of skeletal metastasis. Pain may either be local over the bone affected or radicular if nerve compression has occurred. Pain is insidious in onset. However, it frequently becomes more intense and persistent. The pain is not relieved with rest, is exacerbated with recumbency, and is increased with motion, cough or Valsalva maneuver. Radicular symptoms, pain running down the shoulders into the arms, occur in a majority of patients with cervical spine metastases. The radicular symptoms may be unilateral or bilateral (entry 9). Occasionally, compressive lesions in the cervical spine cause radicular symptoms in the lower extremities (entry 12). Neurologic symptoms which are secondary to spinal cord or nerve root compression by tumor or pathologically fractured bone or by compression of vascular supply to neural structures include muscle weakness, sensory loss or autonomic dysfunction.

§ 4-4(J)(3). Physical Findings.

Physical examination demonstrates pain on palpation over the affected bone. Passive movement of the neck may cause localized pain or radicular symptoms. Tilting of the neck, torticollis, may also occur. Neurologic abnormalities will most commonly be detected in the upper extremities after a careful neurologic examination.

§ 4-4(J)(4). Laboratory Findings.

Early in the course of the lesion, laboratory parameters may be unremarkable. However, subsequent evaluation may demonstrate a myelophthisic anemia, elevated erythrocyte sedimentation rate, and abnormal chemistries including elevated alkaline phosphatase, hypercalcemia and hypophosphatemia. Therefore, initial negative laboratory data should not dissuade a physician from pursuing further diagnostic evaluation in an older patient with severe neck pain.

In patients without a known primary tumor, bone biopsy of the involved vertebra may be required to prove the presence of tumor. Occasionally, biopsy materials suggest the primary location of the neoplasms. More commonly, the histologic features, squamous cells or mucin cells, may be associated with primary lesions in various organs. Some biopsy lesions are so undifferentiated that the pathologic findings offer no clue to the possible source of the tumor. (entry 13).

§ 4-4(J)(5). Radiographic Findings.

Radiographic abnormalities associated with axial skeletal metastases include loss of bone (osteolytic), extra bone (osteoblastic), or a mixture (mixed lytic and blastic). The vertebral body is most frequently affected. This results in a lesion which causes a collapse of an entire body while preserving the intervertebral discs which are more resistent to invasion than bone (entry 7). Rarely, compression by surrounding vertebrae or because of invasive tumor, disc integrity may be lost (entry 10).

Early in the course of a metastatic lesion, plain roentgenographic examination will be unremarkable since between 30% and 50% of bone must be destroyed before a lesion is evident on plain radiographs (entry 5). However, bone scan makes it possible to detect areas of increased osseous activity in 85% of patients with metastases even if they are asymptomatic in that anatomic location (entry 6). Computed tomography may also be useful in detecting changes in vertebral bone which are difficult to identify on plain radiographs (entry 16).

Myelography is the definitive diagnostic procedure for any patient with a metastatic lesion and spinal cord or nerve root compression. Cervical spine injection into the cisterna magna may be necessary to locate potential areas of involvement. Myelography may also identify the location of the lesion to the extradural or intradural space (entry 9).

§ 4-4(J)(6). Differential Diagnosis.

A high index of suspicion for the presence of metastasis is important in the evaluation of the patient with a prior history of malignancy, however remote, or the adult over 50 years of age with increasing neck pain unassociated with trauma. Spinal lesions which occur in the presence of a known primary tumor are diagnosed as a metastatic lesion usually without the need for a biopsy. Patients with no known primary tumor do require a biopsy for tissue diagnosis. Closed needle biopsy can safely yield useful information in a majority of patients (entry 4). Other conditions which must be included in the differential diagnosis of destructive lesions of the spine include primary tumors of bone, infection, Paget's disease, metabolic and endocrinologic disorders, including osteoporosis (entry 14).

§ 4-4(J)(7). Treatment.

Treatment of metastatic disease of the spine is directed toward palliation of pain and reduction of neural compression. A cure is rarely possible since most solitary metastatic lesions are accompanied by a number of silent deposits which only become evident over time. If there is instability in the cervical spine due to marked vertebral destruction, patients should be initially treated with temporary stabilization. Radiotherapy may be used alone as primary treatment to decrease pain and slow growth or as adjunctive therapy after surgical decompression for those patients with neural compression (entries 3, 11). Corticosteroids may help reduce edema and alleviate symptoms in patients with neural compression. Decompressive laminectomy, if helpful, works best when completed in patients who have recently developed neurological symptoms (entry 1).

§ 4-4(J)(8). Course and Outcome.

The course of each patient with skeletal metastasis is dependent on a number of factors: the type of tumor, extent of involvement, sensitivity to therapy, and degree of neurologic symptoms but, in general, the prognosis is poor.

BIBLIOGRAPHY

1. Bansal, S., Brady, L.W., Olsen, A., Faust, D.S., Osterholm, J., Kazem, I. The treatment of metastatic spinal cord tumors. JAMA, 202:686-688, 1967.
2. Batson, O.V. The function of the vertebral veins and their role in the spread of metastasis. Ann Surg, 112:138-140, 1940.
3. Bruckman, J.E., and Bloomer, W.D. Management of spinal cord compression. Semin Oncol, 5:135-140, 1978.
4. Craig, F.S. Vertebral body biopsy. J Bone Joint Surg, 38A:93-102, 1956.
5. Edelstyn, G.A., Gillespie, P.G., and Grebbel, F.S. The radiological demonstration of skeletal metastases: experimental observations. Clin Radiol, 18:158-162, 1967.
6. Fager, C.A. Management of malignant intraspinal disease. Surg Clin North Am, 47:743-750, 1967.
7. Francis, K.C., and Hutter, R.V.P. Neoplasms of the spine in the aged. Clin Orthop, 26:54-66, 1963.
8. Galasko, C.S.B. The anatomy and pathways of skeletal metastases in bone metastasis, Weiss, L., Gilbert, H.A. eds, G.K. Hall Medical Publishers, Boston 1981, pp 49-63.
9. Gilbert, R.W., Kim, J.H., Posner, J.B. Epidural spinal cord compression from metastatic tumor: diagnosis and treatment. Ann Neurol, 3:40-51, 1978.
10. Hubbard, D.D. and Gunn, D.R. Secondary carcinoma of the spine with destruction of the intervertebral disc. Clin Orthop, 88:86-88, 1972.
11. Khan, F.R., Glicksman, A.S., Chu, F.C.H., and Nickson, J.J. Treatment by radiotherapy by spinal cord compression due to extradural metastases. Radiology, 89:495-500, 1967.

12. Langfitt, T.W. and Elliott, F.A. Pain in the back and legs caused by cervical spinal cord compression. JAMA, 200:112-115, 1967.
13. Mirra, J.M. *Bone Tumors: Diagnosis and Treatment.* Philadelphia, J.B. Lippincott Co., 1980, pp 448-454.
14. Nicholas, J.A., Wilson, P.D., and Freiberger, R. Pathological fractures of the spine: etiology and diagnosis. J Bone Joint Surg, 42A:127-137, 1960.
15. Rodriguez, M., and Dinapoli, R.P. Spinal cord compression: with special reference to metastatic epidural tumors. Mayo Clin Proc, 55:442-448, 1980.
16. Wilson, J.S., Korobkin, M., Genant, H.K., and Bovill, E.G. Computed tomography of musculoskeletal disorders. Am J Roentgenol, 131:55-61, 1978.

§ 4-4(K). Intraspinal Neoplasm.

The neural and supporting structures are also at risk of primary and secondary neoplasms as are the bones of the spinal column. These intraspinal neoplasms may be extradural, between bone and the covering of the spinal cord, the dura; intradural-extramedullary, between the dura and the spinal cord; and intramedullary, in the spinal cord proper. Extradural tumors are predominantly metastatic in origin. Intradural-extramedullary tumors are meningiomas, neurofibromas or lipomas. Intramedullary tumors are ependymomas or gliomas. Most severe symptoms tend to be associated with the extradural and intramedullary lesions. More slowly progressive symptoms of sensory loss and motor weakness tend to be associated with intradural-extramedullary tumors. The diagnosis of intraspinal tumors requires histologic examination of the lesion although appropriate evaluation of spinal fluid and myelographic studies may help differentiate patients with neoplastic processes from those with benign ones. Therapy of intraspinal lesions involves the removal of the tumor if possible or the control of its growth with radiotherapy or corticosteroids. Intradural-extramedullary tumors are usually benign and have a good prognosis. Extradural and intramedullary lesions are locally invasive, resistant to therapy and are associated with a poorer prognosis.

§ 4-4(K)(1). Prevalence and Etiology.

Intraspinal neoplasms occur in adults most commonly between the ages of 30 and 50. The extradural space is the predominant site for intraspinal malignant tumors. Metastatic tumors in the spinal canal are extradural in location because the dura is resistant to invasion from lesions which extend from foci in vertebral bone. The extradural space is also the location for Batson's plexus, a valveless venous network which surrounds the spinal cord (entry 1). Meningiomas and neurofribromas are the tumors found in the intradural-extramedullary space since this is the location for the meninges and spinal nerve root which contain the cells which are the origin of these neoplasms. Ependymal and glial cells make up the support structure of the spinal cord and are the primary sources of intramedullary tumors. Metastatic lesions to the spinal cord proper are extremely rare (entry 5).

§ 4-4(K)(2). Clinical Features.

Intraspinal tumors may demonstrate a wide variety of clinical symptoms. Pain is the initial and continuing symptom of extradural metastatic disease. The pain is increased at night and may be exacerbated with activity. Neurologic symptoms including neck weakness, sensory changes and autonomic dysfunction may occur with nerve compression in the cervical areas.

Intradural-extramedullary tumors grow in proximity to nerve roots and are associated with pain down the arms or in the axial skeleton. The slow evaluation of symptoms correspond with the slow growth characteristics of menin-

§ 4-4(K) NECK PAIN

giomas and neurofibromas. Neurologic symptoms also develop more slowly than with metastatic disease. However, neurofibromatosis may be associated with significant complications such as paraplegia or angular deformity of the spine (entries 4, 15).

Intramedullary tumors are painless since there are no sensory nerve endings in the spinal cord. The manifestations of the growth of these tumors is progressive neurologic dysfunction in the form of paresthesias and muscle weakness.

§ 4-4(K)(3). Physical Findings.

Examination of patients with extradural tumors may elicit pain on palpation over the affected vertebra. Neurologic findings in the shoulders and arms correlate with the level and extent of compression on the spinal roots and cord. Patients with intradural-extramedullary tumors demonstrate slowing changing neurologic abnormalities with spinal deformity (entry 14). Patients with intramedullary tumors may have specific sensory changes which correlate with the location of these tumors in the center of the cord. Light touch and position sensation are lost. Hyperreflexia is a result of pressure on the pyramidal tracts. This finding helps differentiate patients with intramedullary tumors from those with herniated disc where hyperreflexia is an unusual finding (entry 10).

§ 4-4(K)(4). Laboratory Findings.

Abnormal laboratory values are most closely associated with extradural metastatic lesions. Refer to the section on skeletal metastases for specific laboratory and histologic findings associated with these lesions.

Intradural tumors do not cause hematologic or chemical abnormalities since they do not metastasize outside of the spinal canal. Evaluation of cerebrospinal fluid obtained by a puncture of the dura may demonstrate marked elevation in spinal fluid protein with intradural tumors.

Histologic findings depend on the cell of origin of the tumor. Characteristic patterns of cells help differentiate metastatic malignant tumors from those of meningiomas, neurofibromas, ependymomas, and gliomas.

§ 4-4(K)(5). Radiographic Findings.

Radiographic abnormalities of extradural tumors are characterized by rapid destruction of bone in proximity to the growing lesion. Intradural lesions are associated with posterior scalloping of the vertebral bodies, a consequence of their location and slow growth (entry 11). Uniform dilitation of a neural foramina is most closely associated with a slow growing neurofibroma which is advancing through that structure.

Myelographic studies are most useful in determining the exact location of an intraspinal tumor (entry 12). Extradural tumors cause a complete block of the column of dye at the site of compression. The spinal contents are displaced and there are irregular edges to the dye column. Intradural-extramedullary lesions produce a sharp, smooth outline since the tumor is in direct contact with the dye. Intramedullary tumors arise in the spinal cord. The myelogram demonstrates fusiform enlargement of the spinal cord with tapering of the column of dye superiorly and inferiorly. Not all fusiform swellings of the cord are secondary to intramedullary tumors. Extradural tumors may flatten the contralateral aspect of the cord. Therefore, films must be taken at 90-degree angles so that intramedullary lesions are not confused with extradural lesions.

§ 4-4(K)(6). Differential Diagnosis.

The definitive diagnosis of intraspinal neoplasms is confirmed by the histologic examination of biopsy material. A high level of suspicion is necessary to make the diagnosis since the initial neurologic symptoms may be overlooked.

Syringomyelia is frequently found in the cervical spinal cord and is an important lesion to differentiate from intraspinal neoplasms (entry 9). Syringomyelia is a fluid-filled cyst lined with benign glial cells which is located in the center of the spinal cord. The cyst grows longitudinally and laterally, first causing loss of pain sensation, then motor weakness in the extremities, spinal curvature, long tract signs (Babinski reflex) and autonomic dysfunction of the bladder and rectum. Diagnosis is made by recognition of characteristic findings discovered on myelogram or computed axial tomography (entry 6). The treatment of syringomyelia is surgical removal of the fluid in the cystic cavity by needle aspiration or myelotomy. Lesions that are allowed to progress, cause increasing disability marked by spasticity, motor weakness, arthropathy, and infections.

§ 4-4(K)(7). Treatment.

Therapy of neoplastic lesions include radiation therapy, corticosteroids or decompressive laminectomy (entries 2, 8). Intradural-extramedullary lesions are usually accessible and are removed by surgical excision. Accessible intramedullary tumors should also be removed with the knowledge that some residual neurologic deficit may result (entry 7).

§ 4-4(K)(8). Course and Outcome.

In general, extradural and intramedullary tumors are malignant while intradural-extramedullary tumors are benign. The course and prognosis of these tumors correspond to their invasiveness, rapidity of growth, and location. Malignant tumors have a poor prognosis while benign tumors which are accessible to surgical removal have an excellent prognosis.

BIBLIOGRAPHY

1. Batson, O.V. The function of vertebral veins and their role in the spread of metastases. Ann Surg, 112:138-149, 1940.
2. Bruckman, J.E., and Bloomer, W.D. Management of spinal cord compression. Semin Oncol, 5:135-140, 1978.
3. Clark, P.R.R., and Saunders, M. Steroid-induced remission in spinal canal reticulum cell sarcoma: report of two cases. J Neurosurg, 42:346-348, 1975.
4. Curtis, B.H., Fisher, R.L., Butterfield, W.L., and Saunders, F.P. Neurofibromatosis with paraplegia: report of eight cases. J Bone Joint Surg, 51A:843-861, 1969.
5. Edelson, R.N., Deck, M.D.F. and Posner, J.B. Intramedullary spinal cord metastases: clinical and radiographic findings in nine cases. Neurology, 22:1222-1231, 1972.
6. Gonsalves, C.G., Hudson, A.R., Horsey, W.J., and Tucker, W.S. Computed tomography of the cervical spine and spinal cord. Comput Tomogr, 2:279-293, 1978.
7. Greenwood, J. Surgical removal of intramedullary tumors. J Neurosurg, 26:275-282, 1967.
8. Khan, F.R., Glicksman, A.S., Chu, F.C.H., and Nickson, J.J. Treatment by radiotherapy of spinal cord compression due to extradural metastases. Radiology, 89:495-500, 1967.
9. McIlroy, W.J., and Richardson, J.C. Syringomyelia: a clinical review of 75 cases. Can Med Assoc J, 93:731-734, 1965.
10. McKraig, W., Svien, H.J., Dodge, H.W., Jr., and Camp, J.D. Intraspinal lesions masquerading as protruded lumbar intervertebral discs. JAMA, 149:250-253, 1952.
11. Mitchell, G.E., Lourie, H., and Berne, A.S. The various causes of scalloped vertebrae with notes on their pathogenesis. Radiology, 89:67-74, 1967.
12. Resnick, D. and Niwayama, G. *Diagnosis of Bone and Joint Disorders*. Philadelphia, W.B. Saunders Co., 1981, pp 432-445.
13. Wetzel, N., and Davis, Surgical treatment of syringomyelia. Arch Surg, 68:579-573, 1954.

14. Winter, R.B., Moe, J.H., Bradford, D.S., Lonstein, J.E., Pedras, C.V., and Weber, A.H. Spine deformity in neurofibromatosis: a review of 102 patients. J Bond Joint Surg, 61A:677-694, 1979.
15. Yong-Hing, K., Kalamcki, A., and MacEwen, G.D. Cervical spine abnormalities in neurofibromatosis. J Bone Joint Surg, 61A:695-699, 1979.

§ 4-5. Endocrinologic and Metabolic Disorders of the Cervical Spine.

Endocrinologic and metabolic disorders are systemic illnesses which affect components of the musculoskeletal system throughout the body. These illnesses include osteoporosis, osteomalacia, parathyroid disease, ochronosis, acromegaly, and microcrystalline disorders. In comparison to the frequency of patients with these illnesses presenting to a physician with an initial or primary complaint of low back pain, patients present rarely with neck pain. Neck pain usually occurs in the setting of generalized musculoskeletal pain affecting many components of the osseous system. Bone pain may be caused by compression fractures of vertebral bodies secondary to inadequate bone stock, extensive degenerative disease of the spine or accumulation of crystals, amino acids or mucopolysaccharides in bone.

The musculoskeletal symptoms of endocrinologic and metabolic diseases may be insidious in onset or acute when associated with vertebral body compression fractures. Frequently, symptoms in other organ systems will occur simultaneously including renal stones, muscle weakness, gastrointestinal malabsorption or change in facial configuration. Physical examination confirms the systemic quality of these illnesses with abnormal findings throughout the musculoskeletal system.

Laboratory evaluation helps confirm a number of endocrinologic and metabolic disorders. Abnormalities of calcium and phosphorous may raise the suspicion of osteomalacia or hyperparathyroidism. Bone biopsy confirms the diagnosis of osteoporosis or osteomalacia. Measurement of parathormone confirms the diagnosis of hyper or hypoparathyroidism. Non-suppressibility of growth hormone during a glucose tolerance test is characteristic of acromegaly. Detection of homogentesic acid in urine is diagnostic of ochronosis. Detection of urate or calcium pyrophosphate dihydrate crystals is essential for the diagnosis of gout or pseudogout, respectively. Radiologic evaluation is not diagnostic but documents the global involvement of the osseous system with these illnesses.

Therapy for these diseases are individualized for each illness. Calcium and vitamin D supplements improve bone metabolism in osteoporosis and osteomalacia. Ablation of the pituitary or parathyroid tumor is the therapy of choice for acromegaly and hyperparathyroidism. Acute attacks of microcrystalline arthritis respond to nonsteroidal anti-inflammatory drugs.

Disability from neck pain is a minor problem compared to the generalized difficulties which occur in the musculoskeletal system. Osteoporosis and osteomalacia, when progressive, are associated with multiple fractures, deformity, and incapacitating bone pain. Patients with acromegaly or ochronosis may develop progressive degenerative disease both in the axial and appendicular skeleton. With most of the endocrinologic and metabolic disorders, it is the extent of involvement in areas other than the neck which determine the limitations on work potential.

For additional information in regard to endocrinologic and metabolic disorders, you are referred to §§ 4-39, 4-40, 4-41, 4-42, 4-43, and 4-44 in *Industrial Low Back Pain* in the Contemporary Litigation Series.

§ 4-6. Hematologic Disorders of the Cervical Spine.

Disorders of the hematopoietic system may affect any portion of the body where bone marrow is located. Since the axial skeleton contains a significant proportion of an adult's bone marrow, disorders which cause hyperplasia of bone marrow or the replacement of normal bone marrow cells with abnormal ones may be associated with pain in the axial skeleton. A characteristic of hematopoietic disorders is that although symptoms are localized to various areas of the skeleton, these illnesses are systemic in origin and cause significant abnormalities in a number of organ systems. Neck pain as an initial or sole manifestation of a hematologic disorder is extremely rare. More usual is the situation where a patient with a hemoglobinopathy or myelofibrosis develops neck pain in the face of generalized skeletal pain including the back and extremities.

The symptom of skeletal pain in a patient with a hemoglobinopathy (sickle cell anemia) occurs during a vaso-occlusive crisis. Sickled red blood cells block small blood vessels which results in infarction of tissue. Patients with myelofibrosis have insidious onset of pain which is the result of the replacement of normal marrow constituents with fibrous tissue.

Physical examination of an adult with a hemoglobinopathy will demonstrate a chronically ill individual with severe pain during a crisis. Abnormal findings may include fever, tachycardia, tenderness to palpation over the axial skeleton and extremities associated with reflex muscle spasm. The patient with myelofibrosis will have pallor, splenomegaly and bone tenderness on palpation.

Laboratory evaluation allows for the specific diagnosis of hemoglobinopathy and myelofibrosis. Hemoglobinopathy is suggested by abnormalities of red blood cells (sickled cells) on a blood smear, and the specific abnormality of hemoglobin is identified by hemoglobin electrophoresis. The blood smear in myelofibrosis contains abnormalities in all components of the blood including abnormal red cell forms, immature white cells, and variable numbers and sizes of platelets. The diagnosis of myelofibrosis is confirmed by the presence of fibrous tissue in the bone marrow and increased osseous tissue (osteosclerosis) in the bone. Radiographic findings associated with hemoglobinopathies include evidence of marrow expansion secondary to hyperplasia which is characterized by loss of trabeculae and cortical thinning, depression in endplates of vertebral bodies, sclerosis and fractures associated with aseptic necrosis of bone. Radiographic findings of myelofibrosis include diffuse osteosclerosis in the axial skeleton and proximal long bones.

Therapy for these hematopoietic disorders are directed towards relief of symptoms. Patients are educated to avoid circumstances which precipitate vaso-occlusive crises. Hydration and analgesic therapy are mainstays of crisis management. Transfusions are reserved for life-threatening complications such as cerebrovascular accidents. Treatment for myelofibrosis is also symptomatic since there is no available therapy which alters the course of the illness.

The disability associated with neck disease caused by hemoglobinopathies and myelofibrosis is minor compared to the severe effects of these illnesses on other organs including the cardiovascular, pulmonary, renal, and musculoskeletal systems. Patients with sickle cell anemia with frequent crises have limited ability to work. Patients with frequent crises may also be at risk for more extensive disease in vital organ systems which may result in premature death. Patients with myelofibrosis also have limited work capability due to symptoms associated with chronic anemia, splenomegaly, and bone pain. Most patients die from the illness within five years of the diagnosis.

For additional information in regard to hemoglobinopathies and myelofibrosis, you are referred to §§ 4-46 and

4-47 in *Industrial Low Back Pain* in the Contemporary Litigation Series.

CHAPTER 5

CERVICAL HYPEREXTENSION INJURIES

Arthur I. Kobrine, M.D., Ph.D.
Michael W. Nabors, M.D.

§ 5-1. Introduction.
§ 5-2. Pathophysiology.
§ 5-3. Symptoms.
§ 5-4. Management.
§ 5-5. Treatment.
§ 5-6. Return to Work.
Bibliography.
Figure 1. Mechanism of Whiplash.
Figure 2. Soft Tissue Injury in Whiplash.

§ 5-1. Introduction.

With increased technology born out of the necessity of World War II, airplanes were often catapulted from carrier take-off decks. Many pilots developed neck injuries during these catapult assisted take-offs, characterized by neck pain, neck stiffness, hoarseness, etc. It soon became apparent that the acute forward acceleration during take-off resulted in a hyperextension of the cervical spine. These symptoms disappeared after the pilots' seats were altered so that head rests prevented the hyperextension.

Following World War II, a booming economy in the United States resulted in a marked increase in the number of automobiles on the highways. With the increase in the number of vehicles came an increase in the number of automobile collisions. Within 10 years after the end of World War II, the rear end automobile collision accounted for 20-25% of all automobile accidents (entry 7).

The rear end collision caused an acceleration hyperextension cervical injury to the driver of the struck car not unlike, in many ways, the airplane pilot who was catapulted off his aircraft carrier. One main difference, however, was the economic ramifications. The airplane pilot was at war serving his country. The automobile driver soon was beseiged by attorneys explaining that the injured driver was, by law, blameless and had a right to litigate. Plaintiff's attorneys considered the rear-end auto collision their "bread and butter" case, since blame was almost always ascribed to the driver of the striking vehicle. In 1928, at a meeting of the Western Orthopaedic Association in San Francisco, California, Dr. H.E. Crowe characterized the acceleration hyperextension cervical injury sustained from a rear-end automobile collision as a "whiplash" injury (entry 1). This rather pernicious label, to the delight of attorneys, allowed the injured party to emotionally as well as physically suffer. In the words of Ian McNab, "Many patients became more disabled by the diagnosis than by the injury" (entry 6).

§ 5-2. Pathophysiology.

Just as a catapult assisted take-off of an airplane acutely accelerates the pilot, the driver of a stationary car that is struck from behind by another vehicle is, likewise, accelerated forward. The driver is usually relaxed and unaware of the impending collision, often stopped at a stop light or stop sign. The sudden acceleration of the struck vehicle pushes the back of the car seat against the driver's torso. This pushes the driver's torso forward and his head is thrown backward, causing hyperextension of his neck (Figure 1). This occurs very quickly, within the first quarter second after impact. If no head rest is present, the driver's head is hyperextended past the limit of stretch of the soft tissues of the neck. The sternocleidomastoid muscle, the scalenes, and the longus coli muscles may be mildly or severely stretched, or at worst torn (Figure 2). Muscle tears of the longus coli muscles might involve injury to the sympathetic trunk unilaterally or bilaterally, resulting in a Horner's syndrome, nausea, or dizziness. Further hyperextension may injure the esophagus, resulting in temporary dysphagia and the larynx, causing hoarseness. Tears in the anterior longitudinal ligament may cause hematoma formation with resultant cervical radiculitis (arm pain) and injury to the intervertebral disc (entry 5). As the driver's head is thrown backwards, the mouth opens since jaw movement lags behind skull movement. This may result in injury to the temporomandibular joint, causing pain on chewing and limited mouth opening. In the recoil forward flexion that occurs when the car stops accelerating, the head is thrown forward. This forward flexion of the head is usually limited by the chin striking the chest and does not usually cause significant injury. However, if the head is thrown forward and strikes the steering wheel or the windshield, a head injury can occur.

In elderly people with pre-existing cervical spondylosis, the sagittal diameter of the spinal canal is compromised at each disc level and a severe hyperextension injury can result in spinal cord compression resulting in paralysis or the central spinal cord syndrome (entry 10).

Clearly from the above discussion, it becomes apparent that the degree of injury depends on the force applied and inertia, rather than the speed of the striking vehicle. The faster the struck vehicle is accelerated forward, the more rapid the hyperextension of the neck and the greater the injury. Therefore, a car struck by a large truck or loaded bus traveling 5-7 mph will be accelerated forward as much as if struck by a small car traveling at a much greater velocity (entry 11). Also, how rapidly the struck car is accelerated forward will depend on road and traffic conditions. If the struck car is essentially bumper to bumper with the car in front, and cannot be catapulted forward, then a strike from the rear might result in significant damage to the struck car, from both forward and back collisions, but the struck car might not be accelerated forward making the resulting injury to the driver slight. In this case the damage to the car might be severe. If, however, the struck car were on an icy street with no cars in front, a rear end collision would accelerate the struck car at a high rate causing very little demonstrable damage to the car but a severe hyperextension cervical injury to the driver.

§ 5-3. Symptoms.

Usually, the driver is often unaware that he has been injured. He suffers little discomfort at the scene of the accident and often does not even wish to go to the hospital. Later that evening or the next day, 12 to 14 hours after the accident, the patient begins to feel stiffness in his neck. Pain at the base of the neck increases and is made worse by head and neck movements. Soon any movement of the head or neck causes excruciating pain. The anterior cervical muscles are often tender to the touch, the patient may have pain on mouth opening or chewing, hoarseness or difficulty swallowing, and now seeks medical care. Often the patient has already contacted an attorney by the time he arrives in the hospital emergency room. Radiating pain may include pain from the neck into one or both shoulders or arms, and up into the base of the skull. Pain can also radiate into the interscapular region and chest, as well as into the vertex of the skull. It should be emphasized that the pain pattern has no localizing value whatsoever as to the site of the lesion.

Patients receiving a whiplash injury of the neck can also suffer from a concussion. Mechanical deformation of the brain occurs during the acceleration-deceleration phase of the injury and concussion can occur without the head actually striking anything. This can account for transient loss of consciousness, as well as post concussion symptoms of headache, photophobia, mild transient confusion, tinnitus, fatigue, and transient difficulty with concentration.

§ 5-4. Management.

A detailed history and physical examination is required of every patient having sustained such an injury. Specific details of the accident, type of vehicles, number of vehicles involved, road conditions, and traffic conditions are important. If the driver wore a seat belt, then the possibility of a seat belt fracture (chance fracture of the lumbar spine) must be considered. A blood alcohol level and a blood drug screen should be performed.

The physical examination must be detailed and complete. Abrasions on the forehead would suggest that forward flexion of the head struck the steering wheel or windshield. A dilated pupil might suggest a Horner's Syndrome secondary to injury of the sympathetic chain along the logus coli muscles or it might be a sign of significant intracranial injury if the patient's level of consciousness is altered. Point tenderness in front of the ear would suggest injury to the temporomandibular joint and tenderness to touch in the suboccipital area would suggest the head struck the back of the seat.

A complete neurological examination is crucial. Any evidence of objective neurologic deficit merits immediate diagnostic tests to determine the cause. Although by definition, hyperextension cervical injury causes damage only to the soft tissue structures of the neck, plain radiographs of the cervical spine should be obtained in all cases. Unsuspected fracture — dislocations of the lower cervical spine, facet fractures, odontoid fractures, or spinous process fractures — might be otherwise missed in the neurologically intact patient. Cervical spondylosis will be demonstrated on plain radiographs as well. Of course, if objective neurologic deficit is present, then further diagnostic aids are necessary, e.g., head CT, spine CT, myelogram, MRI, etc.

§ 5-5. Treatment.

Generally, the patient's symptoms begin after 12-24 hours and this is generally when medical care is begun. Although plain radiographs may demonstrate some straightening of the cervical spine, in the large majority of cases with no neurologic deficit, the cervical spine x-rays are normal. A reasonable medical routine for treatment is based on the premise of resting the involved injured soft tissues. A soft cervical collar helps significantly in relieving muscle spasm and preventing quick head turns. The collar should not be worn for more than 2 to 4 weeks, lest the recovering muscles start weakening from nonuse, and the ground work for a psychoneurosis is laid. Heat is helpful and should be applied by both a heating pad, hot showers, or hot tub soaks. If neck pain is severe, 3-5 days bed rest may be necessary. Mild analgesics, non steroid anti-inflammatory drugs, and muscle relaxants are all helpful and are generally indicated. Narcotic analgesics should be avoided. Activity should be restricted as determined by the severity of the symptoms. Generally, driving should be avoided for the first two weeks. After approximately two weeks of this regimen, significant improvement should be noted. If not, two more weeks of continued conservative care with the addition of home cervical traction should be employed. Generally, cervical traction for 20-30 minutes per day at 7-10 pounds will help alleviate the symptoms. If symptoms persist at 4 weeks post injury, some further testing is necessary before emotional overlay is considered the cause. If headaches persist, a cranial CT scan should be done. If normal at 4 weeks, the patient can be assured that no intracranial abnormality is present. If arm or shoulder pain persist, then a spine CT scan and electromyography can be performed. If these tests are normal, the patient can be assured that no compression of neural structures is present.

If symptoms persist 6 weeks or longer, especially if litigation is pending (often the patient's attorney will accompany the patient to the physician's office), then secondary gain and a compensation neurosis should be suspected. Although symptoms from a severe hyperextension cervical injury can last up to one year, the symptoms should be clearly resolving by 6 weeks and not be incapacitating after that. Physicians should do their best to treat the patient's symptoms without adding to their potential neurosis. There is no indication for cervical braces in the treatment of "whiplash." In patients with a normal neurological exam and normal radiographs of the spine, cervical immobilization should not exceed 2 weeks. To prolong this form of treatment is not good for the patient and feeds any potential emotion of long term disability (entry 3).

In the first paper in the literature concerning "whiplash" injuries of the cervical spine, Gay and Abbott described fifty persons who suffered a whiplash injury of the neck between the years 1948 and 1952 (entry 2). By far, the predominant cause was rear-end automobile collisions. Their patients suffered from the same symptoms described in the present report. According to Gay and Abbott, the most distressing long-term complication was the development of a persistent psychoneurotic reaction, which occurred in 26 cases (52%). It was their opinion that the circumstances inherent in the type of injury made all persons prone to the development of a disturbing emotional reaction. They found that patients who were managed a few hours or days after their injury improved more rapidly and more fully than those patients first seen one to 24 months after their injury. They explained this difference as due to the personal attention, discussion, and reassurance given to the patient. The object of such attention was, according to them, designed to prevent the development of a severe, intractable psychoneurosis that would impede or prevent recovery.

There does appear to be an increased likelihood of patients developing an emotional overlay from cervical soft tissue injuries than from other injuries sustained in the same accident. Often patients with fractured long bones, which require casting from 6-8 weeks will complain much more of their neck pain than any discomfort associated with the fracture. Whether this occurs because the patient infers from his attorney that "whiplash" is worse than a broken bone, or whether the complicated anatomical structure of the cervical regions, i.e., muscles, ligaments, joints, makes injuries to this region less likely to resolve, is difficult to answer. Certainly, all physicians treating patients suffering from hyperextension cervical injuries have seen their symptoms disappear concomitant with legal settlement of the case in their favor. The physician therefore must appropriately treat the patient's symptoms after a history, physical examination, and cadre of diagnostic test do not suggest a diagnosis other than "whiplash." However, he must not overtreat the patient and by so doing encourage the patient to retire from life into a syndrome of chronic incapacitating neck pain.

In a series of 179 patients with soft tissue injuries of the cervical region, Greenfield and Ilfeld found the average length of treatment was 7 weeks, at which time 37% of the patients were asymptomatic (entry 4).

Several studies suggested that whiplash-type injuries accelerated bony changes in the cervical spine which are normally seen as part of the aging process. However, it was pointed out that the appearance of degenerative radiographic changes had no statistical correlation with the presence or absence of symptoms (entries 8, 9).

§ 5-6. Return to Work.

The timing of returning the patient to the work force is, of course, dependent somewhat on the severity of the symptoms and the type of work the patient does. For non-manual labor type of employment, 2 weeks of treatment should yield enough improvement for the patient to return to work. Often busy professional people will return to work after one week. For patients employed in a heavy manual labor position, 3-4 weeks of treatment is often necessary. Generally speaking, all patients should be able to return to employment by 6 weeks and should be encouraged to do so, even if mild symptoms are present. Limitations of work generally include no significant periods of stooping, bending, lifting, or carrying of objects over 50 pounds. These restrictions are often used for the first 1-3 weeks of return to work. Depending on the severity of injury, patients should generally recover totally with no permanent disability. On occasion, a 5-10% permanent partial disability is appropriate.

It is often difficult to assess permanent partial disability in these cases. A very small percentage of patients will have a persistent abnormal finding on physical exam such as palpable muscle spasm. However, the majority of patients who remain symptomatic, which is only about 10-25% of patients having received the injury, will have continued subjective complaints with no objective findings. Many of these patients are employed in a manual labor setting and will state that they are fine as long as they are relatively inactive, but become symptomatic when they are doing heavy labor. In such cases, whether the physician assesses a 5-10% permanent partial disability or not depends on the credibility of the patient. Since objective signs are not present, the physician can only rely on his intuitive feelings regarding the patient's honesty. If the physician feels the patient is truthful, and is symptomatic during hard manual labor, then a 5-10% permanent partial disability is justified. In cases where the physician is not impressed with the patient's credibility, and objective signs are lacking, no permanent partial disability should be assessed.

BIBLIOGRAPHY

1. Crowe, N.E. Injuries to the cervical spine. Paper presented at the meeting of the Western Orthopaedic Association, San Francisco, 1928.
2. Gay, J.R., Abbott, K.H. Common whiplash injuries of the neck. JAMA, 152:1698-1704, 1953.
3. Gotten, N. Survey of one hundred cases of whiplash injury after settlement of litigation. JAMA, 162:865-869, 1956.
4. Greenfield, J., Ilfeld, F.W. Acute cervical strain: evaluation and short term prognostic factors. Clin Orthop, 122:196, 1977.
5. Hohl, M. Soft-tissue injuries of the neck in automobile accidents: factors influencing prognosis. J Bone Joint Surg, 56A:1675-1681, 1974.
6. McNab, I. Acceleration injuries of the cervical spine. J Bone Joint Surg, 46A:1797-1799, 1964.
7. McNab, I. Acceleration-extension injuries of the cervical spine in *The Spine.* Rothman, R.H., Simeone, F.A., (eds). Philadelphia, W.B. Saunders Co., 1982.
8. Rechtman, A.M., Borden, A.G., Gershon-Cohen, J. The lordotic curve of the cervical spine. Clin Orthop, 20:208, 1961.
9. Schneider, R.C., Cherry, G.L., Pantck, H.E. The syndrome of acute central cervical spinal cord injury. J Neurosurg, 11:546-551, 1954.
10. Schott, C.H., Dohan, F.C. Neck injury to women in auto accidents. JAMA, 206:2689, 1968.
11. Severy, D.M., Mathewson, J.H., Bechtol, C.D. Controlled rear end collisions: an investigation of related engineering and medical phenomena. Can Services Med J, 11:727, 1955.

Figure 1

Mechanism of Whiplash

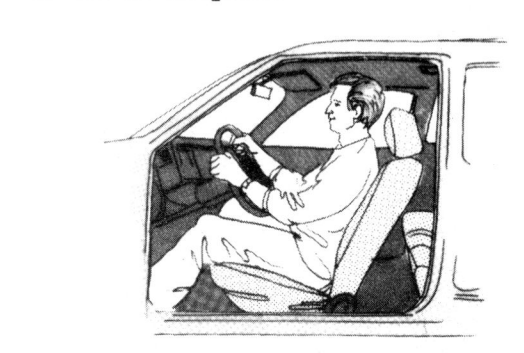

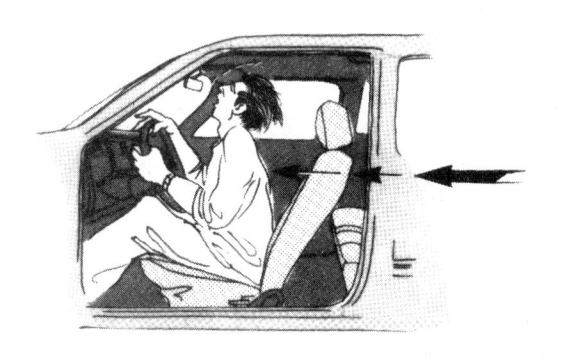

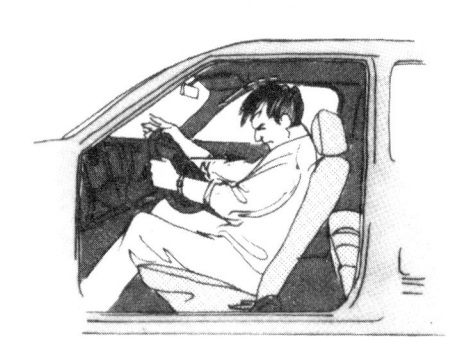

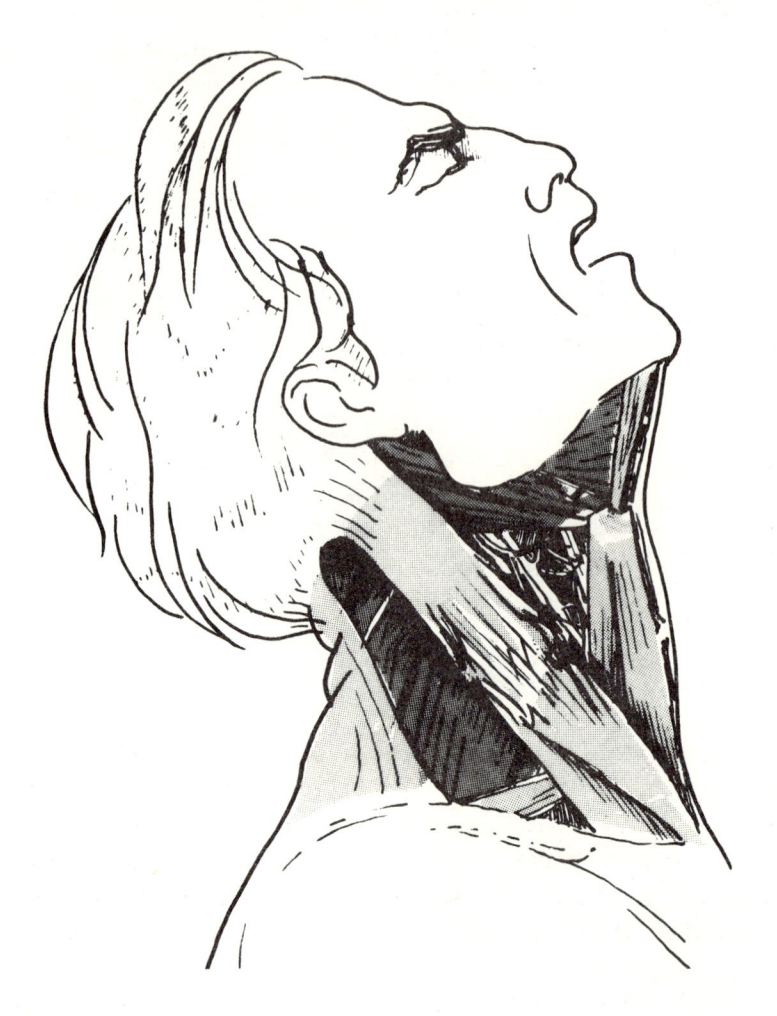

Figure 2

Soft Tissue Injury in Whiplash

CHAPTER 6

ASSESSMENT AND RELATIVE IMPORTANCE OF PHYSICAL FINDINGS AND DIAGNOSTIC PROCEDURES

Rene Cailliet, M.D.

§ 6-1. History.
§ 6-2. Physical Examination.
§ 6-3. The Occipitocervical Segment.
§ 6-4. Injury to the Upper Cervical Segment.
§ 6-5. The Lower Cervical Segment.
§ 6-6. Laboratory Tests.
§ 6-7. X-Ray.
§ 6-8. Myelography.
§ 6-9. Electromyogram (EMG).
§ 6-10. Computerized Axial Tomography.
§ 6-11. Thermography.
§ 6-12. Discography.
§ 6-13. Cervical Disc Distention Test.
§ 6-14. Magnetic Resonance Imaging (MRI).
Bibliography.

The cervical spine can be assessed in terms of the history, physical examination, and special tests which include x-rays and electrical studies. The history and physical examination are performed on every patient upon the physician's first contact. This forms the basis for an initial diagnosis and should dictate what additional tests are necessary.

The history is a detailed story as presented by the patient of what occurred and what subjective problems he/she is having. The physical examination provides objective information about the patient's problem and serves to confirm the physical damage from the injury. Other tests such as x-rays are usually done to objectively document, justify, and clarify the clinical diagnosis reached by the examining physician from the patient's history and physical examination.

The purpose of this chapter is to discuss the relative value of the history, the physical examination, and the diagnostic tests ordered as they relate to the diagnosis and ultimately to the recommended treatment. In neck injuries the evaluation and diagnostic procedures can be uniquely vague, non-precise and difficult to quantitate. It should also be appreciated that there is little understanding as to the mechanism of pain and/or disability production from cervical spine injuries.

§ 6-1. History.

What actually occurred at the time of injury is pertinent and hopefully can be reconstructed by the patient. Many of the patient's voluntary statements are relevant, causative and accurate. Other information can be obtained from questions posed by the physician.

If there has been an impact such as in a motor vehicle accident or a direct body blow in a fall, the exact mechanism of the incident should be reconstructed, particularly in respect to how the head moved during the injury, e.g., flexion, extension, side movement or rotation of the head and neck. Awareness of an impending impact and instinctive "guarding" or tensing of muscles can influence the adverse effects. A minor injury in an unaware person can be substantially more significant than a violent injury to a "prepared" person.

The preinjury mood will also influence the immediate reaction of the injured. Pre-existing anxiety or depression understandably fosters a greater and more distorted reaction, and excessive concern over material damage may influence and aggravate a patient's symptoms.

The location and type of pain the patient is experiencing is particularly important. Pain that is confined primarily to the neck implies localized injury to the ligaments, muscles or posterior joints of the spine. Pain that radiates into the arm below the elbow is usually derived from nerve root irritation. This type of pain will be described as burning in nature and it usually will be associated with some numbness and tingling.

Finally in obtaining the history, it is important to find out if there had been previous attacks, how they occurred, how they affected the patient, how they were treated and how the patient responded to the treatment. The answers to these questions will help the physician determine the severity of the injury, the integrity of the patient and the possible presence of "outside" factors affecting the case.

§ 6-2. Physical Examination.

The physical examination should begin with observation of the cervical spine and upper torso unencumbered by clothing. The physical findings are of two different types. One set can be categorized as non-specific and can be found in most patients with neck pain but will not help to localize the type or level of the pathological process. A decreased range of motion is the most frequent non-specific finding. It can be secondary to pain or, structurally, to distorted bony and soft tissue elements in the cervical spine. Hyperextension and excessive lateral rotation, however, will usually cause pain — even in a normal individual.

Tenderness is another non-specific finding which can be quite helpful and there are two types of tenderness which must be considered. One is diffuse, elicited by compression of the paravertebral muscles, and is found over a wide area of the posterolateral muscle masses. The second type of tenderness is more specific and may help localize the level of the pathology. It can be localized by palpation over each intervertebral foramin and spinous process.

Another set of physical findings, determined by the neurological examination, is quite specific in terms of helping an examiner to accurately diagnose and localize the level of the problem. The neurologic assessment is important not only as a diagnostic and localizing measure in respect to radicular compression, but also as a baseline for the evaluation of myelopathy. Chapter 2 details each of the nerve root patterns and reviews the area of pain, sensory and motor changes, and reflex deficit for each level.

The cervical spine can be separated into three major anatomic areas, each with its unique historical and physical findings (entries 2, 3).

§ 6-3. The Occipitocervical Segment.

Trauma which forcefully moves the head on the neck may initially insult the tissues of the occipitocervical segment.

At this level the head moves in a sagittal direction, that of flexion-extension through a range of approximately 30 to 35 degrees. Saying "yes" is an occipitocervical function. Excessive movement is prevented by ligaments and muscles, both of which can be stressed if flexion-extension is abrupt and excessive.

The nerves emerging from the cervical spine at this level proceed to supply sensation to the head, the base of the skull (occiput) and to the sides (parietal) as well as to the top of the head (vertex). "Headache" ensues.

The usual physical findings are:

1. Limited and possibly painful flexion-extension of the head upon the neck.

2. Tenderness to pressure at the base of the skull.

3. Subjective complaint of headache and often sensitivity over the scalp at the region of the headache.

ASSESSMENT OF PHYSICAL FINDINGS § 6-4

§ 6-4. Injury to the Upper Cervical Segment.

By virtue of the structural anatomy of the upper cervical segment, movement is as follows:

1. Rotation between C1-C2 (atlas-axis articulation) — Persons normally can rotate the head to the left by 45 degrees, to the right 45 degrees with a total, such as in saying "no," of 90 degrees.

There is no intervertebral disc at this level so all restraint comes from the ligaments, muscles and joint capsules. One can expect that excessive movement from trauma will involve those tissues.

Movement between C2 (axis) and C3 is possible in both flexion and rotation but is quite limited. The nerves that emerge at this upper cervical segment join to form the occipitocervical nerve and supplies the head via the superior occipital nerve and can result in headache.

These upper cervical nerves also supply the muscles of the neck and arm and when stretched or injured, they can cause temporary paresis or weakness. This may explain the difficulty a patient experiences in being unable to lift his head from the pillow the morning after an injury.

In as much as the neck muscles in the front are also under the pharynx and esophagus, the patient occasionally may complain of "difficulty swallowing."

The physical findings are:

1. Weakness in lifting the head upon the neck from the supine position.

2. Tenderness over the neck muscles under the mandible (jaw).

3. Pain and limitation of head movement either to the right or to the left.

4. Tenderness either over the base of the skull or in the occipitocervical segment.

§ 6-5. The Lower Cervical Segment.

This is the cervical spine from C3 down to and including T1. All functional units are similar in this segment. A functional unit consists of two adjacent vertebrae along with an intervertebral disc. The posterior joints glide on each other to permit flexion-extension, side flexion, and rotation.

Behind each disc a nerve leaves the cervical spine through a window termed the *foramen*. One division of each nerve supplies the muscles and carries sensation to the neck. The other branch of the division descends into the arm to supply the muscles as well as sensation to the arm, hand, and fingers.

It is significant that when the neck flexes or bends forward, the joints of these functional units glide and open the windows (foramen). As the neck extends (head arches backwards), the foramina close. Normally the foramina open and close without entrapping or stretching the nerves but if movement is excessive, the nerve or nerves can be damaged.

Physical findings from injuries to this segment are as follows:

1. Adequate flexion is limited and there may be pain in the distribution of that nerve. This is termed radiation or radiculation. The pain is referred to a portion of the arm and hand termed *dermatome*. This will be subsequently discussed. If the motor nerve function is impaired, weakness of the muscle it innervates will result. The area supplied is termed a *myotome*.

2. There is tenderness over the precise foramen involved.

3. Pressure over that foramen may cause pain sensation in the distribution of the nerve involved.

4. There is limitation of neck movement, not exclusively but predominantly in the lower cervical segment.

5. Referred pain down the arm to hand or fingers can be reproduced by neck extension or hyperextension as the foramena close on the side *toward* which the neck is turned. This movement also will reproduce pain in the neck and down the arms.

6. With neck extended (bent backwards), firm pressure on the head downward will reproduce or intensify the referred pain.

7. Traction upon the head, which elevates the head and decreases the neck curvature (lordosis), will decrease the pain or momentarily eliminate neurological involvement.

Nerve irritation or nerve damage is the most significant sequela of cervical spine injury. The neurological damage can be to the spinal cord or to an individual nerve root.

§ 6-6. Laboratory Tests.

In evaluating any pathologic process one will usually have a choice of several diagnostic tests. The cervical spine is no exception. This section will deal with the most common ones that are routinely used. In general, all of these tests play a confirmatory role. In other words the core of information derived from a thorough history and physical examination should be the basis for a diagnosis; the additional tests are obtained to confirm this clinical impression. Trouble develops when these tests are used for screening purposes since most of them are overly sensitive and relatively unselective.

§ 6-7. X-Ray.

Radiographic evaluation of the cervical spine is helpful in assessing patients with neck pain and the routine study should include anteroposterior, lateral, oblique, and odontoid views. Flexion-extension x-rays are necessary in defining stability. The generally accepted radiographic signs of cervical disc disease are loss of height of the intervertebral disc space, osteophyte formation, secondary encroachment of the intervertebral foramina, and osteoarthritic changes in the apophyseal joints. This is covered in detail in Chapter 2.

A word of advice is appropriate here in that the identification of "some pathology" on cervical x-rays does not, per se, indicate pathology related to "the accident" nor is it necessarily the cause of the patient's symptoms. At approximately age forty some disc degeneration (narrowing) can be expected, particularly at the C5-6 and C6-7 levels. This is considered to represent a normal aging process. The difficult problem in regard to radiographic interpretation is not in identification of these changes but rather as to just how much significance should be attributed to them. The most careful study in this respect was conducted by Friedenberg and Miller (entry 5) who compared ninety-two matched pairs of asymptomatic and symptomatic patients. It was their conclusion that narrowing of the intervertebral spaces between the fifth and sixth and sixth and seventh cervical vertebra was the most symptomatically relevant radiographic finding. There was no difference between the two groups in regard to changes at the joints of Luschka, the intervertebral foramina or the posterior articular processes. It has also been shown by Brain (entry 1) that large numbers of asymptomatic patients may show radiographic evidence of advanced degenerative disc disease.

Radiographic abnormalities of alignment in the cervical spine may also be of clinical significance but they necessarily need to be correlated with the clinical picture; listhesis or slipping forward or backward (retrolisthesis) of one vertebra upon the vertebra below it is such a finding.

If "instability" is suspected, functional x-rays may be taken. These view the spine from the side with the head flexed (bent forward) or extended (arched back); the spine normally flexes equally at each spinal level. If one vertebral level is "unstable," that particular vertebra moves more or less and disrupts the symmetry of motion. Again, this finding must be correlated with the clinical picture as its mere presence may be asymptomatic.

X-rays, particularly oblique views, depict the adequacy of the foramena. These are the windows through which each nerve root emerges (C3-C8, T1). A narrowing or an encroachment into the foramen by a spur or a herniated disc can compress or impair that *specific* nerve emerging. Again the clinical story will verify the significance of this finding.

It is well accepted that slow progression of osteophytes and arthritic spurs with gradual encroachment upon the nerve permits this vulnerable structure to adapt without damage and unless there is superimposed trauma, the nerve continues to function unimpeded, e.g., without pain, numbness, or weakness.

§ 6-8. Myelography.

A myelogram is performed by injecting a dye into the spinal sac so that the outline of the sac itself as well as each nerve root sleeve, can be evaluated. If there is pressure upon the nerve root or dural sac from either a bony spur or disc herniation it will be seen as a constriction on the x-ray picture.

The myelogram, however, should be used as a confirmatory test to substantiate a clinical impression. It should not be used as a screening test since there are many false positive as well as false negative results. This means that some normal people will have abnormal myelographic findings whereas other abnormal people will be found to have normal myelograms.

§ 6-9. Electromyogram (EMG).

Electromyography, known as an EMG, is an electric test that confirms the interaction of nerve to muscle. The test is performed by placing needles into muscles to determine if there is an intact nerve supply to that muscle. The EMG is particularly useful in localizing a specific abnormal nerve root. It should be appreciated that it takes at least twenty-one days for an EMG to show up as abnormal. After twenty-one days of pressure on a nerve root, signs of denervation with fibrillation can be observed. Before twenty-one days, the EMG will be negative in spite of nerve root damage. It should also be noted that there is no quantitative interpretation of this test. Thus, it cannot be said that the EMG is 25% or 75% normal.

It is important to understand that the EMG like the myelogram is a confirmatory test and in evaluating the routine neck problem, it will rarely come up with any information which cannot be derived from a careful physical examination. This test seems to have developed a certain aura in medical-legal circles and far more importance is given to it than it deserves since many spine centers are able to furnish quality care while limiting the use of the test to very special circumstances. It can certainly be stated that the EMG need not be part of the routine evaluation of neck pain. It is indicated to confirm a clinical impression when there are other objective findings present. It is not a screening test.

§ 6-10. Computerized Axial Tomography.

Computerized Axial Tomography (CAT Scan) permits one to create cross sectional imaging of the cervical spine at any desired level. It lets one look directly into the spinal canal. In addition to the bony configuration in all planes, it also shows the soft tissues in graded shadings so that the

ASSESSMENT OF PHYSICAL FINDINGS § 6-11

ligaments, nerve roots, free fat, and intervertebral disc can be observed as they relate to their bony environment.

The CAT scan has been used with great success in the lumbar spine but has met with considerable disappointment when applied to the cervical spine. There are two main reasons for the poor results in scanning of the cervical spine: One is that the actual anatomic size of the cervical spine is smaller than the lumbar spine and thus the individual structures are harder to distinguish in the former. The second reason is technical and involves the appropriateness of scanning and filming protocols. The protocol in the cervical spine is quite involved and for optimal cervical CAT scan diagnosis the program requires a great deal of flexibility in terms of image manipulation and display options; however, a great deal of effort is now being expended to expand cervical CAT scanning and it should shortly be on the same level as lumbar CAT scanning.

One must remember that the cervical CAT scan should be used to confirm the clinical findings as derived from the history and physical examination. It is not a screening test and should not be the primary basis for a diagnosis. The specificity (false positive) and sensitivity (false negative) for specific diagnostic entities in the cervical spine have not been worked out as of this time.

§ 6-11. Thermography.

Thermography is a pictorial representation of skin temperature. Skin temperature is regulated by sympathetic nerve fibers and these travel with the sensory nerves to the periphery. A change in skin temperature is depicted on a thermogram as a change in color and increased skin temperature is purported to be related to the presence of pain.

There are two basic techniques of performing thermography: electronic, and direct contact (liquid crystal). The electronic technique detects heat emissions from the body by aiming a sensor at the body without direct contact. The direct contact method utilizes the direct application to the patient's body of a rubberized material impregnated with temperature-sensitive cholesteric crystals which change color on contact with the skin. Each technique has its advantages and drawbacks, but results obtained with either seem to be comparable.

Thermography has been suggested for a wide variety of neurologic, vascular, and musculoskeletal problems but there is controversy as to its role in the diagnosis of cervical spine problems. In a double study published in the April 1985 issue of the Journal, Thermology, (entries 6, 7) Mahoney and McCulloch concluded that thermography was of no benefit in the diagnosis of lumbar (low back) disc disease. There have been no direct investigations of the cervical spine but there is no reason to feel that the results would be any different from those in the lumbar spine. The authors feel that thermography does not as yet have a place in the diagnosis of cervical spine problems. However, more work (scientific investigations) needs to be performed before a definite conclusion can be reached regarding the value of thermography in cervical spine disease.

§ 6-12. Discography.

In discography, radiopaque dye is injected directly into the intervertebral disc space and the test is considered positive when dye leaks out of the disc space (entry 4). It is supposed to be indicated when a patient has two or three abnormal disc spaces and the question arises as to which one is causing symptoms. Unfortunately, the leakage of dye on a discogram is not sensitive or specific since a high percentage of cervical intervertebral discs, especially in middle-aged and elderly patients, will demonstrate disc degeneration and dye leakage despite the absence of any clinical symptoms. The test should not play a routine role in the investigation of cervical spine pathology.

§ 6-13. Cervical Disc Distention Test.

The cervical disc distention test requires the injection of physiologic saline solution into the intervertebral disc under investigation. As the disc is distended, the patient is questioned as to whether there is a reproduction of his pain pattern. If the answer is affirmative, it is felt that the injected disc is involved in the patient's symptomatology. This test is particularly helpful when routine roentgenography and myelography demonstrates multiple levels of cervical disc involvement and there is question as to which area is responsible for the patient's pain. The test is not used routinely but only when multiple disc spaces demonstrate disease.

§ 6-14. Magnetic Resonance Imaging (MRI).

MRI is the newest diagnostic test on the horizon for problems in the cervical spine. The MRI gives an image on films which is obtained by measuring the differences in proton density between the various tissues evaluated. With the use of the computer, multiplanar images are obtainable.

MRI is a safer test than either the CAT scan or myelogram since it uses neither ionizing radiation nor contrast agents. MRI technology, however, is still in its infancy and much more research still needs to be done. Once the technology is further refined, there will need to be some large prospective clinical studies evaluating the specificity (false positives) and sensitivity (false negatives) of the MRI as a tool in the investigation of the cervical spine. The MRI does hold great promise with its high theoretical limits in image detail and very low attendant risks. Unfortunately up until now, everyone has been concentrating on the nucleus pulposus, a structure which has been studied to death by all of the other methodology. The real enigma, the nature of "soft tissue injuries" in the cervical spine, probably could be better understood by focusing the MRI investigation on the soft tissue — the muscles and ligaments which cannot really be visualized in any other way.

BIBLIOGRAPHY

1. Brain, W.R., Northfield, D.W., and Wilkinson, M. The neurological manifestations of cervical spondylosis, Brain 75, 187-225, 1952.
2. Cailliet, R. *Neck and Arm Pain,* 2d ed., Philadelphia, F.A. Davis Company, 1981.
3. Cervical Spine Research Society. *The Cervical Spine.* Chapter 2, pp 23-25 Philadelphia, J.P. Lippincott Company, 1983.
4. Cloward, R.B. Cervical discography: a contribution to the etiology and mechanism of neck, shoulder and arm pain. Ann Surg, 150: 1052-64, 1959.
5. Friendenberg, Z.B. and Miller, W.T. Degenerative disc disease of the cervical spine. J Bone and Joint Surg, 45-A: 1171-8, 1963.
6. Mahoney, Z., McCulloch, J., and Csima, A. Relation of thermography to back pain. Thermology, Vol. 1:59-61, 1985.
7. Mahoney, L., McCulloch, J., and Csima, A. Thermography as a diagnostic aid in sciatica. Thermology, Vol. 1:55-59, 1985.

CHAPTER 7

INDICATIONS FOR CERVICAL SPINE SURGERY

Jeffery L. Stambough, M.D.
Richard H. Rothman, M.D., Ph.D.

§ 7-1. Introduction.
§ 7-2. Surgical Indications for a Herniated Nucleus Pulposus.
 § 7-2(A). Neck Pain.
 § 7-2(B). Profound Spinal Cord Impingement.
 § 7-2(C). Progressive Neurologic Deficit.
 § 7-2(D). Unrelenting Radicular Arm Pain.
 § 7-2(E). Recurrent Episodes of Arm Pain.
 § 7-2(F). Patient Factors.
 § 7-2(G). Selection of the Operation for Acute Disc Herniation.
§ 7-3. Indications for Surgery in Cervical Spinal Stenosis.
 § 7-3(A). Selection of the Operation for Cervical Spinal Stenosis.
§ 7-4. Indications for Cervical Spine Fusion.
 § 7-4(A). Neck Pain Only.
 § 7-4(B). Neck and Arm Pain.
 § 7-4(C). Neck Pain and Myelopathy.
§ 7-5. Results of Operative Treatment.
§ 7-6. Complications of Cervical Spine Surgery.
 § 7-6(A). Complications During the Operation.
  § 7-6(A)(1). Complications as a Result of Position.
  § 7-6(A)(2). Vascular Injuries.
  § 7-6(A)(3). Visceral Injuries.
  § 7-6(A)(4). Neural Element Injuries.
 § 7-6(B). Immediate Postoperative Complications.
  § 7-6(B)(1). Pulmonary Atelectasis.
  § 7-6(B)(2). Urinary Retention.
  § 7-6(B)(3). Intestinal Ileus.
  § 7-6(B)(4). Thrombophlebitis and Pulmonary Embolus.
  § 7-6(B)(5). Wound Problems.
  § 7-6(B)(6). Spinal Cord Compression.
 § 7-6(C). Technical Complications Resulting in Persistent Symptoms.
  § 7-6(C)(1). Inadequate Nerve Root Decompression.
  § 7-6(C)(2). Inadequate Spinal Cord Decompression.

§ 7-6(C)(3). Disc Space Infection.
§ 7-6(C)(4). Iliac Crest Pain.
§ 7-6(C)(5). Late Instability and Degenerative Changes.
§ 7-6(C)(6). Foreign Bodies.
§ 7-7. Summary.
Bibliography.
Figure 1. Removal of Osteophytic Spur.

§ 7-1. Introduction.

Surgical intervention, when indicated, provides the patient with cervical spine disease with predictable and gratifying results. Despite areas of minor controversy, the indications for surgical treatment as well as the appropriate surgical procedure have been well established. Unlike the lumbar spine, surgery in the cervical spine is not as easily mastered and the complications when present can be quite serious. With the establishment of strict criteria for patient selection as outlined in chapter 2, the results in the good to excellent category can approach 80 — 95% in most instances.

The purpose of this chapter is not to detail the surgical treatment of cervical spine disorder, but rather to afford the reader a general appreciation for the role of surgery in specific diagnoses with its attendant risks, benefits, and complications. The results from each procedure or diagnostic criterion will be briefly reviewed as well. Where controversy exists or more than one type of procedure is equally successful, it will be indicated.

Surgery on the cervical spine is performed for pain (usually radicular or arm pain), bony instability, and/or spinal cord compression. Thus, most procedures are directed to relieve pain. The procedures performed may be grouped into one of three categories; decompression (with or without disc excision), stabilization (fusion or bony anklyosis), or both. Furthermore, the cervical spine surgeon must decide whether the pathology should be approached from the front or back of the spine; in one or two stages (see Figure 1).

§ 7-2. Surgical Indications for a Herniated Nucleus Pulposus.

When the conservative or nonoperative therapeutic outline in Chapter 3 has proven unsuccessful in managing the patient's symptoms, surgical intervention can and should be considered. This happens in about 10-15% of all cases. A herniated cervical disc presents with variable severity in the degree of symptoms, each with its own surgical priorities. Before discussing these individually, a review of surgery for neck pain is warranted.

§ 7-2(A). Neck Pain.

Failure of nonoperative treatment per se is not an indication for operation treatment. This is particularly true in the case of neck pain. Axial or predominant neck pain responds poorly to disc excision with or without fusion for a variety of reasons. DePalma, Rothman, and associates (entry 5) reviewed a large series of 229 patients who underwent anterior cervical fusion and disc excision for intractable neck pain. Some of these patients had arm pain as well. Follow-up ranged from one to nine years. Good to excellent results were only attainable in 63% of the patients in this series.

One may conclude from this and other studies that cervical fusion for neck pain alone is unpredictable. This relates in part to the lack of correlation between symptoms and radiographic changes previously discussed.

§ 7-2(B). Profound Spinal Cord Impingement.

The most dramatic but fortunately the most rare presentation of a cervical herniated nucleus pulposis is the sudden and profound neurologic loss produced by a large central herniation. This produces a profound or progressive acute myelopathy with quadriparesis or quadraplegia below the level of the herniation. If not decompressed urgently, the potential for lasting weakness, spasticity, loss of bowel and bladder function, as well as sexual dysfunction is increased. In some cases, even the prompt treatment will not reverse the spinal cord damage thought to be the result of lack of blood supply. Once this clinical condition is identified, the patient should undergo myelography and decompression from the front of the spine with anterior interbody fusion. Despite the potential lack of total recovery, the surgery will often prevent further damage to the spinal cord with loss of neurologic function.

§ 7-2(C). Progressive Neurologic Deficit.

If the treating physician can actually document a change or worsening in a patient's neurologic examination, surgery should be seriously considered. Not uncommonly, a patient will present with arm pain radiating into the index and long fingers. A diminished brachioradialis and possibly a diminished biceps reflex will be noted on initial examination. Conservative treatment will be instituted and the patient will be re-evaluated. This might reveal a further loss in the arm reflexes associated with demonstrable motor weakness in the biceps muscle. This constellation of findings represent a progressive neurologic deficit. Since this is not usually reversible with medications and rest, and the surgeon would like to prevent further permanent nerve damage, the appropriate surgical decompression should be done once confirmatory evidence is provided by contrast myelography.

It is more common, however, to find the patient presenting with an acute but stable neurologic deficit. If this is profound with significant motor weakness, for example complete paralysis of the hand intrinsic muscles (C8, T1), surgical intervention is a viable option and most spine surgeons consider it mandatory. While it is often difficult to quantitate, it is generally held for clinical data that the more prolonged and severe the pressure on a spinal nerve, the less likely the nerve is to recover function. Unfortunately, there are no good prospectively controlled series to document the recovery of cervical nerve function. Every spine surgeon remembers cases in which the return was noted within days and those in which it never improved or even worsened. Presently, the recommendations for surgery have to be individualized in each patient based on the clinical picture and the significance of the neurologic findings.

An even more difficult clinical judgment occurs when the patient presents with a partial neurologic lesion (weakness) or the clinical situation is subacute. A stable neurologic finding is not alone a good criterion for surgery because it is unpredictably altered. One must keep in mind the temporal relationship since the acute or subacute pain may not correlate with the patient's neurologic finding. Previous medical records and examination will often be of help in making this decision.

The clinical syndrome of double crush occurs when there is compression of a spinal nerve at two discrete locations in the upper extremity; cervical spine and a peripheral locale. The importance of identifying the dual compression is related to the clinical prognosis. The offending peripheral compression should be relieved (e.g., carpal tunnel syndrome), but if the patient also has involvement of the C6 nerve root in the cervical spine, the results will be inferior. This relates to the altered axonal flow and spinal nerve nutrition which make the particular nerve more susceptible to injury and the recovery less complete (entry 22).

§ 7-2(D). Unrelenting Radicular Arm Pain.

Occasionally an acute episode of brachalgia without neurologic deficit will fail to respond to conservative treatment. The exact timing of surgical treatment will vary from patient to patient depending on the patient's pain tolerance, socioeconomic factors, and emotional stability. In most instances, if the patient has a positive confirmatory electromyogram and myelogram, and has not improved with at least six weeks of nonoperative treatment, the patient should be considered for surgery. Procrastination after a period of several months is ill advised since the development of a chronic pain pattern is more likely to occur, not to mention adverse response to the surgical procedure.

§ 7-2(E). Recurrent Episodes of Arm Pain.

Another small group of patients with arm or radicular pain will develop a recurrent bout of incapacitating pain. Most often the symptoms will be low grade or smoldering between episodes suggesting chronic cervical spondylosis. These periods are tolerable for the patient. If these recurrent acute pain episodes are not too bad and within the patient's pain tolerance, conservative therapy should be rendered. Less frequently, the frequency and intensity of the pain is severe enough to interfere with the patient's gainful employment and avocational endeavors such that surgery should be considered. As a guideline, if the patient suffers four or more episodes in one year, the surgery should be offered if the confirmatory tests are positive.

The relief of the painful condition requires that the surgeon find evidence of a physical or organic cause to the patient's pain. This ideally means that mechanical compression of the suspicious nerve root is demonstrable either from hard or soft pathology. On the contrary, if one undertakes to decompress a nerve root which is not the focus of a mechanical or organic lesion, the results are no better than a placebo and very discouraging. One should avoid at all costs the so-called exploratory spinal operation for pain relief.

Mechanical compression of the spinal nerve is best demonstrated by the pantopaque myelogram. Computerized axial tomography (CT scan) has not proven useful to date in the screening of cervical disc disease. Where the patient with brachialgia is considered for surgery, three criteria should be met if an excellent result is to be anticipated. These are:

1. a neurologic deficit;
2. positive myelogram;
3. positive EMG, shoulder abduction relief sign, Spurling's sign or clearly singular radicular pattern.

The results of surgery cannot be expected to be excellent unless the patient has at least a positive neurologic deficit coupled with a positive correlative myelogram. For example, a patient with arm pain radiating into the middle finger of the hand with weakness of the triceps muscle and diminished triceps reflex, who has a myelogram consistent with a C6-C7 disc herniation, can be expected to have a good and lasting result. The electromyogram, shoulder abduction relief sign, Spurling's sign, or clear radicular pain pattern are added to the decision making, but without the former two criteria surgery is likely to be ineffective in relieving the patient's symptoms. The key to the anatomic confirmation of the lesion causing brachalgia is the pantopaque myelogram, and to date we have no reliable noninvasive substitute.

§ 7-2(F). Patient Factors.

It has been stated that the key to a successful outcome in any surgery but especially spine surgery is patient selection. Even the most expertly performed surgical procedure done in an inappropriate patient is doomed to a poor outcome. The authors have clearly outlined the objective criteria for patient selection, but what about the patient and their emotional, psychologic, and socioeconomic characteristics? This should not be misinterpreted since these factors all inter-relate and even in a difficult patient situation, organic findings and pathology may co-exist.

The emotional factor is hard to quantitate but is a subjective measure best ascertained by the patient interview. Recently, the Minnesota Multiphasic Personality Inventory (MMPI), a questionnaire which measures relative levels of hysteria, depression, hypochondriasis, etc., may be of use preoperatively in predicting the surgical outcome (entry 20). If the patient presents with minor complaints, a paucity of physical findings, and has a significant emotional overlay or even overt depression, continued nonoperative treatment is warranted. If on the other hand, definite physical findings are present (a neurologic deficit) and emotional problems are pre-existing, a psychiatric consultation is recommended. The patient may need to have optimal medical and psychiatric management prior to surgery or as is often the case, once the psychologic overlay is treated, the symptoms improve enough that surgery is no longer needed. As a rule of thumb, the emotional and psychologic factors should be addressed and treated before surgical intervention is rendered.

Socioeconomic factors include the presence of litigation and the work related injury. Patients with cervical spine problems who were involved in an automobile accident (usually minor) or injured at work are some of the most difficult patients to treat successfully. These patients, unlike those with psychologic overlays do not exhibit emotional problems. It is often difficult to pinpoint a reproducible reason for the less than optimal response to treatment in these patients. Unless these patients have profound or progressive neurologic picture with objective findings which would warrant emergency surgery, it is wise to continue conservative treatment until the litigation or compensation is settled. While these problems are not as prominent in cervical spine disease as lumbar spine disease, the presence should not be overlooked or underemphasized. A small group of patients, usually women who have domestic problems, need special mention. These patients may have been injured at home or have spouse related problems, but do not have compensation or litigation claims. These patients have what may be termed "domestic neuroses." The secondary gains which preclude a good response to surgery relate to the patient's home environment or marital problems with varying levels of emotional overlay and depression. Again, unless profound or progressive, neurologic deficits should be treated by nonoperative measures only (entry 16).

§ 7-2(G). Selection of the Operation for Acute Disc Herniation.

Now that we have chosen our patient based on objective criteria, which operation should we do? The goals of surgery for cervical disc herniations are to decompress the spinal nerve by removing what is mechanically impinging on the nerve root. Also, the overwhelming reason for the surgery is to relieve the patients radicular arm pain. Two surgical options of near equal efficacy can be undertaken in these patients. The first involves a partial removal of the offending facet through a posterior approach. This procedure originated by Scoville (entry 18) and popularized by Henderson and Associates (entry 8) is referred to as a "keyhole" foraminotomy. The procedure is successful whether or not a true soft disc herniation or bony spur is causing the patient's radicular pain. A 95% good to excellent result can be expected with only a 3-4% recurrence rate. This procedure is favored by the authors.

The second surgical procedure for one or two level cervical disc disease causing radicular arm pain is the anterior disc excision popularized by Smith and Robinson with or without bony fusion (entry 19). This procedure involves an anterior or front approach to the cervical spine and directly addresses the problem. This procedure is clearly superior in true central disc herniations with acute spinal cord compression. In general, the results provide about 90-95% good to excellent results in relief of radicular arm pain. Despite short term good results without fusion, the authors do not favor the routine exclusion of iliac bone graft in the anterior disc excision (entry 12).

In general, the authors do not favor this procedure for two reasons; the higher risk of complications in the anterior approach, and the problems of donor site pain for autogenous bone grafting. It must be stressed though, that either procedure is perfectly adequate in treating radicular arm pain.

§ 7-3. Indications for Surgery in Cervical Spinal Stenosis.

Cervical spondylosis or chronic cervical disc degeneration produces pathologic changes in the diameter of the cervical spinal canal and/or neural foramina (entry 17). Secondarily the bone spurs or osteophytes may impinge on the esophagus producing dysphagia or the vertebral artery with signs of brainstem ischemia. The latter conditions are rare and respond to the appropriate bony removal or decompression. When the cervical spondylitic spine encroach on the spinal nerves as they exit the spine, signs of radicular arm pain are produced. The management of this problem is discussed in the previous section and further consideration will not be given here.

INDICATIONS FOR CERVICAL SPINE SURGERY § 7-3

Cervical spondylosis leads to the formation of bony ridges or bars that form at the back end of the vertebrae which surround the offending degenerating disc space. This is a result of abnormal or excessive motion and leads to cervical spinal canal narrowing or stenosis. Additional infolding of the ligamentum flavum and/or arthritis changes in the apophyseal or facet joints can further compromise the spinal canal. Cervical spinal stenosis can then compress the spinal cord and either directly or secondarily due to spinal cord ischemia lead to spinal cord damage or myelopathy. The signs and symptoms of myelopathy are discussed in detail in Chapter 2. It should be noted that myelopathic signs and symptoms are often poorly localized unless a clear radicular component and single level disease is seen. The goals of surgery here are to relieve the pressure on the spinal cord and thereby prevent the progression of the myelopathic symptoms. Improvement is harder to achieve and relates to the duration and severity of the spinal cord compression. Neck pain relief is not a goal of the surgery but fortunately not a significant part of the clinical symptoms. Furthermore, the patient and his family must understand that myelopathy unlike radicular arm pain is less predictable in its response to decompression.

Routine x-rays of the cervical spine are quite helpful in cervical spine stenosis revealing degenerative disc space narrowing, spur formation, and a diminished spinal canal diameter. Unfortunately the mere presence of these findings does not explain the patient's clinical picture and further confirmation is required. The CAT scan with small amounts of intrathecal metrizamide will add in the diagnosis but at present cannot substitute for the myelogram.

Although a pantopaque myelogram is usually not required in the decision to operate, it is essential to clearly establish the area(s) of cord compression which are usually multiple. The myelogram is the surgical guide to decompression and there is no less invasive substitute for it.

§ 7-3(A). Selection of the Operation for Cervical Spinal Stenosis.

The goal of an operation for cervical spinal stenosis is to completely remove all pressure from the neural elements, and the type of pathology present will dictate the nature and extent of the decompression required (entry 17). If the process involves encroachment on the spinal canal of a large central soft disc herniation, then this must be removed. More commonly, the process involves anterior spondylitic or bony spurs (called hard discs) which compress the neural elements and are further exacerbated by the posterior changes in the ligamentum flavum and facet joints. Unlike the lumbar spine, complete removal of all the offending elements is not possible or even necessary to provide an adequate decompression.

When the process of cervical spinal stenosis involves four or more levels, the authors favor a posterior laminectomy. If radicular symptoms coexist from foraminal narrowing, appropriate level foraminal decompression is also done. If more than two foraminotomies are required, the procedure may best be done anteriorly despite the need for a large bone graft which may heal and incorporate slowly.

On the other hand, if the spinal canal stenosis involves three or less adjacent vertebral levels, an anterior disc excision without removal of posterior osteophytes and fusion are favored by the authors. Bohlman has shown that the posterior osteophytes or spurs resorb once solid bony fusion occurs and do not need to be removed at the time of anterior decompression (entry 2). The results of the surgery in cervical spinal stenosis are satisfactory in about 80% of cases with the anterior procedures providing slightly better results.

It is not physically possible for a patient with cervical spinal stenosis to return to heavy manual labor after surgery. Most of these patients do not completely resolve their myelopathy and thus some type of job modification will be required. Even in the non-compensatory category, these patients are unable to return to work under these circumstances and usually end up on permanent disability. The aim of the surgeon is to prevent further neurologic deterioration although this is not always possible in moderate and severe cases. The often heard admonition to do a surgical procedure to get the patient back to work is very unrealistic in this case.

§ 7-4. Indications for Cervical Spine Fusion.

In general, spinal fusion is indicated when instability of the spine is symptomatic, painful, or potentially harmful to the neural elements. The cervical spine is the most mobile of all the spinal segments and consequently suffers more degenerative disc disease and late instability. Cervical spine fusion is indicated for tumor, trauma, infection, as well as inflammatory conditions in which angulatory or translateral motion is excessive. The authors apply the criterion of White and Panjabi (entry 23) in assessing cervical spine stability as discussed in Chapter 2, § 2-3(C).

Spine fusion in the cervical spine is performed with autogenous bone graft with wiring of the posterior element to provide early stability. Bony healing occurs over 4-6 months and usually provides a long term stability to the spine. The authors recommend cervical spine fusion in the following clinical situations:

1. Rheumatoid arthritis with intractable pain and neurologic deficits; and
   A. Atlantoaxial subluxation more than 7mm.
   B. Basilar invagination.
   C. Subaxial subluxation with translation more than 3.5mm and angular deformity at adjacent vertebrae of more than 11 degrees.

2. After anterior disc excision for myelopathy or radiculopathy (entry 19).
3. Atlanto-occipital subluxation (more than 1mm) and suboccipital pain (entry 25).
4. After extensive bilateral laminectomy and facetectomy for decompression (especially in a younger patient).
5. Late segmental instability associated with prior anterior fusion or congenital fusion with reversal of the intervertebral angle at the interspace above or below the fusion.

§ 7-4(A). Neck Pain Only.

Although the presence of axial neck pain is not an indication for surgical fusion in cervical disc disease, surgical fusion in conditions such as rheumatoid arthritis or segmental instability will often relieve neck pain. The authors do not advocate fusion primarily as a pain procedure, but as in the case of rheumatoid arthritis the fusion is primarily performed to prevent further neurologic compromise. Cervical spine fusion is not without its late problems. Higher incidence of degenerative disc disease above and below anterior cervical fusion is very common but that may not always be symptomatic. Posterior element fusions frequently tend to extend beyond their intended levels which further compromises neck motion.

§ 7-4(B). Neck and Arm Pain.

Those patients with neck and arm pain with cervical spine instability routinely will resolve their arm symptoms with solid arthrodesis. Decompression is not required and is potentially harmful (e.g., rheumatoid arthritis). When cervical disc disease presents with neck and arm pain, the goals of an anterior surgical procedure is to decompress the nerve roots and a fusion of intervertebral disc space is performed to restore disc space height which also widens the intervertebral foramen. The neck pain when it originates from the involved spine segment will be improved by the surgical procedure and fusion.

§ 7-4(C). Neck Pain and Myelopathy.

Axial neck pain is not a prominent feature in cervical spine disease with myelopathy. Posterior decompressions which are extensive and destroy bilateral facets can lead to late instability with a so-called swan neck deformity which is painful. Cervical myelopathy from a soft central disc herniation is not usually painful once the herniation is complete. Again, the myelopathy symptoms predominate and the surgical intervention is primarily to decompress the compromised spinal cord with fusion of the intervertebral disc space for the reason stated above. Neck pain is often intractable in rheumatoid arthritis with spinal cord compression. In rheumatoid arthritis, the fusion is to maintain spinal alignment. Once reduction is obtained which secondarily decompresses the neural elements, painful, abnormal joint mobility is often relieved as well.

§ 7-5. Results of Operative Treatment.

A general statement regarding the results of cervical spine surgery is not possible. Each category of cervical degenerative disc disease and inflammatory cervical processes have their own peculiar problems which influence the end results. The results of cervical spine surgery for acute herniated disc with radicular arm pain, cervical spondylosis with predominately neck pain, cervical spondylosis with myelopathy and myeloradicuopathy, and for cervical instability in rheumatoid arthritis will be reviewed in the following discussion.

Cervical spine surgery has been performed with regularity since the 1940s. The basic techniques have not been chanced significantly since then, although the results are somewhat better based primarily on more strict patient selection and long term follow-up studies refining surgical indications. The biggest advance in cervical spine surgery has been the routine use of magnification, either loupes or an operating microscope, which allow the surgeon to perform the surgery with the most gentle of techniques. This is especially true when dealing with the spinal cord. Further improvements in surgical result will continue to be based on long-term clinical studies of various techniques and diagnoses, and basic science research which aids in the fundamental understanding of the pathophysiology of the disease process.

Surgery for acute cervical herniated disc has been slowly moving from the anterior disc excision with fusion to the posterolateral "keyhole" foraminotomy. The result of these two procedures are very similar in long term reviews, but the posterior approach and foraminotomy is less risky and easier to perform and does not require bone grafting. Although several authors have advocated simple anterior disc excision without fusion, most surgeons perform anterior interbody fusion to provide stability and to restore disc height. Over one thousand four hundred cases of anterior cervical disc excision with interbody fusion for radiculopathy has been reviewed by Whitesides (entry 24). Although this compilation cannot be strictly compared since the patient populations differed slightly in symptoms and follow-up methods, a total of about 90% good to excellent results were routinely attained. In a specific reference to patients with soft cervical disc herniations only, Aronson reviewed 88 patients who were treated with anterior disc excision with interbody fusion. All but one of the patients were rated as good to excellent with no major complications reported. These results illustrate the response to this treatment method in the proper patient population (entry 1).

In a large review of 295 patients with predominantly radicular pain who were treated with anterior disc excision were reviewed by Lunesford and Associates (entry 12). The patients had either soft or hard disc pathology which did not influence their final result. Overall 84% good to excellent results were reported.

The study population was predominantly male and the ages were between 30 and 60 years. Symptoms were present in the majority for 2 years or less. Patients with soft disc pathology were younger and had a shorter duration of symptoms. Data for the review was obtained from hospital charts, operative and radiographic reports, and follow-up examinations. Follow up was at least 12 months with a mean of more than 3 years.

The results could demonstrate no clear advance to fusion compared to simple disc excision alone. Furthermore, the results did not change depending on the type of fusion. Those patients who had fusion did have a slightly higher complication rate and a longer hospitalization. This study represents a large review which confirms the long term satisfactory results of radicular arm pain treated by anterior disc surgery with or without fusion.

Surgery for cervical spondylosis with only neck pain is less satisfactory. DePalma, Rothman, and Associates (entry 5) presented a retrospective review of patients with intractable neck pain and severe degenerative disc disease who were treated with anterior disc excision and interbody fusion. Some of these patients had radiculopathy but most were treated primarily for neck symptoms. A total of two hundred and seventy-four patients were examined retrospectively by personal examination, telephone interview, and hospital record which included radiographs of the neck. The results of the surgery were graded as excellent, good, fair, or poor. The average age in this study was 42.5 years and follow-up averaged over four years. There were 63% females and 37% males in this review.

The results were satisfactory (good or excellent) in only 63% of these patients. The quality of the result did not deteriorate with time. The authors further analyzed the results to identify correlation between preoperative factors and a successful clinical outcome. In the review, older patients tended to have a higher percentage of satisfactory results. Patients with local neck symptoms tended to have better results than those with vague sympathetic type of preoperative symptoms. Pseudarthrosis nor involvement in litigation seemed to alter the statistical long term results. Additionally, a significant proportion of these patients complained about the anterior iliac crest area where the bone graft donor site was located.

The most serious sequalae of cervical degenerative disc disease occur with spinal cord involvement (myelopathy). When myelopathy occurs with arm pain it is called myeloradiculopathy. The results of treatment of cervical myelopathy depends heavily on the duration and severity of the spinal cord involvement. Permanent changes in the spinal cord regardless of the cause will not be altered by any known surgical procedure. This is illustrated in a classification scheme of cervical myelopathic patients devised by Nurick (entry 14). Basically, as long as the patient is independently ambulatory the prognosis for surgery is good; whereas, once the patient cannot ambulate alone or requires external supports, the prognosis is guarded. The former group will often improve with surgery whereas the latter group will only stabilize and not progress further as a result of their myelopathic surgery.

When the cervical spondylosis results in a diffuse cervical spine stenosis, it is often treated by an extensive laminectomy to decompress the spinal cord posteriorly. The procedure has given between 70-80% satisfactory (good to excellent) results as indicated in a large review by Epstein and Janin (entry 6). These authors reviewed over 700 literature cases of myelopathy treated by cervical laminectomy. The best results were attained with extensive laminectomy, foraminotomy, and excision of osteophytes. The good to excellent result averaged about 85% in a contemporary small series of patients by Epstein and Associates (entry 6) reported in the same review.

Equivalent end results in the surgical management of cervical myelopathy or myeloradiculopathy can be achieved with anterior decompression and fusion (entry 9). Hicks and Associates reported a small series of 15 patients with progressive myelopathy who were treated with anterior decompression and fusion. Most cases required 3 or more levels decompressed. Fusion was 100% with autogenous bone graft. Despite a short follow-up, 10 had improved one Nurick grade, 3 had stabilized and 2 were worse.

Zhang and Associates reviewed a large series of 121 myelopathic patients who were treated with anterior disc excision and fusion (entry 26). There were 107 males and 14 females with the majority between 40 and 60 years old. An average of 3 discs were excised and fused. A total of 98% of patients were either improved or unchanged at a mean follow-up of 22 months. Ninety-one percent of the patients were improved and 73% were able to resume normal activities. The results were judged by a slightly different grading system based on ambulation ability and spasticity. Similar results have been reported by Bohlman in a series of 15 patients with Nurick class IV and V (entry 2).

Rheumatoid arthritis commonly involves the neck but rarely requires surgery. The results of surgery in rheumatoid arthritis are not as good as that for cervical degenerative disc disease. In large part this is explained by the nature of the rheumatoid process. These patients tend to be very sick and the perioperative mortality rate is about 10%. A second attendant problem is the severe bone loss and erosion that is a consequence of the rheumatoid arthritis and disuse osteoporosis. The bones of the neck are weak, do not hold wires well, and fusion fails to occur in 20% of cases.

Ranawat and Associates reviewed a series of 33 rheumatoid patients with deformity of the neck treated by fusion. (entry 15). This represented about 1% of all patients with rheumatoid arthritis in their clinic. The patients all have severe rheumatoid arthritis for an average of 19 years and were over 40 years of age. There were 12 men and 21 women. The patients were followed from 1 to 8 years in the study.

The results were judged as to the rate of fusion, spinal stability, pain relief, neurologic improvement, and complications. Patients were examined, questioned, and radiographs were reviewed. The authors found that 5 of the 28 cases failed to fuse and that atlantoaxial pseudarthrosis was the highest. Pain relief was rendered in 17 patients 90% of the patients either improved or remained the same as to their neurologic impairments (various myelopathic findings). Ten percent of the patients actually got worse neurologically. Complications were most frequent in these rheumatoid patients including pressure sores, sepsis, pin track drainage from the haloapparatus, wound problems, debilitation, and death.

In summary, the long term results in cervical spine surgery for cervical degenerative disc disease and spondylosis, and rheumatoid arthritis has been reviewed and illustrative studies have been given to each use. Surgery for acute herniated cervical discs provided satisfactory results in over 95% of cases; whereas surgery for myelopathy will provide between 70-85% satisfactory long-term results. Myeloradiculopathy will have long-term results similar to the myelopathy group. Surgery for patients with cervical disc disease and only neck pain is the worse with long-term satisfactory results of about 60%. Finally, in rheumatoid arthritic patients, the results are not always satisfactory with high rates of perioperative morbidity and mortality, and pseudarthrosis rates.

Furthermore, we can generalize that cervical spine surgery for the relief of arm pain is very predictable. When the spinal cord is involved as in myelopathy and myeloradiculopathy, the results drop by about 20%. If surgery is performed to alleviate intractable neck pain it drops by yet another 20%. Rheumatoid arthritis represents a special circumstance with most of its inferior results related to the underlying erosive synovitis and bony loss as well as the general medical condition of these patients.

§ 7-6. Complications of Cervical Spine Surgery.

§ 7-6(A). Complications During the Operation.

This section includes complications which may occur from the time the patients come to the operating room until they leave the recovery room.

§ 7-6(A)(1). Complications as a Result of Position.

Anterior spine surgery is performed with the patient supine with the head turned to the left or right. The arms are by the patient's side. If the head of the bed is not angled upward about 40-50 degrees, excessive venous bleeding may obscure the operative field. No specific complications related to this rather natural posture generally occurs.

Posterior cervical spine surgery requires the patient to be prone. Two methods are generally used to hold the head and neck segment; horseshoe ring and the Mayfield headrest with the Gardner three-point vise. The horseshoe ring is a padded U shaped device on which the patient's face rests. Care must be exercised to protect the eyes and nose against pressure or abrasion. The Gardner three-point vise accomplishes the same thing but suspends the head and neck by way of pins in the skull. Even here careful placement is needed to avoid undue pressure on the nasal area once the patient is turned.

Cervical spine surgery is almost always done under general systemic anesthesia. The actual turning of the patient from the supine to prone position can be dangerous. Cases in which severe cervical degenerative disc disease exist with compromise of the spinal canal diameter may result in spinal cord damage when the muscle protective mechanism is rendered ineffective by general anesthesia. To guard against this phenomena, an awake intubation is performed so that the patient's own muscles can help stabilize the neck. The patient is then fully anesthesized once the position is final and they have demonstrated voluntary muscle activity in both arms and legs.

Some surgeons prefer to operate on the cervical spine with the patient in the sitting posture. A low but definite risk of air embolism and cerebral infarction exist and should be carefully monitored by the anesthesiologist and surgeon. The advantage of diminished venous bleeding by this posture can be achieved in the prone position if the patient is angled 45-60 degrees head up. This risk of air embolism is very low to nonexistent. Mayfield reported 3 cases of air embolism which were recognized and treated without sequalae (entry 13).

Attention to these details cannot be overstated. The most expertly and effectively performed surgery is somehow less rewarding if a corneal abrasion, retinal artery occlusion (entry 10) or skin slough about the nose develops postoperatively. Needless to say, a quadraplegic complication from neck manipulation is an extremely unfortunate circumstance.

§ 7-6(A)(2). Vascular Injuries.

Vascular injury as a result of trauma to one of the large arteries of the neck can occur in anterior and posterior cervical spine surgery. Anterior spine surgery despite its relative close proximity to both the carotid and vertebral arteries rarely result in vessel injury. Once the skin and platysma are incised, the dissection of the deep structures of the neck is carried out bluntly. Overzealous manipulation may tear small branches or even the main carotid and are to be avoided. The other potential injury to the carotid can occur by improper traction by an assistant or self-retaining retractor. The carotid artery supplies the major portion of the brain and injury may result in permanent brain damage, stroke, or hemiplegia.

As the anterior dissection continues toward the anterior spine, injury to the vertebral artery can occur. Additionally, branches of the major arteries like the inferior and superior thyroid arteries may be sacrificed when necessary. If the smaller vessels are retracted, care must be taken not to tear those vessels which can cause profuse bleeding which is difficult to control. The vertebral artery lies deep to the longus muscles laterally within the foramina transversarium. Rarely, it is necessary to decompress or operate on the artery which requires magnification and proper lighting. In most cases, one must not stray away from the midline nor dissect into the longus muscle covering the vertebral artery. The vertebral arteries come together in the posterior fossa to supply the brainstem. Disruption of this blood supply can have serious sequalae. The anterior spine is relatively avascular.

Major vascular injury is uncommon in posterior cervical surgery with one very important exception. The vertebral artery is anterolateral to the facet and well away from the operative field until it reaches the atlas (C1). Here the artery turns upward on the cranial portion of the atlas ring before it penetrates the interspinous ligament. It is here that the artery is highly vulnerable. Injuries here to either the vertebral artery or vein can lend to profuse bleeding which is hard to control. Careful dissection starting in the midline and going no more laterally than 1.5 cm in the adult and 1 cm in children is generally safe. Sharp dissection rather than scraping with a periosteal elevator is preferred. Needless to say, prevention of this injury is the key which requires very gentle and meticulous dissection under optimal tightening, magnification, and knowledge of the anatomy.

Venous bleeding and injury is less serious to the patient, but can be difficult to control if the vein is torn or lacerated. Veins larger than 1-2 mm should be ligated with suture and cut to allow access to the areas of surgical interest.

Prevention of vascular injuries is facilitated by gentle technique, a working knowledge of the major branches and their common variants, magnification, and adequate lighting. Strict hemostasis must be obtained layer by layer or else the surgeon finds himself operating in a pool of blood. If injury occurs, the arterial bleeding should be tamponaded by finger pressure and the appropriate help obtained so that primary repair can be undertaken. While rare, these complications have serious implications and must be avoided whenever possible.

§ 7-6(A)(3). Visceral Injuries.

Injuries to the esophagus and trachea are unique to the anterior approach to the cervical spine. These midline structures lie directly on top of the cervical vertebral bodies and are most often injured by improper dissection of retraction. The esophagus is particularly vulnerable since it may be collapsed and cordlike in situ. Placement of a nasogastric tube at the time of intubation is essential to aid in its identification. Additionally, these structures should only be retracted once the prevertebral fascia and anterior cervical vertebral bodies are identified. This places the retractor directly on bone preventing the inadvertent tearing of the esophagus or trachea.

Esophageal fistulae between the skin and esophagus are serious complications. The risk for infection is high and requires the area to be bypassed with nasogastric tube feedings until it heals. These injuries are prevented by careful blunt dissection with good lighting and magnification. The nasogastric tube will aid in esophageal identification too. Only one case of esophageal laceration was reported in 500 cases by Tew and Mayfield (entry 21).

§ 7-6(A)(4). Neural Element Injuries.

Neural injury can involve the spinal cord, nerve roots, or both in the cervical spine. Additionally, there are several important peripheral nerves at risk in anterior neck surgery. Injuries may occur through excessive retraction or manipulation, laceration, or thermal injuries.

Anterior disc excision requires the total removal of the annulus fibrosis to the level of the posterior longitudinal ligament. Some surgeons feel that the posterior spondylitic spurs should be excised. This has the additional risk of traumatizing the anterior spinal cord. Tew and Mayfield (entry 21) reported a single case of spinothalmic tract dysfunction postoperatively in his series of 500 patients. The cervical cord is very sensitive to retraction and permanent, irreversible damage can occur. If the posterior longitudinal ligament is violated, the risk of dural tearing exists which is very difficult to repair.

Anterior disc excision requires meticulous, complete hemostasis. The annulus fibrosis and nucleus pulposus should be excised sharply initially, followed by the use of sharp currettage. The use of small cloward type laminar spreaders facilitate exposure and visualization of the disc space. The authors of this text do not routinely remove posterior osteophytes since they will regress with solid fusion without altering long term results.

Nerve root injuries are rare from anterior surgery but injury to the vagus nerve or laryngeal nerve is possible. Most often these injuries are temporary and recover over a period of weeks. The recurrent laryngeal nerve is particularly important because injury results in vocal cord paralysis. Since the nerve consistently crosses the operative field lower on the left after looping around the aorta, most surgeons approach the cervical spine from this side. Identification of the nerve is greatly aided by loupe magnification (2.5-3.5X). Retraction, when necessary, should be as gently as possible and the nerve should not be excessively dissected. Recurrent laryngeal palsy was the most common neural complication (52 cases) in a review of over 82,000 cases by Flynn (entry 7).

Spinal cord and nerve roots are vulnerable to injury in posterior cervical surgery. The spinal cord may be injured in the removal of the posterior bony covering with the inadvertent plunging of an instrument or excessive retraction. Even the small instrument may be too much in the severely stenotic cervical canal. The authors favor the use of a high speed burr in these cases where the laminae to be removed are first thinned. The laminae are than removed by the upward motion of a currette without placing any instruments under the laminae. Retraction of the cord for any reason is risky. If the posterior vertebral body pathology needs to be addressed, it is most safely done via the anterior approach. Mayfield reported a case where myelopathy was made temporarily worse from cord contusion in a posterior cervical laminectomy (entry 13).

The cervical dura may be torn or lacerated. Any disruption should be sutured once it is found. Great care must be exercised to avoid penetrating the posterior spinal cord. These patients do not require additional bedrest. Mayfield reported no incidence of cerebrospinal fluid fistulae from cervical spine surgery or laminectomy.

Nerve root injury is most common in posterior surgery. The fifth cervical nerve root is particularly vulnerable to any manipulation for reasons not fully understood. The sensory and motor divisions are often separated and the latter can be thinned and splayed by disc herniations. This is subject to injury if disc excision is anticipated and can be prevented by the use of the operating microscope and microinstrumentation. Often the neural foramina is very tight with the nerve root severely compromised. In this situation, the authors will use a high speed burr to thin the facet allowing removal of the residual bone with a currette. Attempting to remove the facet with a cervical punch is likely to result in neural trauma which may cause permanent weakness. In most situations, the hard spurs at the posterior vertebral bodies' edge do not have to be moved.

Prevention of cervical root injuries requires the compulsive avoidance of handling the root. The surgeon should attempt to work away from the root. If one has to work around the root, the use of microinstruments and magnification will prevent excessive retraction. Care should be observed not to retract medially where the spinal cord can be injured as well.

Thermal injuries of the nerve roots can be avoided by the use of bi-polar electrocautery. Microscopic vision is particularly useful in the lateral recesses of the spinal canal. The spinal cord should never be touched with the instrument. Coagulation levels should be carefully set to the least amount of current needed and tested on the subcutaneous tissue before use in the spinal canal.

§ 7-6(B). Immediate Postoperative Complications.

These include pulmonary atelectasis, urinary retention, wound problems, thrombophlebitis, and ileus. These are general postoperative complications and as a result not unique to cervical spine surgery.

§ 7-6(B)(1). Pulmonary Atelectasis.

Pulmonary atelectasis is the result of inadequate ventilation of portions of the lung alveoli. The tiny sac where exchange of gases occur collapse and/or fill with fluid. The complication is more common within 1-3 days after general anesthesia or in a patient with underlying lung disease (e.g., smoker). The clinical picture is one of fever in the immediate postoperative period. Clinical examination and chest radiographs are usually normal although occasionally an area of collapse will be seen. Treatment is directed at mobilizing the patient and reinflating the hypoventilated lung area by coughing and deep breathing. If these measures fail, positive end expiratory pressure breathing or incentive spirometry can be of help.

§ 7-6(B)(2). Urinary Retention.

Urinary retention occurs commonly after any major surgery. The cause is usually multifactorial with age, emotions, outlet obstruction, and neurologic factors acting to a lesser or greater extent. Clearly, the use of narcotics in a borderline situation contribute to the inability to void. Initial treatment should be a trial of voiding with mobilization of the patient. If retention persists, an intermittent cathetarization program 3 to 4 times daily with antibiotic coverage is preferred. Rarely, if the bladder tone is greatly depressed an indwelling foley will be needed. The problem with urinary retention and residual urine has the potential for secondary infection and cystitis.

§ 7-6(B)(3). Intestinal Ileus.

Intestinal ileus is occasionally seen after cervical spine surgery and general anesthesia. The clinical picture includes symptoms of nausea and vomiting, abdominal distention, and hypoactive bowel sounds. The initial management necessitates holding all oral foods and liquids with intravenous supplements. The patient should also be encouraged to move about. Rarely a nasogastric tube with intermittent suction is needed until normal bowel peristalsis resumes.

§ 7-6(B)(4). Thrombophlebitis and Pulmonary Embolus.

Thrombophlebitis and pulmonary embolus are fortunately infrequent complications of modern spine surgery. The routine use of antithrombotic stockings as well as early mobilization undoubtedly contribute. The syndrome of thrombophlebitis consists of pain, swelling, and redness along the course of the involved vein. Rarely, the clinical course will be progressive with embolism of small clots to the lung. The situation is further complicated by the occurrence of pulmonary emboli unheralded by local symptoms of thrombophlebitis. Treatment is symptomatic with rest, heat, and anticoagulation as the cornerstone of therapy. The routine use of anticoagulation in spine surgery is not warranted unless the patient is at very high risk for pulmonary embolus. Even then the risk of wound hematoma and neural compression compared to prophylaxis against thrombophlebitis must be weighed. An incidence of 0.2% fatal pulmonary embolus was reported by Mayfield in a series of 1,402 patients (entry 13).

§ 7-6(B)(5). Wound Problems.

Wound problems can complicate any surgical procedure. Prevention is the best treatment. The skin should be incised sharply not retracted unduly, use of the unipolar electrocautery but to a minimum and not near the skin edge, and use of prophylactic antibiotics. Routine periodic wound irrigation is also recommended with an antibiotic solution.

Wound infection will usually present about one week after the operation with swelling, redness, and pain about the incision. The wound should be cultured with a gram stain if the clinical suspicion exists. If purulence is noted, the wound will have to be opened and preferrably irrigated and debrided in the operating room. Antibiotics are used as the culture and sensitivity dictate.

Rarely, the infection will develop in the depths of the wound and local symptoms except for local pain will be scarce. The patient will have fever and malaise. An epidural abscess must be considered and if substantiated by aspiration of the wound, immediate surgery is mandatory. Surgical debridement and drainage will prevent sequalae like meningitis and even death. Epidural abscesses can occasionally cause a progressive neurologic deterioration with minimal symptoms suggesting infection. Drainage and debridement are an emergency if neurologic function is to be preserved. Wound infections occurred in 1% of the cases in Mayfield's review (entry 13).

§ 7-6(B)(6). Spinal Cord Compression.

Spinal cord compression with acute quadriparesis within the first few hours of surgery strongly suggests an epidural hematoma. If after decompressive cervical surgery the patient is weaker in the recovery room, this must be considered. Other potential causes include spinal cord injury either by manipulation or vascular injury. Hematoma collection must be rapidly drained if neurologic recovery is to be anticipated. The routine use of a closed system drainage system (e.g., Hemovac R) will serve to lesson this dreaded complication.

§ 7-6(C). Technical Complications Resulting in Persistent Symptoms.

Technical complications are problems directly related to the surgical procedure and the surgeon's judgement. Some of the complications are avoidable while others are not depending on the operative procedure.

§ 7-6(C)(1). Inadequate Nerve Root Decompression.

Inadequate nerve root decompression can be the cause of persistent arm pain after surgery. This is unusual after posterolateral "keyhole" foraminotomy but may result after anterior disc excision. The syndrome probably represents compression via the neurocentral joints of Lushka and will respond to a posterolateral foraminotomy. Other causes in the presence of an adequate decompression include traumatic neuritis or unrecognized nerve root compression at an adjacent level. The results of multiple posterolateral foraminotomies are good and should be done if evidence suggests more than one nerve root involved. The presence of a retained hard or soft disc as the cause of persistent symptoms is controversial. At present, re-exploration to find this pathology is not warranted. Disc fragments do not migrate as in the lumbar spine.

§ 7-6(C)(2). Inadequate Spinal Cord Decompression.

Inadequate spinal cord decompression is impossible to define by rigid criteria. The literature is divided as to the amount of lamina to be removed and the removal of spondylitic burs or spurs. The results have roughly been equivalent without clearly demonstrable statistical differences. Coupled with this is the poor understanding of the myelopathic process. One might ask, are the persistent myelopathic findings a result of the disease (irreversible spinal cord compression) or an inadequate decompression? For example, Epstein has stated that no patient over the age of 70 years with myelopathy has improved with laminectomy in his experience (entry 6).

If the patient's symptoms have been progressive preoperatively and continue unabated despite surgery, inadequate decompression is possible. Approaching the disease from the opposite side of the neck of the original procedure is reasonable if the patient's general health and demands permit. The surgical goals of cervical spine decompression should be in most instances a stabilization of the disease (Nurick's Class IV, V) or some improvement (Nurick's Class I-III).

§ 7-6(C)(3). Disc Space Infection.

Disc space infection is a potential cause of persistent neck pain with or without arm pain unique to anterior disc excisions. In the cervical spine, removal of disc material or currettage of the disc from the posterior approach is contraindicated. Therefore, this complication is not seen with posterior procedures.

Disc space sepsis should be considered in any patient who has had anterior cervical disc surgery within one to six weeks, who has a rapid, dramatic occurrence of neck and/or arm pain. The patient will often not demonstrate a high fever but the sedimentation rate will be very high and the technicium 99m diphosphonate bone scan will be very hot in the disc area. Serial radiographs will demonstrate disc space narrowing associated with irregular end plate destruction on both sides of the disc and ultimately, a sclerotic reaction.

The treatment of a disc space infection includes rest, immobilization, and antibiotics. If the patient demonstrates systemic symptoms, or fails to respond to initial conservative courses with antibiotics directed at staphylococcus, an open biopsy of the disc for culture and sensitivity is required. The biopsy is safely done via the anterior approach. Most patients do not have lasting sequalae if diagnosis and treatment are prompt, but chronic osteomyelitis can occur which is exceedingly resistant to treatment.

§ 7-6(C)(4). Iliac Crest Pain.

Iliac crest donor site pain is one of the most bothersome causes of persistent pain after anterior disc excision and fusion. To avoid this, the posterior approach has been used by some, while Brown and Associates (entry 3) favor the use of frozen allograft bone to avoid the iliac crest donor area. Fusion rates are acceptable at 94%, but there is a two-fold increased rate of graft collapse.

If anterior disc excision with antogenous bone graft is planned, preoperative counseling as to the problem will often lessen the patient's pain response. Technically, the authors use a longitudinal incision avoiding the lateral femoral cutaneous and cluneal nerves. Strict hemostasis and a tight closure help to alleviate the acute severe pain. Despite the most careful technique, some residual pain is frequent and unavoidable.

§ 7-6(C)(5). Late Instability and Degenerative Changes.

Late instability or degenerative changes can occur after cervical spine surgery and contribute to persistent pain. Late instability can take two forms; kyphotic deformities after anterior disc excision of two or more adjacent levels without fusion or extensive posterior laminectomy especially in the younger patient (entry 4). Additionally, late degenerative changes above and below an anterior fusion area occur in over 80% of cases (entry 11). Fortunately, these are rarely symptomatic, but tend to be radiographically progressive. When symptoms relate to either late instability or degenerative processes, a cervical fusion is indicated.

§ 7-6(C)(6). Foreign Bodies.

Foreign body retention is rare in the current practice of accurate sponge and needle counts, and radiographic opaque tagging of sponges and cotton pledgets. Unfortunately, on a rare occasion, a pledget can be detached from its string and lost in the wound. These foreign bodies usually cause minimal to no symptoms, but may incite an inflammatory response and should be removed. Other potential irritating substances could include bone wax, antithrombotic agents, and glove powder.

§ 7-7. Summary.

This chapter has outlined the present indications for successful cervical spine surgery. As one reads the voluminous literature on cervical spine surgery, certain precepts, principles, and requirements are evident:

1. Accurate knowledge of the variable normal and abnormal anatomic findings.
2. Precise diagnosis of nerve or spinal cord compression.
3. Understanding of the natural history of the pathologic process.
4. Selection of the proper operative procedure.
5. Skillful execution of the procedure by an experienced spine surgeon.
6. Prompt recognition and treatment of complications.
7. Careful postoperative care.
8. Long term follow-up of the patients.

When patients are treated according to these principles, the results of the surgery are very predictable and gratifying to both the surgeons and their patients.

BIBLIOGRAPHY

1. Aronson, N.I. The management of sott disc protrusions using the Smith-Robinson approach. Clin Neurosurg, 20:253, 1973.
2. Bohlman, H.H. Cervical spondylosis with moderate to severe myelopathy. Spine, 2:151-162, 1977.
3. Brown, M.A., Malinin, T.I., Davis, P.B. A roentgenographic evaluation of frozen allografts versus autografts in anterior cervical spine fusions. CORR, 119:231-236, 1976.
4. Callahan, R.A., et al. Cervical facet fusion for control of instability following laminectomy. JBJS, 59A:991-1002, 1977.
5. DePalma, A.F., et al. Anterior interbody fusion for severe cervical disc degeneration. Surg Gynec Obstr, 134:755-758, 1972.
6. Epstein, J.A., Janin, Y. *The Cervical Spine: Management of Cervical Spondylotic Myeloradiculopathy By the Posterior Approach,* 402-410. Philadelphia, J.B. Lippincott Company, 1983.
7. Flynn, T. Neurologic complications of anterior cervical interbody fusion. Spine, 7:536-539, 1982.
8. Henderson, C.M., et al. Posterior — lateral foraminotomy as an exclusive operative technique for cervical radiculopathy: a review of 846 consecutively operated cases. Neurosurgery, 13:504-512, 1983.
9. Hicks, D.S., Whitecloud, T.S., Gracco, A., LaRocca, S.H. Cervical spondylotic myelopathy: results of anterior decompression and stabilization. Orthop Trans, 4:44, 1980.
10. Hollenhorst, R.W., Suien, H.J., Benoit, C.F. Unilateral blindness occurring during anesthesia for neurosurgical operation. Arch Ophthalmol, 52:819-830, 1954.
11. Hunter, L.Y., et al. Radiographic changes following anterior cervical fusion. Spine, 5:399-401, 1980.
12. Lunsford, L.D., Bissonette, D.J., Janetta, P.J., Sheptak, P.E., Zorub, D.S. Anterior surgery for cervical disc disease. J Neurosurgery, 53:1-11, 1980.
13. Mayfield, F.H. Complications of laminectomy. Clin Neurosurg, 23:435-439, 1975.
14. Nurick, S. The pathogenesis of the spinal cord disorder associated with cervical spondylosis. Brain, 95:87, 1972.

15. Ranawat, C.S., et al. Cervical spine fusion in R.A. JBJS, 61A:1003-1010, 1979.
16. Rothman, R.H., Simeone, F.A. *The Spine,* 440-449, Philadelphia, W.B. Saunders, 1982.
17. Saunders, R.L., Wilson, D.H. The surgery of cervical disc disease: new perspectives. CORR, 146:119-127, 1980.
18. Scoville, W.B. Types of cervical disc lesions and their surgical approaches. JAMA, 196:479-481, 1966.
19. Smith, G.W. and Robinson, R.A. The treatment of certain cervical spine disorders by anterior removal of the intervertebral disc and interbody fusion. JBJS, 40A:607-624, 1958.
20. Southwick, S.M., White, A.A. The use of psychological tests in the evaluation of low back pain. JBJS, 65A: 560-565, 1983.
21. Tew, J.M., Mayfield, F.H. Complications of surgery of the anterior cervical spine. Clin Neurosurg, 23:424-434, 1975.
22. Upton, A.R.M., McComas, A.J. The double crush in nerve entrapment syndromes. Lancet, 2:359, 1973.
23. White, A.A., Panjabi, M.M., Posner, I., Edwards, W.T., Hayes, C.W. Spinal stability: evaluation and treatment. Instruction Course Lectures, Vol. 30:457-483, 1981.
24. Whitesides, T.A. *The Cervical Spine: Management of Radiculopathy and Myelopathy by the Anterior Approach,* 411-423. Philadelphia, J.B. Lippincott Company, 1983.
25. Wiesel, S.W., Rothman, R.H. Occipitoatlantal hypermobility. Spine, 4:187-192, 1979.
26. Zhang, Z., Yin, H., Yang, K., Zhang, T., Dong, F., Dang, G., Lou, S., Cai, Q. Anterior intervertebral disc excision and bone grafting in cervical spondylotic myelopathy. Spine, 8:16-19, 1983.

Figure 1

Removal of Osteophytic Spur

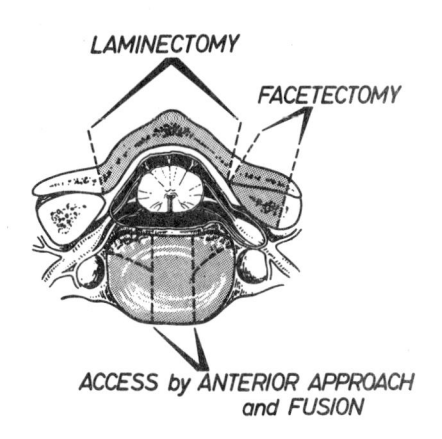

LAMINECTOMY

FACETECTOMY

ACCESS by ANTERIOR APPROACH and FUSION

Removal of osteophytic spur through dowel (Cloward) anterior approach. Through the cylindrical interbody opening, instruments can enter the intervertebral foramen and remove significant portions of the spur and adjacent vertebral body. This is done prior to removal of the anterior longitudinal ligament by fine Kerrison rongeurs.

Rothman and Simeone, *The Spine,* Philadelphia, W.B. Saunders Company, 1982. Reprinted by permission.

CHAPTER 8

PSYCHOSOCIAL PROSPECTIVES ON CHRONIC NECK PAIN

Brian Schulman, M.D.

§ 8-1. Introduction.
§ 8-2. Pain and the American Worker.
§ 8-3. Illness and Disease.
§ 8-4. Acute and Chronic Pain.
§ 8-5. What Is Chronic Pain?
§ 8-6. Psychosocial Affects of Chronic Pain.
§ 8-7. "The Patient in Pain" Versus "The Pain Patient."
§ 8-8. Is Chronic Pain Really a Variant of Depression?
§ 8-9. Are Chronic Pain Patients Depressed?
§ 8-10. The Complications of Treatment.
§ 8-11. The Failure of Traditional Treatment.
§ 8-12. The Adverse Effect of Pain Treatment on Pain Patients.
    § 8-12(A). Polypharmacy and the Overutilization of Analgesics.
    § 8-12(B). Loss of the Ability to Work.
    § 8-12(C). Experiencing the Loss of a Future Sense.
    § 8-12(D). Disruption of Social and Family Situations.
    § 8-12(E). Inappropriate Surgery and Hospitalization.
§ 8-13. Understanding the Pain Complaint.
§ 8-14. Pain as a Four Component System.
    § 8-14(A). Stage I: Nociception.
    § 8-14(B). Stage II: The Pain Message.
    § 8-14(C). Stage III: Suffering.
    § 8-14(D). Stage IV: Pain Behavior.
    § 8-14(E). Summary: Implications for the Treatment of Pain.
§ 8-15. The Importance of the Meaning of Pain.
§ 8-16. Doing and Not Doing.
Bibliography.

§ 8-1. Introduction.

What is pain? This is an age old question which has troubled philosophers and scientists since before Aristotle's time. Varieties of this complex sensory sensation have been recognized from 200 A.D., when Galen separated sensory nerve fibers and delineated the particular pain nerves. Since then, our understanding, as well as our ability to treat pain has expanded. Yet, we are still a long way from a satisfactory solution.

Most physicians agree that pain is still one of the most difficult and complex medical conditions to understand and treat. Pain is an enigma, it describes the feeling of getting a toe stubbed, as well as the sensation of losing a loved one. It is at once an extreme physical response to a noxious stimulus, as well as the emotion of suffering. Pain has as many meanings as there are people who complain of suffering from it.

In medicine, pain has many qualities, it is described by its intensity, location, duration and radiation (the course it follows). Pain creates a state of discomfort that is clearly distinguishable from touch or other tactile sensations. And, that "discomfort" is highly regulatory — that is, pain has an enormous power to influence and determine behavior. A patient in pain is quickly, and rather dramatically preoccupied by the experience of being in pain. Pain has a way of wiping out all other emotions, thoughts and feelings from conscious awareness. While pain may not be the most important thing a person experiences, it very quickly becomes the only thing that really matters.

§ 8-2. Pain and the American Worker.

Pain is a major factor in occupational disability. Recent polls indicate that pain causes a loss of about four billion sick days per year — or 23 days per worker. By extrapolating data, statisticians have shown that in 1984, 97 million American backs "went out" and 127 million complained of suffering with headache (entry 18).

Surprisingly, age was inversely related to pain. Younger people were more likely to suffer most types of pain, especially headache and backache. Other demographics showed more women experienced pain than men; and white Americans are far more likely than blacks or Hispanics to complain of a pain problem.

The data, taken by pollsters, makes us aware of how common a problem pain is and how much of an effect it has on the utilization of health benefits, as well as job attendance and productivity. Although two workers may suffer the same injury, their response to that injury may be traumatically variable. There are those stoic people who find illness intolerable and resent being sick, especially if the illness interferes with their work or daily activities; and will struggle, often in pain or with significant restriction of movement, to resume their particular level of activity.

Others are not so motivated and are incapacitated by even a mild injury, such as whiplash or cervical strain syndrome. Where as the normal course of events tells us that the cervical strain should be self-healing, and the pain and stiffness ameliorate within a week or two, there are those individuals who will go on for months, even years, complaining of constant unremitting pain that evolved from a simple cervical strain injury. How does one go about explaining this paradox? In general, the emphasis has been on trying to discover what disease lies beneath the cervical strain. If a worker is unable to return to work following an uncomplicated injury, the assumption is that maybe something else is wrong. The assumption is that underlying all impairment is some major disease.

It may come as a shock to the medical layman, that doctors and medical researchers can (and often do), disagree as to whether a disease is really a disease. A good example is chronic pain syndrome. Whereas in acute pain, pain is the body's alerting sensation that warns of danger and initiates the body's healing response; in chronic pain, pain is itself the disease. Dr. Wilbert Fordyce, of the Rehabilitation Medicine Department of Washington School of Medicine, believes that learning and conditioned response play an important role in the disease chronic pain (entry 8). For example, *primary emotional factors* (the need for punishment, the desire to be cared for, etc.), the issue of *secondary gain* (such as monetary judgments, the *avoidance of stressful or dangerous work,* the attention of family), and the habituation to pain-killing medications may all play ideologic roles in the so called "disease" of chronic pain. At this time, there is considerable disagreement as to whether chronic pain is a unique disease, or simply a nonspecific form of chronic illness behavior.

§ 8-3. Illness and Disease.

It is important to distinguish between two often interchangeable, but distinct concepts — illness and disease. Although these items are used interchangeably by lay public, and many physicians, they are not similar. Disease is defined as an anatomic deformity or pathologic process that can be objectively demonstrated by either clinical, laboratory or radiographic examination.

Disease is generally associated with tissue damage, and/or changes in the mental status, and is usually related to a specific etiology such as infective agents, trauma, toxins, degenerative changes or specific psychosocial changes. Disease may be psychiatric and purely subjective, or at least determinable only by the clinical mental status examination or other psychological testing. In these cases, disease is demonstrable by virtue of changes in mental status, alterations in cognition, changes in emotional responsivity and distortions or disruptions in interpersonal relationships. Additionally, all disease is predictable. That is, disease has a demonstrable progression (pathogenesis), as well as a defined response to specific treatment.

Illness is a much more encompassing concept than disease involving not only the biologic, but the social, occupational, familial, and volitional state of a person. Frequently, the illness, as manifest by a person's symptoms and behavior, does not parallel the course of disease.

Illness can be influenced by any factor that effects the well-being of a person. Therefore, illness takes into account the personal nature of suffering (entry 6), the response to life change (such as separations, loss, financial changes) (entry 17), stress (entry 14), and the loss of vocational stability and social support system. Also, of great importance, is the nature of the doctor/patient relationship. Unfortunately, many physicians trained to emphasize the scientific aspects of medical care may neglect the fact that disease is only one aspect of an illness.

Thus, illness encompasses all aspects of a person or his behavior, that deals with his being sick or alternatively, not being well. To correctly measure the severity of an illness, and the concomitant impairment of the person who is ill, one must assess all aspects of an individual's biology, behavior, and psychology. For example, the amount of time a person spends resting in bed, the use of medication, the number and type of physician consults, are objective measures of the *amount of illness behavior.* Additionally, the frequency and intensity of complaints, the amount of perceived impairment, and the limitations on activity are related examples of subjective evidence of illness behavior.

In monitoring the progress of an ill person, one appreciates a "Gestalt" or overall picture of how a person is doing. This general impression — a summation of a host of perceived behaviors — is global and nonspecific. Nonetheless, on balance the observer pictures a certain relationship between *illness behaviors* and, conversely, *healthy behaviors.* The whole — the impression left by the summation of illness and healthy behaviors — is the "state of a person's health," generally described as "healthy" or "sick," a shorthand way of saying a person is either "better" or "worse."

When evaluating occupational injuries of the neck and cervical spine, one must appreciate the distinction between illness — as a biopsychosocial process — and disease, which is an anatomic and pathophysiologic process. All too often, medical evaluation and treatment, subsequent litigation, including compensation determination, focuses too narrowly on the physical objective evidence of disease (the bioscientific-finding) and ignores the consequences of illness.

This over-emphasis on the hard science of disease does not comprehensively address the injured worker's level of impairment; i.e., the factors that are actually inhibiting his recovery and preventing a return to work. Indeed, overemphasis on disease and evidence of disease creates distortions in the process of health care delivery, as well as prejudicial patterns for compensation of injured workers. The facts — i.e., the biopsychosocial reasons for a worker's impairment — are subordinated or ignored. Instead, tunnel vision focused solely on discovering evidence of organic disease predominates, leading patient, doctor, and compensation carrier into the maelstrom of "find it and fix it medicine" (entry 1).

The outcome can be disastrous. Some victims of "back pain" have a history of as many as 40 operations, running from nerve blocks to the removal of spinal disks and the fusion of vertebrae (entry 24). These patients have been through courses of medicine, including muscle relaxants, pain killers (narcotic and non-narcotic), tranquilizers, antidepressants and more. They have gone on to paramedical treatment, such as chiropractic manipulation and adjustments of the spine, to acupuncture and eventually holistic healing. In the end, after all the searching, seeking and scarring, they are clinically discarded, the majority labeled "crocks," "masochists," or "malingerers." Simultaneously, medical science concedes as the patient retreats into a permanent state of nihilistic regression. The chronic complaints continue. Nothing they have tried has managed to *persuade* them to feel any better. They are "abused" patients. A conglomeration of well-versed complaints without even the dignity of a disease.

§ 8-4. Acute and Chronic Pain.

The effective treatment of pain requires one to distinguish between acute and chronic forms.

Acute pain is a consequence of a primary physiologic or pathologic event or process. The stimulation of nocireceptors (specialized sensory nerve endings that communicate the experience of pain) by crushing, stretching or inflammation initiates the experience of acute pain. The pain message is instantaneously communicated to the brain through a series of specialized nerve fibers. There, the pain is localized, measured and identified as an emotional experience. Adaptive homeostatic mechanisms are initiated. The muscles surrounding the injured site contract, moving the body away from the painful stimulus and protecting the injured area. A sympathetic response may occur as hormones and chemicals are released initiating the body's healing process.

Acute pain is self-limited. Once the offending pathology abates (i.e., the displaced disk is removed, the inflammation of bursitis is reduced), acute pain subsides.

Psychologically, neck pain is particularly disturbing as it "strikes close to home." It's all in the spinal cord and its plexus of nerves passes through the neck, neck pain can have far reaching and devastating effects in the body as a whole. The pain can radiate up the spine and become a headache, or down the back into a backache. It may shoot into the arms, the hands or radiate down the spine into the legs creating sensations ranging from intense lightning-like sensations to wavering periods of weakness.

The acute pain of cervical strain leaves that person restricted and in distress. He seeks relief, usually in the form of analgesics and a variety of "conservative" treatments (heat, physical therapy, possibly traction). The patient in acute pain seeks reassurance and confidence from his physician. If good communication is established and a reasonable treatment plan initiated, the acute pain patient will be able to endure the pain until the body's natural recuperative powers take over and promote healing.

§ 8-5. What Is Chronic Pain?

The term chronic pain syndrome is clinically applied to a large group of heterogenous patients who have regular and persistent complaints of pain. Their pain persists for six months or more and is refractory to the usual and customary medical treatment. These patients often lack a physical organic basis for pain, but have often sustained a musculoskeletal injury that heralds the advent of pain. In all cases, their impairment exceeds what one would expect from the physical findings alone.

Diagnosing the chronic pain syndrome is fraught with uncertainty as there are few hard signs of organic pathology. In the past ten years, this syndrome has been extensively described in the medical literature (entries 25, 26). Criteria for diagnosis are largely based on demographic and clinical characteristics of patients studied at major university medical centers specializing in pain treatment (entry 5).

The hypothetical chronic pain patient is approximately 45 years of age and may either be male or female. In general, he has suffered with pain from anywhere from three to five years.

A speculative gross psychological profile would include the following characteristics: This person comes from a large family with no history of any major psychiatric disorder, but an increased likelihood of a family chronic pain disorder. Typically, the person describes his early years (prior to the onset of pain) in glowing terms — free of any health related problems. Characteristically, there is an early acceptance of responsibility, possibly causing premature termination of education and training, and the undertaking of pronounced responsibilities in early adult life (entry 22).

The patient suffers from pain despite limited diagnostic findings and what appears to have been adequate medical treatment. Consequently, they seek multiple consultants, undergo a broad variety of therapies, ranging from physical therapy to acupuncture and spinal manipulation. By age 45, they have undergone an average of 2.2 surgical procedures, 6 hospitalizations and have a 75% likelihood of having suffered some significant episode of drug or substance abuse requiring pharmacologic withdrawal and/or hospitalization. Approximately 50% use narcotics on a regular basis. Codeine and oxycodone are the most commonly abused drugs. Many common pain patients use both tranquilizers and pain-killing medications. Fifteen to twenty percent use alcohol on a regular basis to cope with pain.

The most consistent finding in the chronic pain syndrome is the subjective complaint of pain, and the degree to which that complaint produces psychological, social, and vocational impairment (entry 20). The core symptoms appear to be excessive for physical findings (and often cannot be explained by physical findings alone), the issue of *pain* as a purely monosymptom is common. A finding that has led some authorities to conclude "that whereas in acute pain, the pain is the symptom of the disease; in chronic pain, the pain is the disease itself" (entry 10).

§ 8-6. Psychosocial Affects of Chronic Pain.

Patients with chronic pain syndrome are in continual pain. Often, a definitive pathologic diagnosis is lacking, and the physical findings are either absent or inconclusive. Patients with chronic pain syndrome "suffer" — they genuinely agonize in despair about their condition. They often lose interest in their life activities, feel helpless about their future, and retreat from responsibilities.

The family dynamics are strained. Initially, family members generously respond to the growing needs of the patient. However, over time, the confusion surrounding the diagnosis and the persistent state of disability, despite adequate care and treatment engenders some sense of frustration. As the syndrome progresses, and the patient regresses, the social and familial sequelae begin to take effect. Family members become irritated. The primary concern is the patient's preoccupation with pain and the increasing use of pain behavior and pain language to communicate with and manipulate family members. Healthy members become frustrated and lose patience. Eventually, resentment becomes a primary characteristic of the family dynamics. One readily available target of the pent-up anger and frustration is the physician (and health care system in general) viewed as "not helpful," "indifferent," or simply "ineffectual." In essence, the fault lies with the medical care giver who has failed to rescue the chronic pain patient and his family.

§ 8-7. "The Patient in Pain" Versus "The Pain Patient" (entry 25).

In the early 1970s, Dr. Richard Sterbach distinguished the "patient in pain" from the "the pain patient." Essentially, this is the difference between acute pain and the chronic pain syndrome. He pointed out that the "patient in pain" experiences a number of recurring acute painful events. During the episodes of pain, the predominate psychophysiologic state is *arousal*. The heart rate and cardiac output increase, breathing increases, and muscles tighten. The body prepares to "fight" the pain. The patient feels anxious and acutely distressed. The pain is an interruption and variance from the routine and expected. The "pain state" is perceived as alien and undesirable. In a psychological sense, the pain state is called ego-dystonic.

The "pain patient" or the one with chronic pain syndrome is another matter. *Pain is the central organizing feature of their lives.* They are always thinking, talking or acting out a feature of their pain. Pain is integrated into all aspects of living.

The psychophysiologic effects of pain are primarily regression and anergia (the loss of energy). Subjectively, these people experience a loss of initiative, poor appetite, cognitive dullness, mental blocking, as well as feelings of low self-esteem and sad mood. "Being and living in pain" is now a way of life, simply the way things are. Psychologically, it is said that their pain is ego-syntonic.

§ 8-8. Is Chronic Pain Really a Variant of Depression?

Because the psychophysiologic response to chronic pain is so similar to depression, many clinicians have considered chronic pain a variant of depression (entries 19, 2). Additionally, the clinical course of depression in chronic pain share many common "biological" features including anhedonia (the inability to experience happiness), anergia (the loss of energy), as well as a wide spectrum of appetite and sleep disturbances, cognitive and motor disturbances.

The view that chronic pain and depression are biologically similar disorders is fueled by the following evidence:

1. The discovery, in 1977, of beta-endorphins in the human brain, as well as the existence of an endogenous opiate system. This system, considered to be intimately involved with the internal regulation of well-being and pain is also intimated as contributing to schizophrenia, mania, and depressive symptomatology. Beta-endorphin has been suggested as a "biologic link" and as a common pathologic link between pain and depression.
2. Tricyclic antidepressant medications, a mainstay in the treatment of depression are commonly used, often with considerable benefit in the treatment of chronic pain states (entry 3). The reported clinical improvement of improved sleep, decreased fatigue, decreased preoccupation with pain, and a subjective feeling of energy and enthusiasm are found to be symptoms often associated with the clinical improvement from depression.
3. Patients with depression and chronic pain syndrome show an increased incidence of resistance to dexamethasone suppression (entry 9). This clinical test finding is suggestive of abnormal cortisol regulation and possible abnormalities in the pituitary adrenal axis — a finding often associated with biologic depression.
4. Various researchers have attempted to prove that chronic pain syndrome is a variant of depression through clinical studies. Such studies often focus on elevated depression subscales found on psychological testing (MMPI) or conclusions of structured interviews for depression. Other clinical studies show increased incidence of depression or depressive spectrum disorder in the first degree relative to the patients with chronic pain (entry 19).

Most studies attempting to prove that chronic pain is a variant of depression produce equivocal findings. Among experts, there is considerable disagreement over the degree of "overlap" between primary affective illness (depression) and the syndrome of chronic pain.

§ 8-9. Are Chronic Pain Patients Depressed?

The incidence of depressive symptoms is high among chronic pain patients (entry 11). Specifically, they complain of sleep disturbance, particularly difficulty falling asleep and staying asleep; hyperphagia (overeating with consequent obesity), motor agitation and restlessness, loss of concentration (increased distractibility, thought blocking, mental dullness), and excessive brooding and subjective sadness. Characteristically, this symptom complex is circumscribed around the "pain complaints." Typically, the pain patient states that the onset of all the psychological disturbances occurred following the "advent of pain."

Swanson (entry 22), reporting on the accumulative psychological test findings at the Mayo Clinic Pain Clinic, found that chronic pain patients are "convinced their pain is *caused* by organic (bodily) pathology, and that it is serious whether others concur or not." There is a firm rejection of psychological factors, or that the patient is in any way responsible for his problems. These patients admit to problems in expressing their feelings, such as anger, and acknowledge the presence of anxiety and depression, which they attribute completely to their pain problem. Yet, they deny life problems apart from their pain and illness.

Swanson speculatively concludes that benign, nonprogressive chronic pain can be conceptualized as a chronic emotional disorder, not unlike the syndromes of anxiety or depression, but distinct from either (entry 21).

While many chronic pain patients are depressed, the majority vehemently denies symptoms of depression, except as they relate to the suffering associated with coping with unremitting pain. Pilowsky and Associates (entry 16) examined a series of 200 consecutive admissions to a pain clinic and found only 10% of them had a depressive syndrome. Pilowsky (1979) (entry 15) considered the apparent depression of chronic pain patients, to be more a demoralization than depression. Maruta (1976) (entry 12), in comparing chronic pain patients to those with depression, found that chronic pain patients showed less acceptance of psychological concepts and "dealt with their current life stresses through the medium of somatic complaints rather than emotional distress." It is my feeling that chronic pain is not necessarily a progenitor of depression. Clinically, many chronic patients are so overwhelmingly preoccupied and focused on "pain" and the "relief of pain" that they are unable to experience depression, a far more subtle and ambiguous emotional state.

§ 8-10. The Complications of Treatment.

Often, in the management of chronic pain states, the physician (or other health care provider) renders treatment that may make the patient worse. Conflict invariably arises when the goal of providing effective care is frustrated by an unresponsive patient, particularly when the patient complains about the persistence of pain in the absence of objective organic findings. This typical case results in a confrontation between physician and patient that ultimately leads to certain complications. These are inevitably found in the treatment of chronic pain patients.

§ 8-11. The Failure of Traditional Treatment.

The "failure of treatment" and the "persistence of pain" evokes a subtle struggle between physician and patient.

Often, both the physician and the patient are unwitting participants in what becomes a circle of futile treatment and negative response to medical care.

The following events routinely occur:

1. The physician persists in his therapeutic efforts despite evidence that the treatment is ineffective. Common examples include excessive and overextensive efforts at physical therapy including diathermy, ultrasound and the application of transcutaneous nerve stimulation. When these procedures fail to produce the intended response, the physician is left with a sense of frustration and the patient begins to believe that efforts at physical rehabilitation including thermal modalities are useless.
2. The application of frequent analgesic trigger injections of corticosteroids and anesthetic agents when the efficacy is minimal and the duration of pain relief is short-lived.
3. The repetition of neurodiagnostic procedures (EEG, EMG, Cat scans, myelography) in the absence of objective clinical signs which would indicate the appropriateness of confirmative diagnostic tests. The use of neurodiagnostic procedures as a process of discovery as opposed to a means of confirmation leave the patient with a sense of uncertainty about the nature of his care. Often, the chronic pain patient believes that something inside of him is "broken" or otherwise "damaged" and that the failure of medicine is the failure of "discovering the cause." This leads to the extensive and often inappropriate use of diagnostic procedures as a means of "fishing" for the answer.
4. The revolving referral of pain patients from specialist to specialist. This process is enhanced by the current treating physicians developing a strong negative attitude toward their recalcitrant pain patients.

Frustration leads to impatience and a desire to rid themselves of noncompliant patients whose complaints are grossly out of proportion to the degree of known organic illness. The chronic pain patient thus enters the "pain-go-round" (entry 20). The loss of a primary care physician is an inevitable consequence of over-referral. This leads to the poor integration of care, repetitious procedures and multiple medications. There is a lack of integration and orchestration.

5. The failure of therapy has a natural escalating effect on the type of treatment rendered. As more conservative, benign treatment, such as analgesics, muscle relaxants, and physical therapy fail, there is a tendency to prescribe more aggressive and ultimately invasive procedures. First, the patient is hospitalized for prolonged periods of traction, often with minimal relief, and ultimately surgical interventions, which, at first deferred, are ultimately considered and implemented.

6. Patients with chronic pain typically shun psychiatric treatment, even when that treatment is conducted in the "pain clinic" (entry 21). Although much is said about the efficacy of a biopsychosocial approach to pain management, few centers can actually alter the traditional medical hard science approach to health care sufficiently to avoid the stigmatization of a mind versus body pain. Thus, in what remains a dichotomized health care delivery system, a psychiatric referral is viewed as a delegation to second-rate treatment and has a pejorative and negative implication — that the pain is really "self-created." There is little doubt left in the patient's mind that the examination of psychosocial issues is a direct consequence of the failure to find a real organic basis for pain; thus, the perceived pain is viewed as a deficiency of mind. Compliance with and the acceptance of psychiatric treatment is severely affected.

§ 8-12. The Adverse Effect of Pain Treatment on Pain Patients.

In the course of treating pain patients, certain adverse consequences are often encountered. I will enumerate some of the more common problems:

§ 8-12(A). Polypharmacy and the Overutilization of Analgesics.

Typically, chronic pain patients are prescribed a wide range of analgesics. In chronic pain states, analgesics may serve to aggravate an already complicated problem. This is particularly true of narcotics which invariably complicate and prolong the pain condition. In fact, many authorities believe that analgesics are contraindicated in all chronic pain conditions with the possible exception of cancer pain (entry 25).

As chronic pain states are long-term conditions, the ability of narcotics to manage these states is extremely limited — with high potential for dependency, habituation and abuse.

In a study conducted at the Mayo Clinic's Pain Clinic in 1979, the extent of the drug habituation was found to be enormous. Of 144 patients with chronic pain of nonmalignant cause, 35 (25%) were drug-dependent, 59 (41%) were viewed as drug abusers, and 50 (35%) were nonabusers (entry 23).

Fully two-thirds of all clinical pain patients were either dependent or abusers meaning that many of these people had no medical explanation for the sustained use of the drug and were experiencing the need for increasing daily doses of a narcotic.

§ 8-12(B). Loss of the Ability to Work.

Typically, the occupationally injured worker is *sent home* to get well. In chronic pain states, this process may last anywhere from a few weeks to twenty years. The loss of wage-earning ability is only one of the many stressors the home-bound worker faces. More significant in extending disability, is the loss of occupational role and the absence of a daily structure for time and activity. The injured, "pained" worker sits home. With children in school and spouse at work, the injured worker confronts a role reversal and the absence of specific tasks and responsibilities.

The consequences include — disrupted wake/sleep patterns. Sleeping during the day (often to relieve ennui and boredom) combined with decreased physical activity, causes sleep difficulties at night such as difficulty falling asleep or staying asleep.

With increasing time to "think" or "worry," the pain patient begins to focus on his pain and to become increasingly aware of its distressing qualities. The pain patient begins to experience an increased feeling of social and occupational impotence. The *idea of working* becomes stressful and overwhelming. Further, workers with dangerous jobs ponder the likelihood of some catastrophe (such as roofers "freezing," bus drivers being "assaulted," or glazers "falling"). The high-risk worker may, in the process of *resting* at home, "lose his nerve" and unconsciously fear returning to work. The likely expression of this mental conflict is in the form of increased pain perception.

§ 8-12(C). Experiencing the Loss of a Future Sense.

Commonly, the injured, pain-afflicted worker is advised to assume modified duty to facilitate a return to work. Often, the imposed restrictions obviate the job function and leave the worker perplexed as to what, if anything, he can do to earn a living. In most manual trades, there is no perceived limited or modified duty, i.e., a bricklayer is expected to lay "x" number of bricks per day, a roofer must agilely climb, the bus driver must be 100% vigilant and attentive.

While modified duty can often facilitate early return to work, many times the restrictions leave the worker psychologically fearful of not being able to perform adequately at his previous level of competence. Further, workers take great pride in their acquired skills and the advice to simply "be retrained" or assume "another occupation" is fraught with high levels of anticipatory anxiety. Many people are unable to conceive of doing anything other than their perceived occupational role.

§ 8-12(D). Disruption of Social and Family Situations.

The regression often associated with chronic illness behavior creates considerable role distortion. The adult pain patient undergoes a transactional crisis in the family as chronic "invalidism" becomes an erosive force among family and friends.

The fear of not performing — either sexually or emotionally — leads to abstinence and social withdrawal. Studies show that there is a high incidence of sexual problems in men and women with chronic pain (entry 19). Up to 80% of patients in a particular study experienced a deterioration in sexual adjustment with decreased quality and frequency of sexual experience.

§ 8-12(E). Inappropriate Surgery and Hospitalization.

The persistent chronic pain complaints, as well as the preoccupation with pain, lead responsible and competent physicians to pursue more invasive means of treatment. Surgical procedures that are equivocal are pursued with the hope of establishing some type of permanent amelioration of the pain problem. Patients are perceived as being desperate and unresponsive to any other treatment; thus, a more dramatic form of therapy appears to be indicated and warranted.

This leaves the patient with a state of residual disability that is a direct consequence of some type of therapeutic intervention. Whether this is in the form of substance dependency or the residuals of a failed back syndrome, the ultimate outcome is persistence of chronic pain and continued disability.

§ 8-13. Understanding the Pain Complaint.

In 1977, Dr. George Engel proposed a biopsychosocial approach to medical care (entry 7). Borrowing heavily from general systems theory, the biopsychosocial approach proposes to see the patient in dynamic equilibrium with his total environment. The biology of a person is composed of intricate microsystems of chemical and cellular reaction. This biology adapts to the demands of the "environment" — one that includes psychological as well as social, occupational, political, and economic variables. A person is constantly seeking adaptation within this environment — a state of health poised somewhere along a continuum between "health" (i.e., good health) and illness.

In the biopsychosocial model, *everything* counts, a consideration which has made its implementation in the hard science milieu of 20th century American medicine a formidable task. In teaching this model to medical students, I have found considerable resistance and confusion. "If *everything* matters, how do I know what to do for the patient . . . how do I know what is *really* important?"

The modern physician's dilemma has its roots in the technologically hard science origins of modern medical practice — origins heavily biased toward a biologic model of disease and pathology. The model assumes that all disease is caused by some infective agent, anatomic malformation or injury, or a pathophysiologic process (such as headache caused by muscle contraction in the neck and shoulder girdle). Biologic evidences of disease are called signs and can be identified by physical laboratory or x-ray examination. These findings are commonly considered medically determinable evidence because they have a *biologic* basis and can be objectively identified.

Chronic pain experiences defy the limitations of a strictly biologic approach. Psychosocial variables, however complex and subjective, are inextricably linked with the progression of the syndrome. To successfully treat the "patient in pain" or more commonly, the "pain patient," one must apply some form of reductionistic analysis to the pain complaint. Such delineation will clarify much of the enigma that chronic pain states create.

§ 8-14. Pain as a Four Component System.

To understand the psychosocial consequences of pain, it is helpful to divide the pain complaint into four components: nociception, pain message, suffering, and pain behavior (entry 4).

Nociception involves the chemistry of pain perception. Components of nociception are almost entirely biological, the reactions are chemical and physiological. The *pain message* involves the neurological transmission of perception into the central nervous system. Here the neurological and orthopedic systems play critical, but not exclusive roles. As the message enters the thalamus, limbic system of the brain and higher cortical centers, psychological and emotional variables influence the pain experience. *Suffering* is the third component, it compasses the person as a whole, his experience of pain and the meaning of that pain as it pertains to the present and future of the person. Finally, the *pain behavior* is the totality of pain-regulated behavior, the manifestation of pain on the thought, feeling, planning, and lifestyle of a person.

§ 8-14(A). Stage I: Nociception.

Nociception refers to the mechanical, thermal or chemical stimulation of nerve fibers. When nociceptors are stimulated, pain is evoked. The stimulation is effected by certain chemicals (amines, peptides, and derivatives of lipids) coming into contact with the nociceptor nerve fibers. One common feature that precedes the stimulation of nociceptors is inflammation — a complex event involving increased blood flow, increased permeability of blood vessels and the interaction of certain blood cells. For example, arachidonic acid (a breakdown product of a lipid cell constituent), and its metabolites, the prostaglandins and the leukotrienes, excite the nociceptors. The effect of the analgesic aspirin — and other anti-inflammatory agents — is felt to act in part by inhibiting the metabolism of arachidonic acid to prostaglandins. Thus, aspirin is effective in relieving pain *associated with inflammation,* but is not effective when pain is unrelated to inflammation (entry 9). Thus, it is likely that prostaglandins are mediators for nociceptive activation only in the presence of inflammation and that other as yet unidentified chemical intermediaries are involved in noninflammatory pain.

What we are learning is that the chemistry of pain perception is quite complex, but very specific to the interaction of nociceptors with their chemical environment.

§ 8-14(B). Stage II: The Pain Message.

Impulses from pain receptors are communicated along special nerve fibers from the body into the spinal cord. Shortly after entering the spinal cord, neurons synapse at a point in the cord called the dorsal horn. The synapse is a chemical communication that occurs at the site of the neural junction — the point where individual nerve cells (neurons) connect with each other.

The pain message may be transmitted through several different synapses as it is communicated to the brain. At the first synapse in the dorsal horn of the spinal cord, the pain message is divided into separate and distinct tracts, which travel to the brain. Simultaneously the message follows the spinothalamic tract to the thalamus (where the neuromessage is perceived as pain and then into the cortex where it is somatopically organized (given location, intensity, and character). Pain travels along fast and slow pathways into the brain, thus giving the opportunity to have an acute pain response as well as a more chronic protracted pain experience.

To experience pain the message must be received by the nervous system and be recognized as a negative signal of distress. Simply stated, to feel pain you must recognize the sensation as pain. The experience of pain must have been previously coded into the nervous system. Presumably, a memory bank for pain exists that mediates each new experience of pain.

However, not all pain is perceived as pain. The medical literature is replete with case histories of soldiers who suffer incredibly severe injuries, yet continue to fight unaware of any pain, or the soccer player with a fractured clavicle, who does not "feel pain" until hours after the athletic contest.

Thus, just having a nociceptive stimulation and a pain response (the reporting of pain into the central nervous system) does not guarantee the experience of pain. Factors such as intense attention to alternate activities (i.e., fighting for survival) can inhibit or dramatically modify the pain experience.

§ 8-14(C). Stage III: Suffering.

The third component of the pain complaint is *suffering* or a negative emotional response which is generated by higher brain centers. Pain has the capacity to evoke suffering and suffering can persist long after the cessation of a provoking pain.

Cassel (entry 6) has noted that suffering is distinct from physical distress . . . "that suffering is experienced by persons, not merely by bodies, and has its source in challenges that threaten the intactness of the person as a complex social and psychological entity. Suffering can include physical pain, but is by no means limited to it."

Reasonably, one can suffer from pain and the meaning of that pain. Especially the effects of that experience and one's appearance and ability, as well as the perception one has of his personal future. In one basic sense, suffering is the experience of threat to the intactness of a person and as such, the pain associated with suffering can be perceived as extraordinary and unremitting, regardless of the extent of the organic injury or illness.

§ 8-14(D). Stage IV: Pain Behavior.

Finally, the pain complaint involves *pain behavior* — all the thoughts, actions, activities, feelings, and possibilities of the pain patient are classified as pain behaviors. These behaviors either reinforce or aggravate the pain experience or serve the opposite effect and minimize the pain response and reduce the level of suffering. When pain behavior predominates and the activities of a person are circumscribed around the experience of "being in pain" he/she may exhibit a chronic illness behavior. Essential to the effective management of patients who exhibit severe self-reinforcing pain behavior is the recognition that behavior is very much a function of the degree of suffering — which may or may not be related to any original injury.

Factors that influence pain behavior may include things such as *primary gain* or unconscious drives, conflicts, and feelings that are motivating one toward behaving in a certain way. For example, dependency needs, unresolved infantile conflicts are influential in affecting pain behavior, as are *secondary gains,* or financial, social or occupational advantages that are incumbent in the pain illness experience. Factors such as job opportunities, compensation benefits, attention of family members, avoidance of certain unpleasant activities are all aspects of a person's lifestyle and environment that may influence the type of pain behavior he manifests.

§ 8-14(E). Summary: Implications for the Treatment of Pain.

By emphasizing the importance of suffering on the resultant chronic pain behaviors, the ambiguity and diagnostic uncertainty of chronic pain syndromes can be permanently avoided. Understanding the four-component theory of the pain complaint avoids the pejoritive connotation invariably associated with dividing pain into physical and psychological components.

It can be argued that the aim of medicine should more precisely address the relief of suffering. Over attention to the "objective" elements of pain, that is the site of injury, the nature of the disease, and the pathogenesis of disease processes, may be therapeutically restrictive.

Unfortunately, a pure biologic approach fails to adequately or even accurately address the source of a person's distress. Managing the biological determinence alone is necessary, but not sufficient, to control chronic pain. For example, the state of nociception, where the chemistry of inflammation stimulates the pain perception mechanisms, is dramatically responsive to anti-inflammatory agents. The efficacy of aspirin has stood the test of time, and remains a mainstay in the management of acute and episodic inflammatory disorders. The new generation of prosaglandins sythetase inhibitors more specifically affects pain relief by inhibiting the initial reaction in the genesis of pain — actually preventing the stimulation of nociceptors.

The use of traction, bed rest, and physical therapy modalities are critical when one is managing problems related to pain message disorders, especially those where excessive muscle contraction, physical deconditioning and fatigue play instrumental roles in amplifying the pain experience; of course, the utility and effectiveness of surgical intervention, where nerve entrapment, encroachment, or compression are pathologically active and pain producing.

The relief of suffering is a different matter. Medicine has been overly restrained in its attention to the relief of suffering, often delegating this seemingly ubiquitous task to the supporting family, friends, clergy, and other paraprofessionals. When directly addressed in the medical milieu, the relief of suffering is much more the responsibility of nurses than physicians. Even social workers, technicians, and paramedical personnel are more often consciously committed to this goal than the attending physician. When the goal is delegated to the psychiatrist member of the treatment team, his effectiveness is easily obscured by the more academic appeal of doing psychotherapy or exercising some form of psychiatric diagnosis. Thus, the delegation of treating the "suffering component of the illness" is fraught with the risk of disenfranchising the relief of suffering from the mainstream of medical care and pain control. It is no wonder that the psychological component of the "chronic pain syndrome" has such a perjoritive and threatening connotation for the patient with chronic pain.

It is necessary to re-emphasize that suffering is not pain per se. Suffering may encompass, but is not limited to, experience of pain. As Cassel has noted, and as his observation is validated by my experience with pain patients "suffering occurs when an impending destruction of the person is perceived; it continues until the threat of disintegration has passed or until the integrity of the person can be restored in some manner (entry 6)." While suffering can occur in the presence of physical pain, it extends beyond the physical. It is not limited to the presence of a nociceptive stimulation or the active state of a pain message. Suffering can, and does, occur in relationship to any aspect of a person, body, mind, social role, occupational status and perhaps most significantly, his perceived future or the anticipated dread of what that future bodes.

§ 8-15. The Importance of the Meaning of Pain.

When a person experiences pain in the neck, it implies to him that there is something wrong with the neck. When the physician cannot find evidence of disease in the neck, he may suggest that the pain is "psychological." What the physician *means* is that there is no disease (at least none that he or the tests that he performed can detect). What the patient hears is that *"the pain is not real,"* that, in fact, he is faking. In the presence of pain and suffering, the word "psychological" has a pejorative connotation. The reality is that suffering can, and does occur even when a physician does not find the source of a patient's pain. Thus, the patient with chronic pain is in conflict; feeling "pain," but threatened by the lack of confirmation from "medical science." He thus must rely on behavior to demonstrate "how much I hurt."

Above all else, one must avoid the pejorative implication that "psychological" pain places on the pain patient. It effectively shifts the "burden of proof" to the patient. He may become distrustful and suspicious, especially needful of convincing the doctor of the reality of his pain. The advent of "pain behaviors" are manifestations of this very process — the conscious desire and, in part, the unwitting intention to behaviorally act out the experience of distress. This is not "faking" or "malingering" but a behavioral intention to demonstrate pain in a living form.

Pain behavior can vary in form, style, and intensity. All pain behavior is characterized by a central preoccupation with the experience of being in pain. Movements may be guarded and dramatized, overprotecting the affected painful area or suddenly invested with the restraints of pain, showing in deliberate and emphatic gesture the effect of the pain. It is the kind of pain that draws attention to itself. Typically, the display of pain is intensified by observation and scrutiny. It is pain that is meant to be witnessed and shared.

Thus, dealing with pain behavior requires an understanding of the meaning of that pain behavior and how that pain behavior is part and parcel of the underlying illness.

§ 8-16. Doing and Not Doing.

To successfully treat chronic pain requires awareness and restraint. Particularly, the ability to question and investigate the multiple complaints of pain and to tolerate the uncertainty of "not knowing all the answers."

It is noted in the literature, that chronic pain patients have found their entire belief systems violated and shattered by their experience with the injury, pain, and failure of the medical compensation and legal system (entry 26). Perhaps this disappointment is the function of unrealistic expectations, perhaps poor education, perhaps lack of reality testing prior to the advent of injury. Nonetheless, they find themselves perpetually disappointed and frustrated. Their expectations for cure are, at first, a challenge of ambitious, zealous physicians, but later the bane of their frustrated therapeutic efforts.

The "pain patients" are especially vexing. They are difficult patients for psychiatrists as well as other physicians. It is suggested that these patients are simultaneously dependent and rebellious; an intolerable combination of traits. Thus, while demanding "everything," they are noncompliant and embittered, seeking to project their failure and disappointment on external courses. Their mistrust and need to externalize their difficulties borders on overt paranoia.

Thrown into the context of this interpersonal struggle, the physician seeks expedient solutions. Diagnostic procedures, polypharmacies, physical therapy and analgesic injections are convenient, but short-lived solutions. Invariably the futility of their efforts comes back to haunt them.

To successfully manage the pain patient requires the dual ability to see everything and do only what is absolutely necessary. Rebuilding the belief system of the pain patient is critical. Slow, progressive understanding, an emphasis on self-reliance and increased tolerance of pain are critical. Reducing the reliance on analgesics, tranquilizers, and other marginal therapies is similarly important. Establishing trust requires avoidance of unnecessary treatment and inappropriate investigation. Above all else, the physician's restraint is the expression of genuine understanding and compassion. If nothing else, it affirms the Hippocratic principle to *"do no harm."*

BIBLIOGRAPHY

1. Acute Pain vs. Chronic Pain. Moving Away from "Find it and Fix it," *Topics in Pain Management,* Vol. 1 No. 4, September 1985.
2. Blumer, D., Heilbronn, M. Chronic pain as a variant of depressive illness: the pain prone disorder. J Nerv Ment Dis 170:381-406, 1982.
3. Blumer, D., Heilbronn, M. Antidepressant treatment for chronic pain: treatment outcome of 1,000 patients with pain prone disorder. Psychiatric Annals, 14:796-800, 1984.

4. Bouckoms, A.J. Recent developments in the classification of pain. Psychosomatics, 26:637-645, 1985.
5. Brena, S. Chronic Pain States. A Model for classification. Psychiatric Annals, 14:7 78-7 82, 1984.
6. Cassell, E.J. The nature of suffering and the goals of medicine. NEJM, 306:639-645, 1945.
7. Engel, G.L. The need for a new medical model: a challenge for biomedicine. Science, 196:129-136, 1977.
8. Fordyce, W.E. Learning processes in pain, in the *Psychology of Pain.* R.A. Sternbach (E.D. Editor), New York, Raven Press, 1978.
9. France, R.D., Krishnan, K.R., Houpt, J.L. Differentiation of depression from chronic pain with the dexamethasone suppression test and DMS-III. Am J of psychiatry, 141:1577-1579, 1984.
10. Haward, L.R. The stress and strain of pain. Stress Medicine, 1:41-46, 1985.
11. Hendler, N. Depression caused by chronic pain. J Clin Psychiatry, 45:30-36, 1984.
12. Maruta, T., Swanson, D.W., Swenson, W. Pain as a psychiatric symptom: comparison between low back pain and depression. J of Psychosomatics 17:123-127, 1976.
13. Maruta, T., Osborne, D. Sexual activity in chronic pain patients: J of Psychosomatics, 19:531-537, 1978.
14. Mechanic, D. Effects of psychological distress on perceptions of physical health. J Human Stress, 4:26-35, 1978.
15. Pilowsky, I., Bassett, B.L. Pain and depression. Br J Psychiatry, 141:30-36, 1982.
16. Pilowsky, I., Chapman, C.R., Bonica, J.J. Pain, depression and illness behavior in pain clinic population. J of Pain, 4:183-192, 1977.
17. Rahe, R., Ranson, A.J. Life change in illness studies. J of Human Stress, 4:3-15, 1978.
18. Research Briefing. Pain and Pain Management. National Academy of Science, Institute of Medicine, Committee of Science, Engineering and Public Policy. May 22, 1985.
19. Schaffer, C.B., Donlon, D.T., Bittle, R.M. Chronic pain and depression: a clinical and family history survey. Am J Psychiatry, 137:118-120, 1980.
20. Smoller, B., Schulman, B. *Pain Control,* Garden City, N.Y., Doubleday, 1983.
21. Swanson, D.W. Chronic pain as a third pathologic emotion. Am J of Psychiatry, 141:210-215, 1984.

22. Swanson, D.W. Some psychiatric observations on the chronic pain patient. Psychiatric Annals, 14:7 83-7 86, 1984.
23. Swanson, D., Maruta, T. Patients complaining of extreme pain. Mayo Clinic Proceedings, 55:563-566, February 1980.
24. Swanson, D.W., Swenson, W.M., Maruta, T., et al. Program for managing chronic pain. Mayo Clin Proc, 1952:401-408, 1976.
25. The Chronic Pain Syndrome. Distinguishing the "Patient in Pain" from the "Pain Patient," *Topics in Pain Management,* Vol. 1 No. 5, October 1985.
26. Whittington, H.G. The Biopsychosocial Model Applied to Chronic Pain. J of Oper Psychiatry, Vol. 16 No. 2:2-8, 1985.

CHAPTER 9

PHYSICAL THERAPY, ERGONOMICS, AND REHABILITATION

Thomas M. Welsh, R.P.T.

§ 9-1. Introduction.
§ 9-2. Modalities Used in Physical Therapy.
 § 9-2(A). Heat.
 § 9-2(B). Cold.
 § 9-2(C). Electrical Stimulation.
 § 9-2(D). Ultrasound.
 § 9-2(E). Traction.
 § 9-2(F). Joint Mobilization.
§ 9-3. Impairment of Functional Ability.
§ 9-4. Assessment of Cervical Musculoskeletal Disorders and Treatment Plan.
 § 9-4(A). Assessment.
 § 9-4(B). Treatment Plan.
§ 9-5. Specific Cervical Pain Syndromes and Physical Therapy Treatments.
 § 9-5(A). Whiplash.
  § 9-5(A)(1). Ligament Sprain.
  § 9-5(A)(2). Muscle Strain.
 § 9-5(B). Spondylosis.
 § 9-5(C). Nerve root (Radicular) Pain.
 § 9-5(D). Postural Pain.
Figure 1. Posture.
 § 9-5(E). Temporo-Mandibular Joint Dysfunction.
§ 9-6. Cervical Collar.
Figure 2. Cervical Collar.
§ 9-7. Exercise: Therapeutic, Postural, and Preventive.
Figure 3. Therapeutic and Postural Exercise.
Figure 4. Postures for Preventing Neck Strain.
§ 9-8. Ergonomics and Prevention.
Figure 5. Incidence of Impairment in the Neck Related to the Neck-head Angles of 57 Accounting Machine Operators.
Figure 6. Adjustment Features of an Ergonomic Work Seat.
Figure 7. Adjustment Features of an Ergonomic VDT Work Station.

Figure 8. Recommended Approximate Dimensions (in centimeters).
Figure 9. The "Mean Body Posture" Under Practical Conditions at Preferred Settings of the VDT Work Station.
§ 9-9. Returning the Injured Worker to the Job.
§ 9-10. Summary.
Bibliography.
Table I. Limits and Representative Values of Range of Rotation.
Table II. Mean Percentage.
Table III. Approximate Percentage Restriction.
Table IV. Flexion and Extension.
Table V. Human Factors and Task Redesign.
Table VI. Work Place Redesign Considerations.
Table VII. Postural Efforts at VDT Work Stations.
Table VIII. Medical Findings in a VDT Field Study.
Table IX. Model for Prevention and Return to Work.

§ 9-1. Introduction.

The purpose of this chapter is to present current physical therapy and rehabilitation techniques in the management of specific cervical pain syndromes based on the author's clinical experience and literature review. Concepts of prevention and ergonomics, therapeutic exercise, and work evaluation are also discussed.

§ 9-2. Modalities Used in Physical Therapy.

Several investigators believe that reflex reactions occur within the structures beneath the surface when heat, cold, and irritants are applied to the surface (entry 54). It has been stated that "the efficiency of physical therapy in the treatment of disease depends both on the direct reflex effects of the stimulating agents employed and the influence of these agents exerted through the higher autonomic centers" (entry 31). The modalities and procedures of physical therapy which may be prescribed in the management of cervical pain are heat, cold, electrical stimulation, cervical traction, ultrasound, massage, mobilization, and exercise.

Exercise and its recommended use will be discussed in § 9-7 of this chapter.

§ 9-2(A). Heat.

Moist heat is the most commonly prescribed modality in treating musculoskeletal pain. It is applied for its relaxing effect on the pathological tonic activity of skeletal muscle. The pain so often connected with these conditions is not only temporarily relieved, but in many patients repeated heat treatments effects more or less permanent improvement apparently by breaking up a vicious cycle, in which pain reinforces reflexly the abnormal muscle activity (entry 32).

Moist heat is often used during cervical traction and before mobilization, massage or therapeutic exercise. Usually, it is applied by means of a hydrocollator or moist hot pack for a fifteen to twenty-minute time period to relieve muscle spasm and promote relaxation.

In a home, self-administered, therapeutic program, the individual patient may use a hydrocollator, hot shower with a thick towel around the neck, or an electric moist heating pad. Cervical hydrocollator packs can be purchased at most pharmacies for under fifteen dollars but these are troublesome to prepare and most patients will not use them daily because of this. The Thermophore electric moist heating pad is more expensive (forty-five to fifty dollars), but more convenient to use at home or at work. A dry electric heating pad is usually not recommended because of its comparatively ineffectiveness in producing desired results. It is also not recommended that any heat treatment be applied for a longer period than one-half hour due to the possibility of increased congestion of blood flow and resultant stiffness.

There are conditions in which the application of moist heat may be contraindicated. These are: deficient vascularity due to organic disease of the blood vessels, deficient sensation, malignant neoplasms in the area being treated, bleeding, active tuberculosis, open wounds on burned areas, and certain arthritic conditions that are inflamed (entries 58, 45).

§ 9-2(B). Cold.

Cold is applied to relieve pain and spasm and most commonly indicated within forty-eight hours of the injury to stop bleeding and reduce the amount of swelling in the damaged tissue. It should be a frequently used modality in physical therapy. In addition to it being a vasoconstrictor of the peripheral vessels of the skin, promoting an increased blood flow to the deeper vessels and tissue, cold increases muscle tone, reduces swelling, increases the patient's tolerance to deep massage, and enhances voluntary motion. Its temporary anesthetic effect also helps the patient to better tolerate stretch to chronically, painful, contracted muscles by the physical therapist to restore normal movement in the neck structures.

In the clinic, cold may be applied by ice packs, ice blocks or a vapor-coolant spray. Either flouromethane or ethylchloride sprays are used with the former being preferred. The spray technique involves using a pressurized bottle of the spray and applying it to a local trigger point or individual muscle, most commonly the upper trapezius or sternocleidomastoid muscles in the neck. A spray period of three seconds is usually sufficient followed by massage and active motion. Care must be taken to consider the patient's skin reaction to cold. If the skin reddens after massage, the patient's circulatory reaction is normal; if the skin stays white, then prolonged ice application may be contraindicated. Ice packs and ice massage have the same precautions and the application time is dependent upon the patient's tolerance and should be monitored.

In the home or at work the patient may be instructed in using cold applications and muscle stretch techniques. Ice packs, frozen wet towels, ice pops or even a cold soda can can be used for temporary relief of muscle pain and spasm.

Contraindications for the use of cold modalities are similar to those of heat applications. These include impaired circulation, peripheral vascular disease, loss of thermal sensitivity and psychological opposition to this type of therapy (entry 45).

§ 9-2(C). Electrical Stimulation.

Transcutaneous Electrical Nerve Stimulation (TENS) is a common electrotherapy prescribed in treatment of acute and chronic cervical pain syndrome. The device is a small electrical generator which stimulates soft tissue superficially with a low-intensity, direct or alternating, pulsed current. Application is via skin electrodes attached to the stimulator which is then adjusted in mode, frequency, pulse width, and intensity dependent upon the patient's diagnosis and desired effect.

Electroanalgesia by means of TENS has been shown effective in both animal studies and in controlled clinical studies (entries 37, 51, 52). An explanation of the actual physiology of pain and its relief is not available. Three theories have been suggested. The Specificity Theory maintains that pain is a special modality like vision or hearing with a fixed, direct-line communication system from the skin to the brain. The Pattern Theory suggests that the nerve impulse pattern for pain is produced by intense stimulation of nonspecific receptors. The Gate Control Theory proposes a mechanism at the spinal level which affects the perception of pain by the comparative activity of large diameter A-beta fibers and specific pain fibers (A-delta and C) in cutaneous afferent nerves. All of these theories are contradictory, in part, by some clinical observations (entry 42).

Because of this uncertainty of the mechanism of TENS analgesia there is some skepticism in the medical community about its use. In this author's experience, TENS has been used only if indicated as another modality to be employed in treatment of pain when more conservative and less expensive methods have failed to produce effective pain relief. Several clinical studies have shown that the practical use of TENS is widespread, convenient, safe, and effective (entries 11, 34, 36, 48).

In the treatment of cervical pain syndrome involving head and neck pain, TENS may be appropriate in selective treatment of whiplash injury, headaches, chronic and acute neck pain, temporomandibular joint pain, and muscle spasms. The preferred electrode placements are bilateral upper and mid-trapezii muscles. To be most effective, a thorough explanation of the technique must be made to the patient, instructions in using the machine and placing the electrodes must be understood and the patient must comply with the therapists' directions.

Placement of electrodes is usually best applied at painful site or proximal to the area in the cases of nerve injury (entry 12). The stimulation parameters are left to the clinical experience of the physical therapist and the manufacturer's recommended guidelines. Relatively high frequencies (80-1000 H_2) and low pulse width are preferred by this author for clinical application for brief analgesic effect within five to ten minutes. Other acceptable parameters are a brief intense mode with maximum pulse width and pulse rate for immediate relief of pain; a low rate mode with minimal pulse rate and moderate pulse width for long duration of relief; a burst mode with the minimal rate and moderate pulse width for long duration of relief; and a modulated mode with moderate pulse rate and low pulse width for an intermediate duration of relief.

TENS does not result in pain relief for all patients, therefore, a trial of its effectiveness should be tested in the clinic before considering the home use of it by the patient. These machines are expensive ($80-100/mo. rental; $580-625 purchase). This author recommends rental rather than purchase unless the device is used for more than three months. Care must be taken not to allow the patient to become dependent upon the device and to establish from the beginning a decreased usage with increased comfort and physical conditioning.

Precautions for using TENS are few. The device should not be used unless there is a diagnosis of the cause of the pain syndrome. Also, patients should be instructed in proper skin preparation and care to prevent skin irritation at the electrode site. The only contraindications to TENS at this time are in cases of pregnancy and with individuals using demand-type cardiac pacemakers (entry 13).

§ 9-2(D). Ultrasound.

Ultrasound therapy is another very frequently prescribed modality when local deep heating is indicated. Sound is a form of vibrating energy propagated through a medium in the form of waves. Ultrasound is simply sound at frequencies higher than audible range with 20 kH_2 usually chosen as an arbitrary lower limit (entry 53). Sound waves travel through soft tissue and are reflected by hard tissue (entry 50). As the sound wave travels through tissue at a penetration depth of 5 centimeters or more some of the energy is lost and some of the energy is absorbed (entry 56). It is the absorbed energy that promotes tissue healing by producing local changes in tissue temperature, blood flow, and oxygen uptake (entry 2). There is much less known about the non-thermal bioeffects of ultrasound such as cavitation, radiation forces, acoustic microstreaming, and there are many unanswered questions for some phenomena caused by ultrasound therapy and phono-phoresis (entry 39).

An ultrasound machine consists of a generator of a high frequency current and a sound head transducer, which converts the electrical energy to mechanical energy. This sonic energy is transmitted through a coupling medium, such as gel, oil, or water, to the local tissue. To prevent heat build-up to underlying tissue the sound head applicator is continuously moved over the skin with light pressure either in circular or stroking patterns.

Prescription for ultrasound is usually 0.5 to 2.0 watts per centimeter squared for five minutes although at present there are no established guidelines other than careful observation by the physical therapist for adverse side effects. Overdosage of ultrasound destroys tissue. Some patients complain of burning or aching pain sensation during the treatment which may be due to tissue accumulation of heat. Pulsed ultrasound versus continuous frequency may prevent this, however, some of the deep heating effect may be lost.

A treatment series is considered to be six to twelve applications applied daily or every other day (entry 45). It is this author's experience that ultrasound will be helpful in relieving symptoms after two treatments or it will not and should be stopped if it is not. As with any other heat treatment, it should also be followed by massage and/or therapeutic exercise, active or passive, to promote circulation.

There are few contraindications for ultrasound in physical therapy, however, caution should be exercised when treating a patient with a diagnosed malignancy and when the individual complains of any adverse side effects.

§ 9-2(E). Traction.

Cervical traction is prescribed for many clinical entities, including symptoms arising from pressure on nerve roots, from degenerative joint disease, and from cervical spine injuries (entries 33, 23). Due to a lack of substantial clinical studies the beneficial effects of traction are questionable (entries 43, 44, 10). Traction generally is considered an empirical form of physical therapy and should be employed only when more conservative treatment is not effective. In this author's opinion, the effectiveness of any procedure depends upon accurate diagnosis, clinical assessment, method of application, and therapist skills. No traction should ever be prescribed by a physician unless x-rays have been taken to rule out fractures or other pathology.

Review of the literature reveals a wide ranging statement of effects from the application of traction to the cervical spine. The effects reported are: prevention and freeing up of adhesions within the dural sleeves, nerve roots and adjacent capsular structures; relief of nerve root compression and irritation within the intervertebral foramen; separation (distraction) of the articular surfaces of the apophyseal joints; improvement of the circulatory status within the epidural spaces of the spinal and lateral nerve root canals; decompression of the intervertebral joint with reduction of derangements of the disk; reduction of the inflammatory response, pain, and subsequent muscle spasm (entry 44).

The methods employed in traction vary. It can be applied manually or mechanically, intermittently or continuously, and in a vertical or horizontal direction.

Intermittent traction is indicated for acute facet injury, osteoarthritis and sub-acute strain of spondylosis. Relief of symptoms is thought to be accomplished by the rhythmic, intermittent pull improving circulation and preventing the formation of adhesions between the dural sleeves of the nerve roots and the adjacent capsular structures (entries 22, 9). However, some studies show that there is no significant differences in myoelectric activity or relaxation of the upper trapezius muscle during or after intermittent traction (entry 24). In some chronic cases intermittent traction may even aggravate the symptoms at which time it should be discontinued. The most advantageous intermittent traction is that which can be tolerated in both force and duration in a supine position with minimum discomfort to the patient's chin and jaw. The forces applied may vary from 5 to 35 lbs. for fifteen seconds on and seven seconds off for a five to twenty-minute time period dependent upon the patient's tolerance. The amount of force and time may increase with each treatment.

Continuous traction is prescribed for treatment of chronic conditions with muscles and ligament tightening and postural faults. It is thought to be less comfortable to the patient because of constant pressure to the chin and jaw. If correctly applied it may straighten the cervical spine and enlarge the intervertebral foramina to relieve compressive or irritative forces upon the nerve roots (entry 22). In an acute stage up to a maximum of 5 lbs. of traction is recommended for a brief duration of five minutes or less. Up to 35 lbs. for fifteen minutes may eventually be endured with small increased increments with each treatment dependent upon patient tolerance.

The traction force and duration of pull varies from patient to patient. Clinical effect and assessment should determine the parameters. In general, vertebral separation is the desired effect and the literature agrees that this occurs somewhere between 25 and 45 lbs. (entry 44). It is also reported that the separation of the vertebrae posteriorly is also related to the angle of the rope pull — the greater the angle of neck flexion (20-30 degrees), the greater the elongation (entries 7, 8).

Manual traction is the preference of this author because it allows a continuous assessment of the muscle spasm and joint movement while applying a controlled amount of force with the hands under the occiput at varying angles of cervical flexion, extension, and rotation. It can be used to identify specific involved segments which may later be treated with mechanical traction, massage, or mobilization techniques. The position of the patient is always supine and moist heat is applied prior to treatment to promote maximal relaxation. It is the author's clinical experience that patients also prefer this technique of traction over mechanical traction.

The contraindications to cervical traction are many (entries 49, 43). These include malignancy, cord compression, infectious disease, osteoporosis, hypertension or cardiovascular disease, rheumatoid arthritis, pregnancy, old age, inflammatory disease, disc prolapse, joint hypermobility, structural scoliosis, or marked kypholordosis. Special care should be taken when there is acute torticollis or temporo-mandibular joint dysfunction. It is recommended that when a force is applied to the chin that a resting mandibular splint (which may be as simple as a wad of gauze or moldable wax) should be used either as correction of abnormal mechanics or as a prophylaxis (entry 44).

§ 9-2(F). Joint Mobilization.

Special examining techniques must be learned before any attempt at joint mobilization is made. Joint play movements are for the most part less than 1/8 inch in extent. This tiny range is difficult for the average physician or physical therapist to accept when they are accustomed to thinking of movements through an arc of up to 180 degrees. But, recognition of the fact that the movements to be restored by manipulative therapy are very small is prerequisite to the safe and effective use of this treatment modality (entry 58).

The most important factor in achieving effective mobilization is learning to sense or "feel" movement. Until this is learned by clinical practice, treatment by mobilization will not be fully successful and could be harmful. There are two forms of mobilization — articulation and manipulation, and various schools of thought on their application.

Articulations are techniques whereby a joint is passively taken through its available range and at its limit has applied gentle stretch and progressive oscillations to relieve the restriction in movement. Manipulation involves more of a sharp, short thrust for the same purpose. These techniques may be accompanied by a "snap" signifying the breaking of an intra-articular adhesion, a "pop" signifying a temporary alteration in the fluid/gas state within a synovial joint, or by a "sliding sensation" where a joint fixed for a time in a certain position is now able to move to its neutral or rest position (entry 41).

In articulation the purpose of treatment is to relieve pain through mild, repetitive, small-amplitude movements. There is no intention to stretch tight tissues, break adhesions, restore displaced material or increase the range of movement. It is this author's experience that severe manual manipulations should be avoided for potential harm to the patient such as additional tissue trauma, mobilizing unprotected joints, and stretching the wrong joint or tissue. Rules of procedure should be followed at all times: (a) careful examination, (b) economy of vigor in technique, (c) treatment guided by assessment and reassessment throughout, (d) discontinuing treatment which begins to produce deterioration in the signs and symptoms (entry 19). Special care should be taken in presence of radiculopathy. Due to the lack of clinical studies and pathological knowledge in this area, practitioners are forced to adopt an empirical approach. There are, however, two distinct approaches. One is based on relieving nerve root pressure and the other is based on restoring mobility (entry 41). Chiropractors claim to move vertebra for relieving nerve root pressure and they are specific; Dr. Cyriax moves the disc for this purpose and he is mildly specific. All manual therapists who base their approach on restoring segmental mobility are specific in their treatment. Osteopathy manipulates to correct the mobility of joints and soft tissues; Maigne manipulates into the direction of least restriction of movement and believes that no manipulation should hurt; Maitland principally uses articulation into the direction of limitation and believes there should be no resultant pain or muscle spasm; Minnell articulates or manipulates with an emphasis on joint play and its restoration; Paris uses articulation and manipulation into the direction of limitation and will manipulate through pain in selected cases (entry 41).

Absolute contraindications to mobilization are: malignancy involving the vertebral column; spinal cord involvement or involvement of more than one spinal nerve root on one side, on two adjacent roots in one limb; rheumatoid collagen necrosis of vertebral ligaments; active inflammatory arthritis; bone disease of spine; hypermobility; dizziness (entries 19, 35).

§ 9-3. Impairment of Functional Ability.

The neck is strained more frequently than any other structure of the body and an injury may often lead to chronic symptoms such as headache, painful "cricks," decreased mobility and stiffness. A cervical pain syndrome, either of old or recent onset, can be aggravated by muscular strain or stretch, trauma, or emotional stress. During each recurrent episode familiar symptoms of pain and stiffness may be experienced and feared. Residual symptoms of late origin may occur from cervical spondylosis, and marked osteoarthritic changes in the interlaminar joints may give rise to symptoms later in life. After an acute whiplash injury, for example, a patient may relate any painful symptoms, even if resultant from other underlying causes, to that particular accident no matter how long ago it occurred. It may be months or even years.

Functional ability may be impaired if not properly treated and avoidance of any tasks associated with exacerbation of symptoms may make everyday movement, working, and social enjoyment difficult. If residual, uncomfortable symptoms are present in the neck, shoulders, or upper back, then efforts involving carrying, lifting, driving, typing and like, manual tasks may aggravate the condition. Reading, writing, sewing, and other desk/table activities may be curtailed if the symptoms involve headache or pain when flexing the neck forward or laterally. In occupations where a high degree of concentration or stress is involved, frequent, short rest periods may be necessary. When restricted rotation of the neck to the left or right is involved then simple acts like sleeping prone or turning the head while driving to change lanes or to reverse direction can be uncomfortable and causative. Just walking up and down stairs can cause pain by the compression of the head on the neck. Any type of activity that requires extending the neck and looking up is usually omitted entirely from activities of work and daily function (e.g., ceiling work, tree work, and other awkward, high positions).

In other cases when the residual symptoms involve less pain and stiffness but more weakness and limb numbness, the complaints from patients about their feelings of impairment may not be as great. But, these symptoms could be more hazardous depending upon the individual's work and lifestyle. Objects could easily be dropped with poor grip strength and paresthesia in the upper extremity can be especially dangerous when working around sharp or hot objects.

When the symptoms are caused by trauma and there is evidence of degenerative joint disease, goals of treatment are to relieve pain and improve mobility. Plans to return to normal activities should await the final outcome of the course of treatment. When there is no history of degenerative joint disease or frequent recurrence, then the functional goals of treatment are to return the person to the same level of performance experienced prior to the accident as soon as possible. In both cases, the patient will benefit from appropriate physical therapy and education in a daily exercise program, job ergonomics, and postural habits in daily living. More of this is presented in §§ 7 and 8.

§ 9-4. Assessment of Cervical Musculoskeletal Disorders and Treatment Plan.

§ 9-4(A). Assessment.

The physical therapist's role in assisting in the medical treatment of any patient is to assess the nature and severity of the symptoms and dysfunction. In a neck pain syndrome, the musculoskeletal functional evaluation should not be confined to the cervical spine and soft tissue structures of the neck, but should also include the whole back and upper extremities. This assessment is recorded and reported to the physician who has made the diagnosis, established the goals, and recommended any precautions in treatment. Together, a treatment plan is developed with goals to relieve pain, restore function, promote relaxation, and reduce the risk of recurrence.

The subjective evaluation includes relevant information about the site, description, behavior, and onset of symptoms with recollection of any previous physical treatment. Other important questions which may help in deciding any contraindications of any physical therapy modalities or procedures may concern history of dizziness, blackouts, temporo-mandibular joint dysfunction, rheumatoid arthritis, or other inflammatory diseases, and any symptoms presenting in the extremities.

In the objective examination, the physical therapist is guided by the history and seeks to clarify the abnormalities of function and joint-play movements. Active, passive, neurological, and special tests are used for measuring the severity of the symptoms. Observations of posture, gait and willingness to move head and neck, trunk, and shoulders should be made. The movements of neck and trunk include flexion, extension, lateral flexion, and rotation (see Table I) (entry 57). The quality of movement should be observed and any asymmetry or expression of discomfort at any particular range should be recorded. Shoulder flexion, extension, abduction, and adduction should also be evaluated and noted.

Mild resisted movements may be used to provoke pain or demonstrate weakness to rule out muscle involvement. Good judgment must be practiced in the amount of resistance applied.

Gentle passive movements are used to test restricted range of motion and evaluate ligament and joint tension. It should be noted whether the pain is elicited at end of motion with or without overpressure.

Upon completion of the subjective and objective evaluation, an assessment is made. Based on their correlation and the physician's diagnosis, an appropriate treatment plan for the involved body parts of that individual can be made.

§ 9-4(B). Treatment Plan.

Many physical therapy treatment modalities and procedures may be used dependent upon the type of tissue involved. After each session the effects of the treatment should be assessed. If the effects are not achieved as planned for relief of pain within an expected time period, then the physician's re-evaluation of the diagnosis or the physical therapist's reassessment of the treatment, or both, should be made. To continue to use any modality or procedure of physical therapy for an unpredicted period of time without measurable improvement is poor medical management. It is the author's experience that often times physical therapy services are overused, and sometimes abused, when there is continued therapy prescribed with no positive results. There are also occasions when the services billed as physical therapy are performed by untrained and unlicensed people in a physician's office.

If a modality of physical therapy is prescribed for any reason other than for the reasons of principle, namely, (1) to prevent morbidity, (2) to maintain as normal a physiological state as possible in parts only secondarily affected by the primary pathological condition, (3) to effect rest from function in the anatomical structure in which the primary pathological condition is situated, and (4) when healing has occurred, safely to restore any lost function, then physical therapy is being abused (entry 58).

When indicated, many modalities and procedures of physical therapy may be considered:

(1) Manual Therapy: massage, traction, joint-play mobilization.
(2) Traction: intermittant, continuous, or manual.
(3) Heat: hydrocollator, ultrasound.
(4) Cold: ice packs, ice massage, vapocoolant spray.
(5) Electrotherapy: transcutaneous nerve stimulation.
(6) Exercise.
(7) Patient Education.

Each will be mentioned throughout this chapter and described in §§ 9-2 and 9-7.

The goals of treatment ultimately are to return individuals to their prior level of function, both socially and economically. It is very important from the onset of treatment to set a reasonable time frame for goals to be achieved. Given that most cervical strains and sprains will recover in six weeks or less, it is largely a measure of clinical experience when the person with more severe and out-of-the-ordinary symptoms can return to normal function. In general, muscle and ligaments should be free from pain, but not necessarily from stiffness which can cause restricted range of motion. Also, the joint-play movements of any segment of the cervical spine should be normal and pain-free if the patient is expected to resume normal function with reduced risk of recurrence. This clinical presentation can change on any given day and requires close attention by therapist and physician. When the patient is ready, normal functional activity should begin the next day. The patient can be taught self-mobilizing exercises, relaxation exercises, and active-rest immobilizing techniques which can be performed at work or home without having a great impact on productivity.

If unsatisfactory progress is being made or there are frequent recurrences then it is good practice to discontinue the physical therapy for one or two weeks. Sometimes it is helpful to resume only treatment if the patient reports "feeling better." A return to the physician is appropriate if the symptoms are unchanged or are worsening. In these cases, motivation of the patient must also be considered and the treatments by the therapist evaluated.

§ 9-5. Specific Cervical Pain Syndromes and Physical Therapy Treatments.

§ 9-5(A). Whiplash.

The mechanism and severity of this acceleration-deceleration injury are discussed more completely in Chapter 5 of this text. In this section, the mechanics of injury and subsequent symptoms which are of most interest in planning the physical therapy treatment will be presented based on this author's clinical experience and current literature search.

When a violent hyperextension injury occurs to the head and neck the anterior cervical structures are consequently stretched and so may be the temporo-mandibular joint ligaments and muscles. Because of the usual sitting posture with the head and neck slightly flexed and protruding forward, it can be assumed that the anterior nuchal muscles (i.e., sternocliedomastoid, longus colli, and scalenii muscles) are relaxed prior to the rear-end collision. The loss of tone of the anterior muscles is complete so that only the ligaments are able to resist hyperextension. Possible injured parts are: (a) anterior longitudinal ligament tear, (b) anterior herniation of the intervertebraldisc, (c) chip fracture of vertebral body, (d) facet encroachment into foramen, and (e) acute facet impingement (entry 4).

In the less frequent flexion injury, the movement of the neck is limited by the chin contacting the chest or steering wheel (entry 6). However, possible injuries are: (a) acute synovitis due to subluxation of the articular facets, (b) capsular tear of an articulation, (c) posterior nuclear herniation, and (d) posterior longitudinal ligamentous tear (entry 4).

In both cases the nerve root may be impinged and cause neck and arm pain. Also, the lack of balance between the weak anterior muscles and strong posterior structures may be a predisposing factor to the frequency of cervical injuries (entry 3). This is an important consideration in rehabilitation and treatment.

Some clinical factors that have been associated with poor prognosis following soft-tissue injuries of the neck are: numbness and/or pain in the upper extremity, sharp reversal of cervical lordosis, restricted motion at one interspace (radiograph, flexion/extension), need of cervical collar for more than twelve weeks, need of home traction, or need to resume physical therapy more than once due to symptom exacerbation (entry 20).

§ 9-5(A)(1). Ligament Sprain.

The history of the sprain invariably has a traumatic onset. Patients may complain of a dull ache, which is worse after immobility or rest and aggravated by a directed force, either passively or actively. A burning ache may also be reported after prolonged tension on the posterior neck structures. The patient usually presents with poor posture and upper shoulder and interscapular pain in posterior ligament sprain. There is no complaint of pain on manually resisted neck movements in a short range but pain is elicited when the ligament is stretched.

In mild sprains, physical therapy treatment can begin immediately with application of moist heat (hydrocollator or shower), followed by gentle, soft tissue massage, and isometric exercises. Range of motion exercises may begin after the patient's discomfort to stretch becomes tolerable, usually within ten days time. Instruction in a home-treatment program of warm shower (or wet towels) and progressive exercises are usually sufficient for recovery. Only two or three physical therapy visits for assessment, progressing the exercise program, and ergonomic/postural education are necessary. The course of recovery is two to three weeks, but the patient may function during that time at work and home with minimum restriction in lifting and reaching overhead, as determined by the physician.

In more severe cases, it is usually two or more weeks before the initiation of physical therapy. In that time the patient may wear a soft cervical collar to relieve pain caused by mechanical stress on the injured neck structures. This acute phase is usually characterized by a gradual worsening of symptoms. Muscle spasm is commonly present and any neck movement is restricted and painful. During this early period of recovery, the frequent "office or clinic visit" for more application of heat, be it moist heat, ultrasound, or other modalities, is inadvisable. The travel

THERAPY, ERGONOMICS, REHABILITATION § 9-5(A)

time, the discomfort, and anxiety of traveling, the usual delay in the waiting room, and so forth, all nullify any possible benefit from the treatment proffered there (entry 4).

The purpose of the physical therapy treatment in a severe sprain is to relieve pain, reduce muscle guarding, and encourage movement. Moist heat followed by gentle massage to the spasmodic muscles is usually effective, and, if pain is very severe, then transcutaneous nerve stimulation may be tried for a brief period. The patient can be instructed in performing gravity eliminated rotation exercises with the head supported in a neutral position by a pillow. The exercise should not cause pain. This program should be performed at home at least three times per day and preferably after a warm shower. After two days of the self-administered therapy, the patient should return to the physical therapist for reassessment of pain and functional mobility. Usually, symptoms are less severe and more localized with some increased movement. At this treatment session, gentle, manual traction may be applied followed by mild pressure over the spinous process and transverse process of any cervical or upper thoracic vertebra which may have tenderness or paraspinal muscle spasm associated with it. Traction in this manner is applied for one minute, assessment is repeated, then traction again, and repeated up to five times. The patient is cautioned that painful symptoms may flare up initially, but if muscle guarding is decreased and mobility increased especially in flexion and extension, then the treatment is producing positive effects. The course of physical therapy is four to six treatments over two weeks. Other techniques in addition to manual traction, massage, and heat include rhythmic stabilization and active exercises. Rhythmic stabilization is a form of isometric exercise, is safe, and is well-tolerated. The patient exerts an equal muscle force to that of the therapist's hands which permits no active neck movement. This promotes relaxation of the guarding muscle spasm and may permit freer range of motion afterwards. Also, during this two-week period the patient is instructed in a progressive self-treatment program which may be performed at home and/or at work. Return to work status is determined by the physician.

Instruction in postural awareness, exercises, and work ergonomics can be helpful in reducing the risk of recurrence. By learning to relieve the neck stiffness and muscle spasm by isometric and range-of-motion exercises, the patient may also prevent the development of subacute and chronic conditions of pain and disability.

§ 9-5(A)(2). Muscle Strain.

Pain and stiffness may be present hours or days after the injury. Headache may be one symptom, delayed or intermittent, and radiating upward and over the cranium to the frontal area. There is commonly present palpable hypertonicity and tenderness over the posterior cranial and nuchal muscles which may also radiate downward and across the shoulders and scapular regions. In patients with muscle strain, pain is reproduced by isometric contraction or contraction against mild resistance in a shortened range of neck movement. These effects are more pronounced in an evaluation before any heat treatments. The nature of the discomfort may be a weary ache and it may worsen with fatigue. The symptoms may be bilateral or unilateral with measurable loss of range of motion. Palpable trigger points are usually located in the cervical paraspinal muscles, the upper trapezius, levator scapulae, rhomboids, teres minor and teres major, and lateral deltoid muscles.

In minor strains, when pain is diffuse and spread over a large area, warm showers and range of motion exercises are usually effective treatments. These may be instructed along with postural and ergonomic recommendations in one or two physical therapy visits. A follow-up visit may be scheduled for increasing the exercises and reassessing the program after one week.

In more severe cases, the physical treatment may be more involved. Again, it is unwise for the patient to drive to an office or clinic for a simple treatment that can be performed at home during the initial phase of the acute injury. For some patients who experience progressive worsening in pain and muscle guarding, a soft collar may be worn while they are not resting. When at rest the individual should be encouraged during the first two weeks or so to begin specific, active movement exercises if they do not cause increased pain. Preferably, these should be performed three to four times daily after a warm shower or other application of heat.

If severe symptoms still persist after two weeks, more frequent physical therapy is appropriate. Moist heat followed by gentle massage to the involved musculature may be administered and assessed for effectiveness. If muscle spasm is not relieved then continuous cervical traction may be applied at the same time as moist heat. The technique of aligning the traction is left to the choice of the clinician. This author prefers the supine position with the head in neutral position for upper cervical conditions and in flexion for lower cervical conditions. If the physician indicates that there are also radiological degenerative changes present, then intermittent cervical traction may be used. In either traction method, a starting force of five percent of the body weight will be used and increased up to fifteen percent for twenty minutes. Occasionally, the patient may complain of increased muscle tension in the neck and upper shoulders. This is normal, but should be observed closely. No more than four consecutive traction treatments should be performed if ineffective each time.

Adjunctive treatments of cold spray, TENS, ultrasound, or pressure massage to the spasmodic muscles can be helpful. Again, these treatments should be evaluated individually for effectiveness and not applied all in one visit. It is very difficult to determine what helps and what hurts with overtreatment.

After each treatment the therapist should reassess the appropriateness of the modalities and procedures administered. If after two weeks or four visits (whichever comes first), the patient shows no progress, an appointment with the physician should be made for re-evaluation. More ineffective physical therapy will not make the treatment more effective. However, if the patient is gradually improving, decreasing the number of visits or discontinuing physical therapy might also be considered. Instruction to the patient regarding progressive exercises and job/home related ergonomics should be given prior to discharge. Also, a home-care program should be advised. When home-traction units are prescribed by the physician, the apparatus should be set up by a physical therapist in the individual's home initially to insure effective, safe use. The soft collar should be removed after the initial two to three weeks and may be used at night if the patient has pain and/or stiffness upon awakening. The collar may also be used intermittently for fifteen to twenty minutes to rest strained posterior neck muscles during the day.

In both the muscle strain and ligament sprain injury, physical therapy may be resumed if symptoms worsen which happens in many cases. Some simple suggestions can be made for reducing risk of recurrence and these will be discussed in the ergonomic section (§ 9-8) and exercise section (§ 9-7) of this chapter.

§ 9-5(B). Spondylosis.

Spondylosis is a diagnosis which indicates that there are degenerative changes in the intervertebral discs of the cervical spine and its adjacent structures. Nerve root irritation may result, or in more advanced cases, spinal cord myelopathy. The nerve can become squeezed and deformed by a slowly growing osteophytic protrusion, without any clinical evidence of irritation or dysfunction. Reactive fibrosis may also involve the root-sheaths and peri-articular tissues, obliterating the root pouches, yet the root remains functionally intact. Such changes, however, always make the root extremely vulnerable to all kinds of stress and pain (entry 14).

The immediate precipitating cause of symptoms may be some slight trauma or stress on the neck structures (e.g., sleeping on a high pillow, an unusual bumpy car ride, ceiling painting, an auto accident, reading in an awkward position, etc.). Symptoms are commonly unilateral, may vary from diffuse to severe neck pain and stiffness, and may be aggravated by any movement of the neck. Rotation towards and lateral flexion of the neck away from the pain is usually the least aggravation.

When the pain is localized to the mid-cervical region and there is no distal pain, the symptoms are usually relieved by rhythmic manual traction or mechanical, intermittent traction and massage of the involved and lower segments and paraspinal musculature. The prognosis for short term recovery (two weeks) after two or three physical therapy treatments is good.

In most patients who present with unilateral symptoms with no neurological signs in the upper extremity, the treatment is usually the same for the involved segment of the spine which appears stiff and tender. Prognosis is generally good in these cases and the treatment course is short. The patient is instructed in a home-exercise program for strengthening the neck muscles for increased support and range of motion exercises for increased mobility and function. If the patient complains of periodic achiness during the day or upon awakening, then a soft collar may be recommended to be worn briefly during the day (twenty-minute rest periods, three or four times per day) and during sleep.

§ 9-5(C). Nerve Root (Radicular) Pain.

The symptom of radicular pain to the upper extremity can be caused by irritation or compression of the nerve root. Factors which can produce this condition include disc protrusion, osteophytes from the uncovertebral or facet joints, swollen capsule of the facet from traumatic inflammation, ligamentous thickening and vertebral subluxation (entry 22). Paresthesia, objective numbness, muscle weakness, and a depressed or absent reflex may also be present.

The treatment of choice is mechanical traction, continuous or intermittent, depending upon severity. Positive effects should be tried to be achieved with minimum duration and poundage. Manual techniques can be applied during the same treatment session if appropriate. Patients should be supine and the neck flexed to 25 to 40 degrees. Initial poundage should not exceed five percent of patient's weight. Apply a continuous pull at this weight for five minutes. Reassess signs and symptoms. Alter weight and time only if there is no positive effect. Then add two to three-pound increments until a maximum of fifteen percent of body weight is attempted. Add increments of time of five minutes up to one hour. Moist heat may be applied during traction for relaxation followed by gentle massage. As symptoms improve intermittent rhythmic traction may be initiated. Long periods of hold (15 seconds) and rest (7 seconds) should be set with the same weight tolerated in continuous traction. As the condition improves, set shorter duration of hold and relax to encourage more movement. The twenty-minute traction session should be followed by reassessment and exercises as tolerated.

Course of treatment is variable from two to twelve weeks dependent on response. Physical therapy is prescribed two to three times per week for that time period and discontinued if two weeks pass without improvement. Patients should be re-evaluated by a physician at that time for further recommendation.

§ 9-5(D). Postural Pain.

Cervical muscle imbalance can cause postural changes which may have adverse effects on the head and neck. Patients who complain of chronic achiness in the neck and upper back often have a deformity of neck posture. One important environmental factor is that many occupations and activities require that the arms and head be positioned more anterior to the trunk than is comfortable and often for prolonged periods. This anterior positioning may eventually change the length/tension relationship of the anterior, lateral, and posterior cervical musculature. With the head positioned more anterior to the center of gravity, the strong posterior cervical muscles contract, hold, and exert a backward bending force on the occiput (entry 27). To compensate for downward vision in this posture, the lower cervical and upward thoracic portions of the spine extend forward, producing an observable cervical thoracic kyphosis. This adapted position allows the eyes a horizontal field of vision (see Figure 1) (entry 28).

NECK PAIN

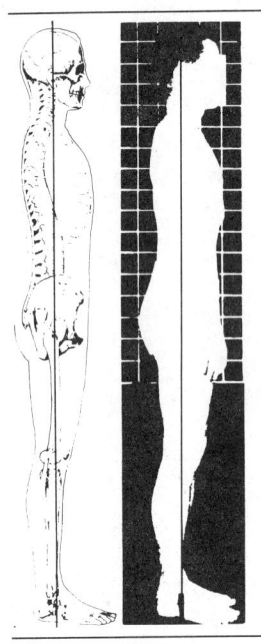

Figure 1
POSTURE
Side View

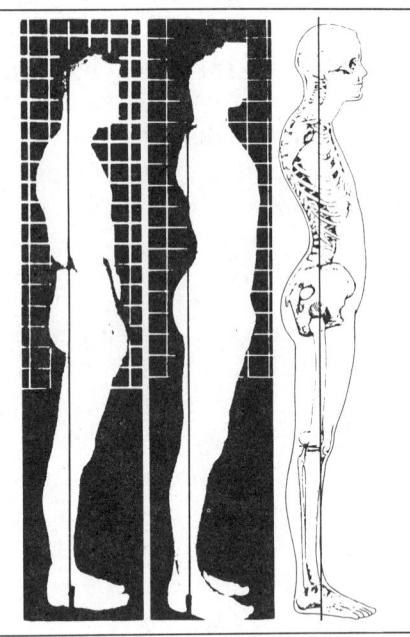

Good	Faulty		
Head erect, chin in	Head forward	Head tilted back slightly	Head forward
Chest up, but not exaggerated	Upper back and shoulders, too round	Shoulder blades slightly "winged"	Upper back round (kphosis)

Normal curves of the spine:
  Neck, slightly forward
  Upper back, slightly backward
  Lower back, slightly forward
  Hip region, slightly backward
	Chest depressed		Chest depressed

	Lower back tends to be too flat	Lower back arched	Abdomen protruding Lower back arched (lordosis)
Neutral position of the pelvis, not tilted forward or backward	Pelvis tilted slighlty back	Pelvis titled forward	Pelvis tilted forward
Knees "easy," neither bent nor pushed back	Knees pushed back	Knees slightly bent	Knees pushed back
Proper alignments of the body in relation to the perpendicular line which passes through the arch of the foot (indicated in the photographs by the suspended plumb line)	In relation to plumb line, head and hips, forward; upper trunk and lower legs, back	In relation to plumb line, body is too far forward, throwing weight over the balls of the feet	In relation to plumb line, head and mid-trunk, forward; upper trunk and knees, back

372

The structural stress on the cervical spine from these postural adaptations can contribute to early degenerative and spondylogenic changes, especially in the weight-bearing, zygoapophyseal joints. Forces from altered posture may also lead to the formation of traction spurs, which may encroach upon nerve roots or supporting ligamentous structures (entry 22).

Another problem associated with forward head posture is with shoulder girdle protraction or "round shoulders." This may cause irritation to the dorsal scapula nerve as the scalenii muscles become more tense and to the suprascapular nerve which may lead to symptoms of weakness and/or pain in the shoulder structure (i.e., glenohumeral and acromioclavicular joints) (entry 29). Tightness of the pectoralis muscles and overstretch or weakness of the rhomboids and levator scapulae are often present in this type of patient.

Abnormal postures with slight neck rotation or lateral head tilt with one sloping shoulder are observations frequently made. There may be an increased lordosis of the lower cervical spine, rigidity of the upper cervical segments, and lack of rotation in the upper thoracic vertebrae during range of motion testing (see Table I).

With the above predisposing structural factors, an onset of more severe pain may be elicited by trauma, a "crick" in the neck, reading in bed with a high pillow supporting the head only, talking on the telephone with the receiver resting between ear and shoulder, etc. In these cases, a brief course of physical therapy is appropriate for a thorough evaluation and assessment of the muscular and ligamentous imbalances in strength, tension and length. These imbalances are usually asymmetrical. When there is muscle tightness in one direction, muscle and ligamentous stretch is usually observed in the opposite direction. The evaluation should also include the thoracic and lumbar spine.

The treatment for postural faults includes specific, individualized exercises for stretching or strengthening as indicated. It may also address patient education in cause and symptoms of poor posture and how to prevent the problem. Postural habits at work and at home should be reviewed with special attention to body mechanics during activity and at rest. Moist heat (hydrocollator or warm shower) may be helpful in relieving muscle achiness from fatigue or strain. The course of treatment should be no more than two to three visits over a four-week period. The prognosis is good that postural pain can be relieved with good patient compliance to the exercise program and maintenance of good postural alignment throughout the day. Figure 4 includes a list of some common activities and correct postures.

§ 9-5(E). Temporo-Mandibular Joint Dysfunction.

Functionally, the cervical spine and the temporo-mandibular joint are closely related. Posture, trauma, and similar symptoms are also common to the problem.

A forward head posture can affect proper occlusion by changing the mandibular alignment. Muscle balance between the flexors and extensors of the neck can be associated with proper function of the masseter, suprahyoid and infrahyoid muscles of the TMJ.

A whiplash injury can cause trauma to the joint as can any injury to the head and neck. Usually, the head rest is just high enough to act as a fulcrum below the occiput. On impact the jaw drops forward, head goes backward and TMJ discs and ligaments are stressed.

Many of the symptoms are not related to function of the TMJ. Pain and/or tenderness are often seen in specific areas of the head such as temples, posterior part of zygomatic arch, angle of jaw, occiput, or muscles of mastication. Related pain may be felt in the dorsum of the neck, sternocliedmastoid muscle, or trapezius muscle (entry 15). Generalized headache is also a common complaint of patients with this disorder. These are similar to symptoms in an upper cervical spine pain syndrome.

It is important to rule out TMJ syndrome before beginning any treatment for the cervical spine. They may coexist, but treatment technique would be changed.

Treatment in physical therapy for TMJ may include cold/heat, ultrasound, massage, electrical stimulation, and postural exercises. Cervical traction with occiput-chin harness would be contraindicated and the use of a cervical collar in the initial phase of injury would have to be reconsidered because of the pressure it would place on the chin.

The treatment team includes a dentist, in addition to an orthopedist and a physical therapist. A special mouth prosthesis may be required.

§ 9-6. Cervical Collar.

A collar is prescribed in an attempt to immobilize the neck. It has two criteria: (1) it should prevent some of the motion at the various cervical levels, although this is only in degrees; and (2) the collar must be comfortable and not cause the wearer added discomfort. The collar furnishes a means of support for the head so that the cervical structures may rest during the initial stages of the injury.

It is important that the collar fit properly to the individual patient to hold the head and neck in flexion and not extension (Figure 2). The slightly flexed position is encouraged since it places the neck in a relaxed position. No cervical orthotic device completely immobilizes the cervical spine. See Tables II, III, and IV; (entries 16, 21, 25, 26).

For most cervical spine injuries which do not involve a fracture, dislocation, or subluxation, a soft collar is used most frequently. It does not appear to be immobilizing, but if there is a minor muscle spasm or pain associated with spondylosis or mild trauma, the soft collar can be comfortable. In more severe cases the other collars listed may be indicated.

Figure 2

Cervical Collar

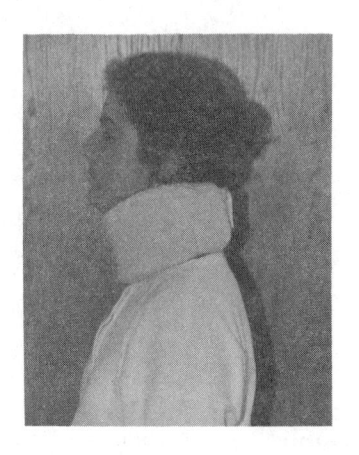

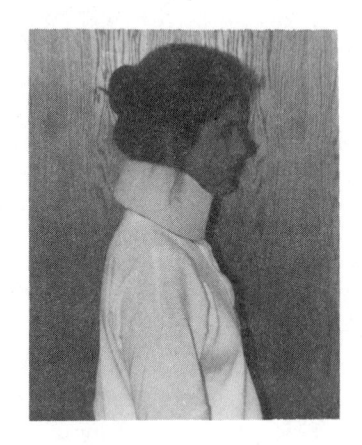

Incorrect: Neck is Extended   Correct: Neck is Flexed

Before the collar is applied it should be explained to the patient that it is only temporary and should be worn for only two weeks. It may be worn occasionally after that for long rides in the car or bus, walking long distances, etc. It can be used anytime that proper posture positioning needs reinforcing. The patient may wear it to bed if achiness and stiffness in the neck is experienced in the morning.

§ 9-7. Exercise: Therapeutic, Postural, and Preventive.

The purpose of these therapeutic and postural exercises is to relieve pain or discomfort and to regain normal movements in the neck. The first three exercises are recommended to be started during the initial phase of recovery. That is, when the symptoms of pain are still present, but the inflammatory process of the injury is decreased. These may be performed during the time period that the patient is wearing a soft collar. Patients should remove the collar and carry out the exercise instructions in Stage 1 (Figure 3).

The patient may progress to Stage 2 when the pain becomes more tolerable and less extensive. In these three exercises, the patient should actively exert the neck structures to the point of pain, then release and return to the starting, relaxed position. If stiffness instead of pain is present than an overpressure can be manually applied when flexing the neck toward the chest in Exercise 6.

When the symptoms are not exacerbated by Stage 1 and Stage 2, the patient may progress to Stage 3. Again, if stiffness is the major complaint, then overpressure may be carefully applied manually and within a comfortable tolerance.

The last stage includes postural exercises which, with Exercise 5, should be performed forever in order to reduce the risk of recurrence of neck pain and stiffness.

The objectives of any of the exercise stages is the gradual relief of symptoms and improved movement. Exercises should be stopped if they are increasing the severity or radiation of pain other than the expected discomfort or stiffness associated with normal exercise. It is a good idea to add only one new exercise per day in order to assess the effect it will have on the injured neck structures. The program should be kept brief in Stages 2, 3, and 4 involving no more than five minutes per session. All exercises should be performed carefully without causing excessive pain. It has been this author's experience that some patients are overaggressive and should be cautioned as a common practice.

The postural exercises should be performed five to six times per day for one month or until posture has improved. Afterward, twice per day has been found to be sufficient for promoting postural awareness.

General exercises such as walking, cycling (with head in good alignment), and swimming (with face in water, use snorkel) are enjoyable exercises. In each, however, continuous extension of the neck must be avoided. These may commence after the severe pain and associated discomfort are relieved. When resuming any athletic activity it is advisable to warm up with Stage 3 and begin slowly.

Figure 3. Therapeutic and Postural Exercises

Stage 1 (#1, #2, #3)
1. Lie on back, face-up. (May be performed with or without pillow. Should progress to using no pillow). Tuck chin downward toward collar bone and at same time force the back of the head to be in contact with the mattress or pillow. Perform gently and do not hold the contraction. Repeat 10 times, three times per day.

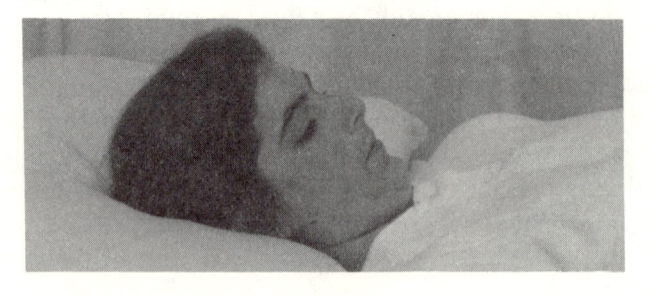

Stage 1 Position.

THERAPY, ERGONOMICS, REHABILITATION § 9-7

2. Lie on back with small flat pillow under head. Tuck chin downward and gently rotate head and neck to right, return to neutral, then repeat to same side five times. Perform same procedure to opposite side. Do not overturn and cause added pain. Perform three times per day.

Starting Position.   Finished Position.

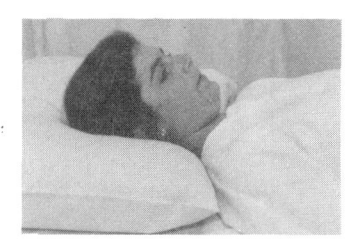

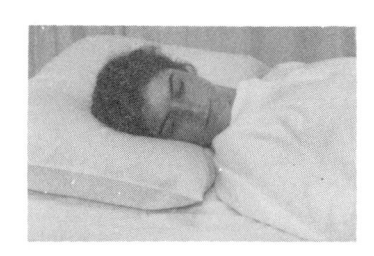

3. Lie on back with or without pillow. Take a deep breath with upper chest and keep shoulders back. Slowly inhale through nose and exhale through mouth. Repeat ten times, three times per day.

Position without pillow.

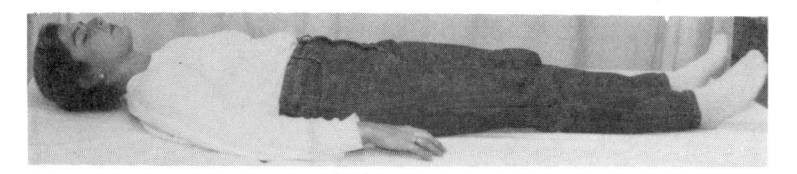

Position with pillows in more acute situation.

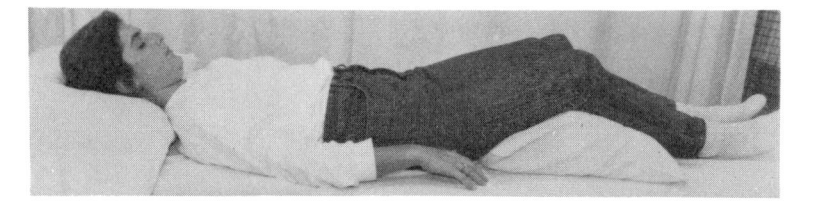

§ 9-7   NECK PAIN

Stage 2 (continue Stage 1 exercises with these)

4. In sitting position with head in good posture, perform shoulder shrugs by raising shoulders up toward ears. Hold for a three count, rest, and repeat ten times. Repeat hourly.

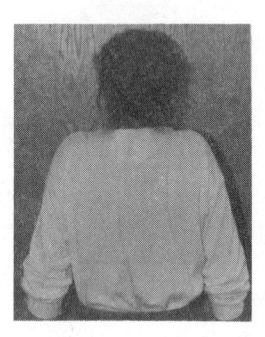

5. In a sitting or standing position perform isometric exercises for the anterior, posterior, and lateral neck muscles. Do not be overaggressive. Repeat three times per day. Place one or both hands in front of forehead and apply equal forces of pressure from hands against the forward motion of the head and neck. Hold for a count of five, relax for count of three, and repeat five times.

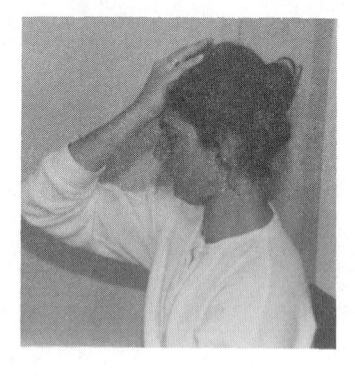

THERAPY, ERGONOMICS, REHABILITATION § 9-7

Place both hands behind head and apply equal forces of pressure from hands against backward motion of the head and neck. Hold for a count of five, relax for count of three, and repeat five times.

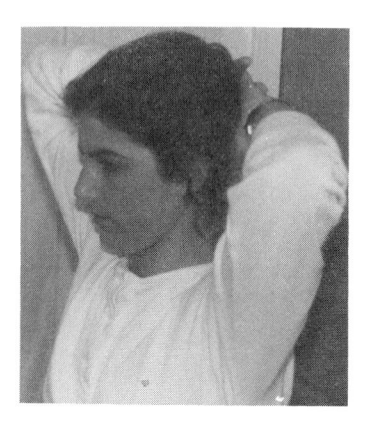

Place the right hand against right side of face and apply equal forces of pressure from hands against the lateral bending with rotation of the head and neck. Hold for a count of five, relax for a count of three, and repeat five times. Perform same procedure to left side.

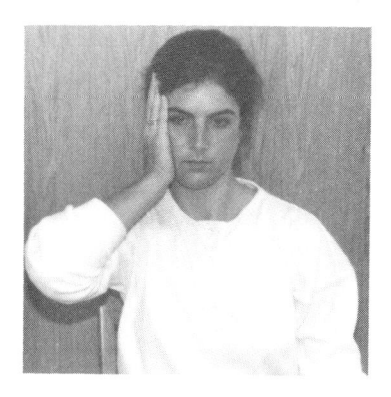

6. In sitting position, bend the head and neck toward chest without forcing the movement if there is pain. If there is stiffness and no pain, apply overpressure with hands at end of movement. Repeat ten times, hourly.

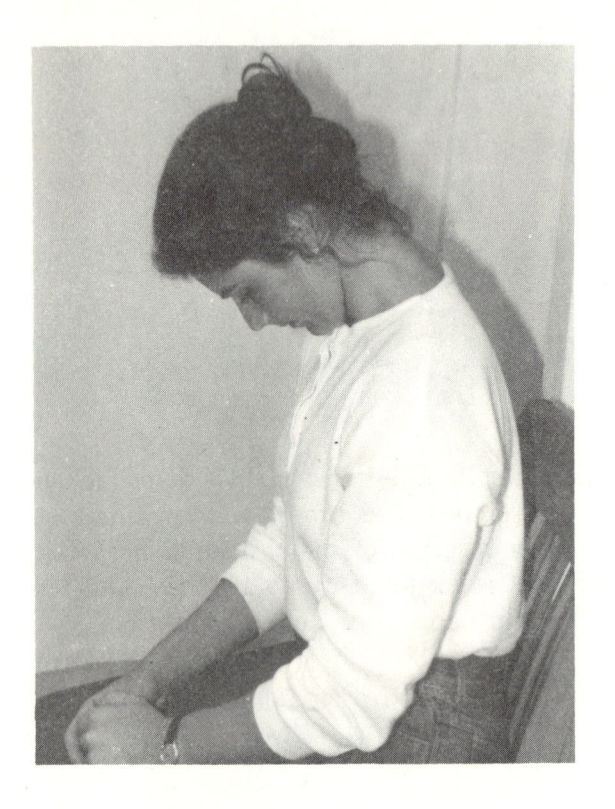

<u>Stage 3 (Stop Stage 1, continue Stage 2 and add one of Stage 3 exercises daily as tolerated).</u>

7. Lie on back with small, flat pillow under neck. Raise head off pillow and bring chin to chest.

Try one time and assess pain. If too difficult, do not bring head up as far. Try one time again, assess discomfort. If tolerable, repeat five times. If there is no added pain the next day add one more repetition until ten repetitions can be performed comfortably. Perform three times per day.

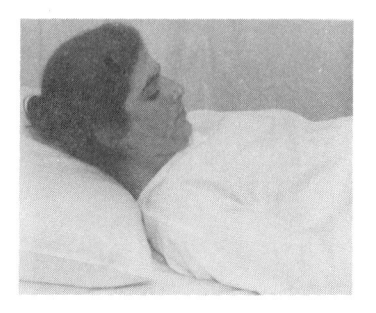

8. In sitting position keep chin in and rotate the head to look over the left shoulder within pain tolerance, hold for a three-count, and return to center. Perform same procedure to right side. Repeat ten times, hourly.

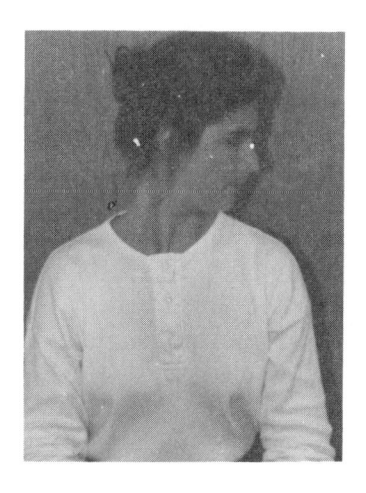

9. In a sitting position, keep chin in and laterally bend head and neck so that left ear is moving toward left shoulder. Do not raise shoulder. If there is stiffness and no pain, gentle overpressure may be applied with left hand. Perform same procedure to right side. Repeat ten times, hourly.

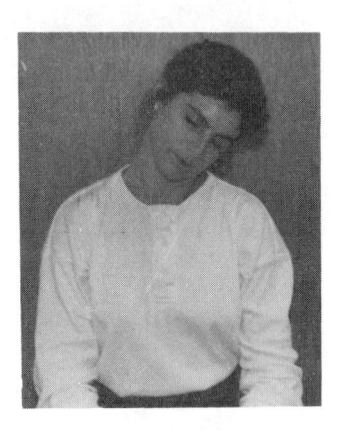

Stage 4: Postural and Prevention Exercises (stop all exercises in Stages 1, 2, and 3, except exercise number 5).

10. In a sitting position, tuck chin in and rotate head and neck toward right shoulder. Then, bend neck laterally so that right ear is directed toward chest. Apply overpressure with right hand if comfortable. Hold for a three-count,

THERAPY, ERGONOMICS, REHABILITATION § 9-7

relax three-count, repeat five times. Perform same procedure to opposite side.

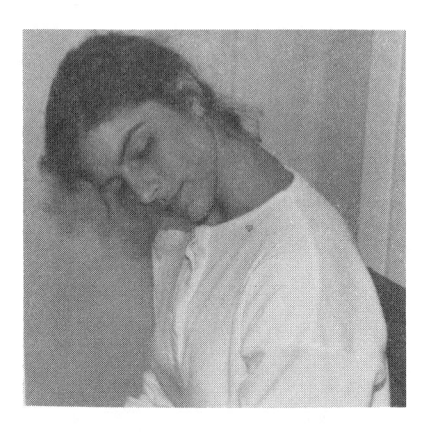

11. In a standing or sitting position raise arms straight toward ceiling. Do not look up. Take notice of posture of head on neck. This is good alignment. Hold arms up for a three-count and repeat ten times.

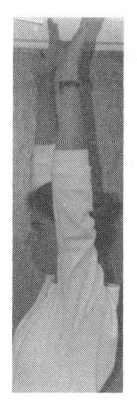

385

§ 9-7 NECK PAIN

12. In sitting or standing position, tuck chin in and hold head and neck in good alignment. Bend elbows and raise both arms out to side so that they are parallel to ground. Rapidly, move arms backwards with elbows moving toward each other behind back. Perform these movements for ten seconds.

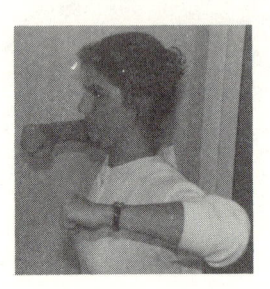

13. In standing position with back to a wall, tuck chin in and try to flatten the back of the neck against the wall. Hold for a three-count. Perform ten repetitions.

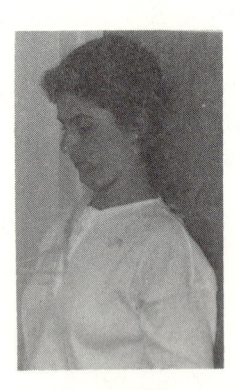

THERAPY, ERGONOMICS, REHABILITATION § 9-7

Figure 4. Postures for Preventing Neck Strain

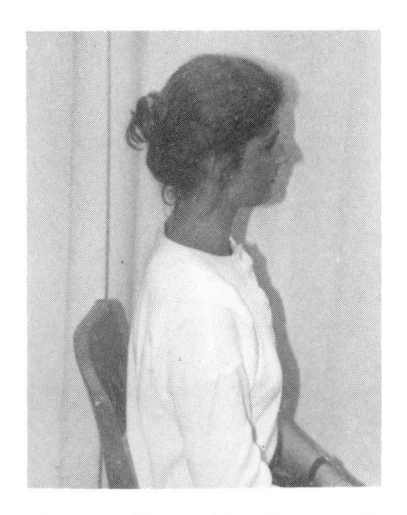

1. <u>Sitting</u>:

Correct: Keep chin down and head drawn back.

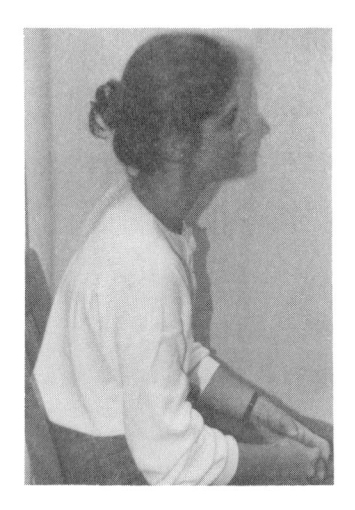

Incorrect: Do not keep your chin up and head back. Avoid sitting up close in theater environment.

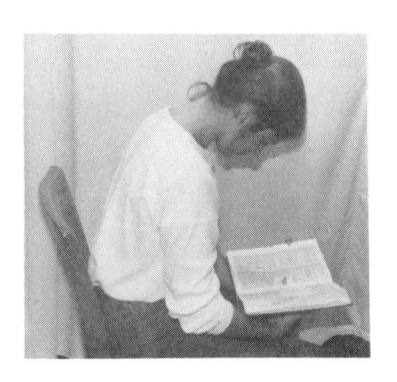

Incorrect: Avoid reading position which encourages prolonged forward head posture.

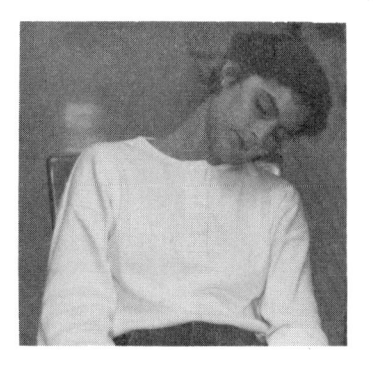

Incorrect: Avoid slouching and prolonged stretch to neck.

§ 9-7   NECK PAIN

2. <u>Driving</u>: Keep chin tucked in before rotating neck to look behind you. Use mirrors frequently. Sit up straight and use a pillow to sit on if the seat is too low. Adjust headrest to align with the middle of head and not just below the base of the skull.

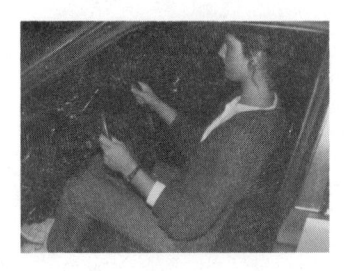

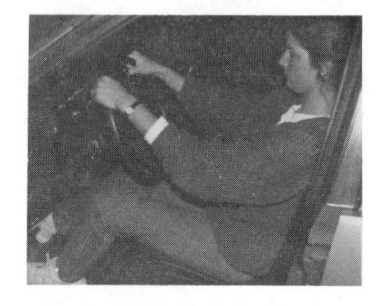

Correct: Sit up close to wheel with elbows at side. Keep chin down and head drawn back.

Incorrect: Do not sit with head resting forward. Do not keep elbows away from the body for prolonged periods.

3. <u>Drinking</u>: Do not tilt head backward when drinking from container. A bottle is easier than a can and a glass is better than both. Use a straw when necessary.

4. <u>Overhead work</u>: Avoid prolonged reaching and looking overhead. Use a ladder or stool to keep work at chest level. Use an extension pole when painting overhead areas or washing windows.

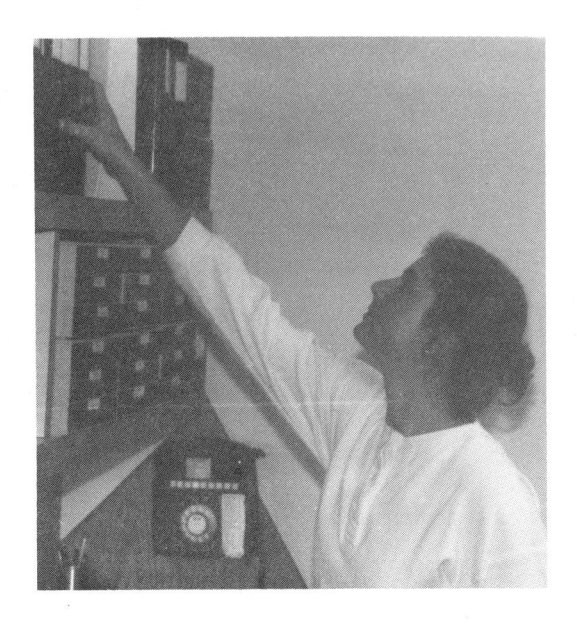

Incorrect: Avoid continuously reaching overhead and extending neck to look up. Reorganize work area to keep objects at chest level or use stool or step ladder.

§ 9-7 NECK PAIN

5. <u>Stooping and Lifting</u>:

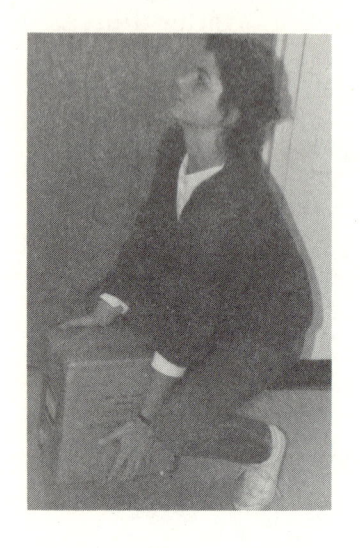

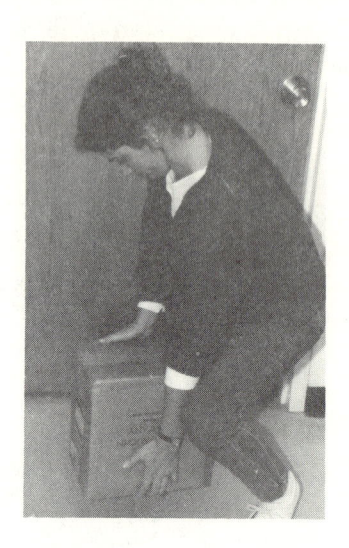

Incorrect: Avoid extending neck and lifting quickly.

Correct: Keep chin down and neck muscles fixed. Lift with your legs and shoulders.

6. <u>Reading</u>: Position should be comfortable with head, shoulders or arms supported and close to body. Use reading

THERAPY, ERGONOMICS, REHABILITATION   § 9-7

glasses instead of bifocals to avoid tilting the head backwards under close viewing conditions.

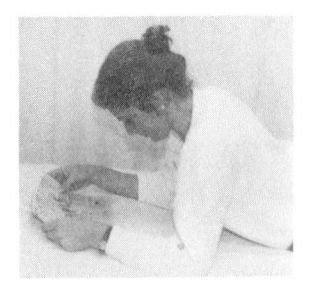

Incorrect: Do not read while in this position. It encourages too much extension and muscle activity in posterior neck.

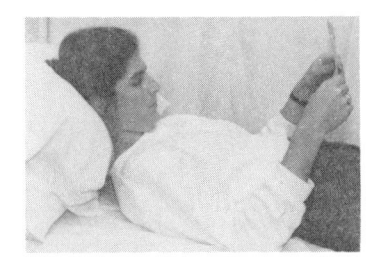

Incorrect: Do not read in bed with several pillows under head alone. This position promotes stretch in the posterior neck structures. Pillows should support both head and shoulders.

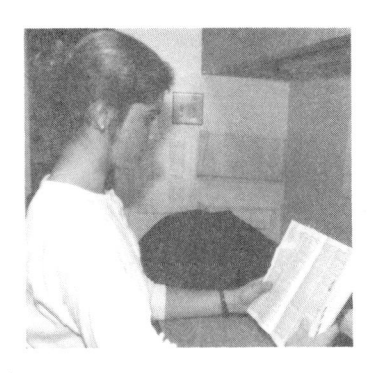

Correct: Read at desk with arms supported, material held up toward eyes and head erect. Low back should be supported by chair backrest.

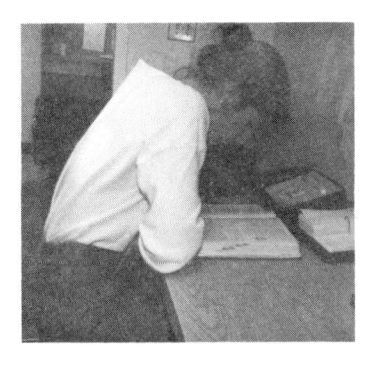

Incorrect: Avoid this position of head forward and eyes downward.

7. Telephone:

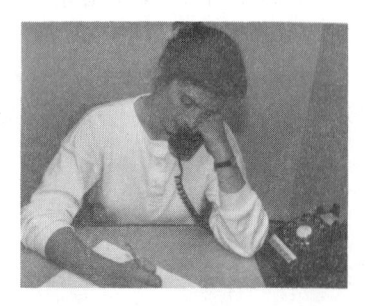

Correct: Hold receiver to ear with free hand with head in midline position. Use a headset if both hands are frequently busy with desk material.

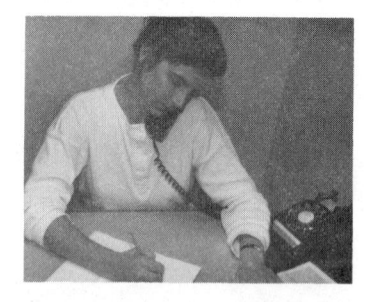

Incorrect: Avoid cradling the receiver between shoulder and ear. Use of a receiver cradling device is absolutely necessary on a headset.

8. **Typing or Word Processing**: Adjust copy material or video screen to be in line of vision without placing head forward and hyperextending the cervical spine. It may be helpful to use a special stand for typing material.

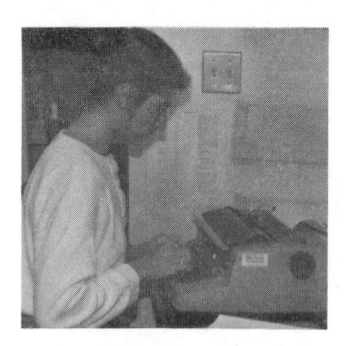

Correct: Chin down, head erect with elbows resting comfortably at sides. May or may not use arm rests. Keep low back supported.

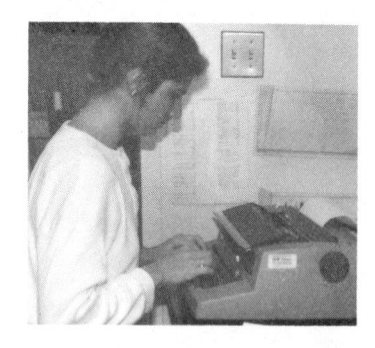

Incorrect: Avoid head forward posture and unsupported low back.

THERAPY, ERGONOMICS, REHABILITATION § 9-7

9. <u>Sleeping</u>: Proper pillow should fill space between back of head and round of upper back without flexion or extension of the spine. When sidelying the pillow should fill the area between the ear and mattress without encouraging side-bending of the neck. Pillows made of feathers or small pieces of foam are more adaptive than those of foam rubber or felt.

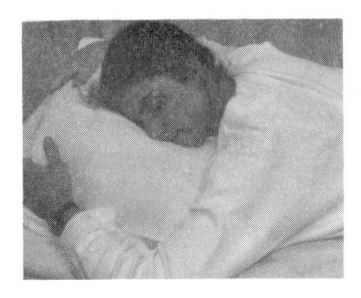

Incorrect: Avoid stomach lying with neck rotated and extended.

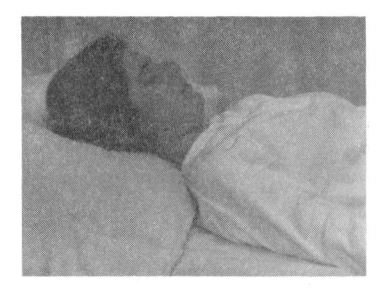

Correct: A flat pillow to hold the neck in neutral position. A special cervical pillow may also be used.

10. <u>Couch and television viewing</u>: Assume position where head, neck, and shoulders are properly supported.

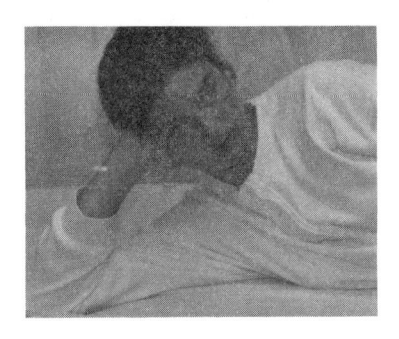

Incorrect: Avoid prolonged use of this position.

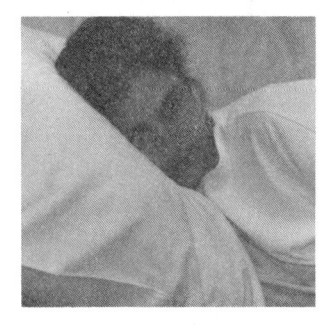

Incorrect: Avoid sidelying with neck in sidebend position.

§ 9-8. Ergonomics and Prevention.

Ergonomics (often referred to as human factors or human factors engineering in the United States) is a multidisciplinary activity concerned with ensuring that machine, task operations and work environment are designed in order to match human capacities and limitations (entry 46). Typically, the individual interested in initiating ergonomics activities in a production organization is a member of the industrial engineering, occupational safety, personnel selection and training or industrial medical group within the corporations. Often times, regardless of the effectiveness in design of equipment or work stations, the worker may still experience fatigue, muscle tension, and postural discomfort. A physical therapist may be another member of the ergonomic team who has the educational and clinical background to improve human physical capacities and decrease the worker's functional limitations by evaluating and treating the individual's body and not redesigning the machine. The individual may need specific instructions concerning which equipment adjustments are adaptable for a particular body type. Simple, brief postural exercises (Figure 3, Stage 4) may also be taught and performed at the job station.

In this author's experience, it has been found that people are more often the limiting factors in ergonomics rather than the equipment. Occupations which require visual, hand tasks and a high degree of concentration or stress often give rise to postural pain problems involving the neck, shoulders, upper and lower back. These individuals may complain about fatigue or muscular aches during the day and voice dissatisfaction with the work place and the work itself. This can create a stressful environment which can be contributive or predisposing to a chronic pain condition.

When evaluating the worker at the job site (e.g., video display terminal operator, secretary, materials handler, ceiling or tree worker, dentist, motor vehicle operator, etc.) the physical therapist observes and assesses the individual's muscular effort, both dynamic and static, required to perform the task. During dynamic muscular activity (work when in motion) the muscles contract and relax rhythmically (entry 17). Examples of dynamic efforts are walking, climbing stairs, turning a wheel, loading boxes, pushing a cart, etc. Static muscle activity supports a given weight without movement but with a steady consumption of energy. This requires a sustained effort with muscles being maintained at a constant length and contraction (entry 17). Examples of static tasks are standing at attention, neck and head forward posture while sitting, neck overflexed laterally to hold phone receiver between ear and shoulder, etc. There are, of course, combinations of static and dynamic muscular activities. Some examples may be a mechanic working under the car, looking up and painting a ceiling, looking downward and laying bricks, typing with head and neck rotated to read material, etc.

With excessive static activity demands in a job, overfatigue and strain are more likely to occur. Both are contributing factors to discomfort and stiffness of the neck and upper shoulders. However, dynamic muscular activity can be carried out for hours without the same degree of fatigue and consequences. One part of an explanation for this difference may be the blood circulation during each separate activity. During static muscular efforts the blood flow is decreased into the muscle and other soft tissue. This leads to diminished supply of oxygen and a build-up of wasteproducts. This build-up, particularly carbon dioxide and lactic acid, brings about a painful state of fatigue. In dynamic muscular efforts, the blood flow is increased, replenishing the oxygen supply and energy-producing substances and at the same time eliminating the waste-products (entry 17). A brief set of exercises, which may be performed at the job station, can also help stimulate blood circulation.

When a potential problem job is identified either by injury rate or employee complaints, it may be worthwhile for any member of the ergonomic team to evaluate the situation. In Table V a sample of a questionnaire to determine a need for an ergonomic assessment and indicators for task redesign is presented (entry 1). See Table VI for some indicators of the need for work place redesign and special considerations in the working environment (entry 1). Usually, changes can be kept to a minimum if the employer is well instructed in effective working postures, exercise, and body mechanics.

In the literature there are many investigations by ergonomists relating to jobs that require sitting, typing, and word processing (entries 5, 18, 38, 55). No studies were found associating painful neck syndromes with blue collar and other white collar jobs. Since society is becoming more service and information oriented, this desk-sitting, computer-adapted, work population is an appropriate target for prevention of neck injuries.

Ergonomists cannot reach agreement that proper posture is directly related to a decrease in incidence of neck, shoulder, and back pain (entries 5, 18, 47). They do, however, support the concept that ergonomic design could help reduce muscle fatigue and incidence of neck and shoulder pain (entries 5, 38, 40). This author's clinical experience is that posture, pain, and ergonomic design considerations are areas that correlate well in the assessment of an individual's pain syndrome. One study reported that electromyographic studies of the upper trapezius record lower electrical activity when there is an arm rest versus no arm rest on the chair. The subjective feelings of tension and pain in the neck, shoulders, and back were also reported to be lower for the same reason (entry 55).

In a field study of 119 accounting machine operators it was reported that the incidence of stiffness and pains in the neck increases with the degree of prolonged forward bending of the head and neck (see Figure 5) (entry 18). In another field study 159 VDT operators and 133 other office employees were examined by a physician. In Table VII the results of reported "almost daily pains" are shown for all examined groups (entry 18). Medical findings in a VDT field study revealed painful pressure points at tendons, joints, and muscles in various operators (Table VIII) (entry 18).

§ 9-8 NECK PAIN

Figure 5

Incidence of impairments in the neck related to the neck-head angles of 57 accounting machine operators.

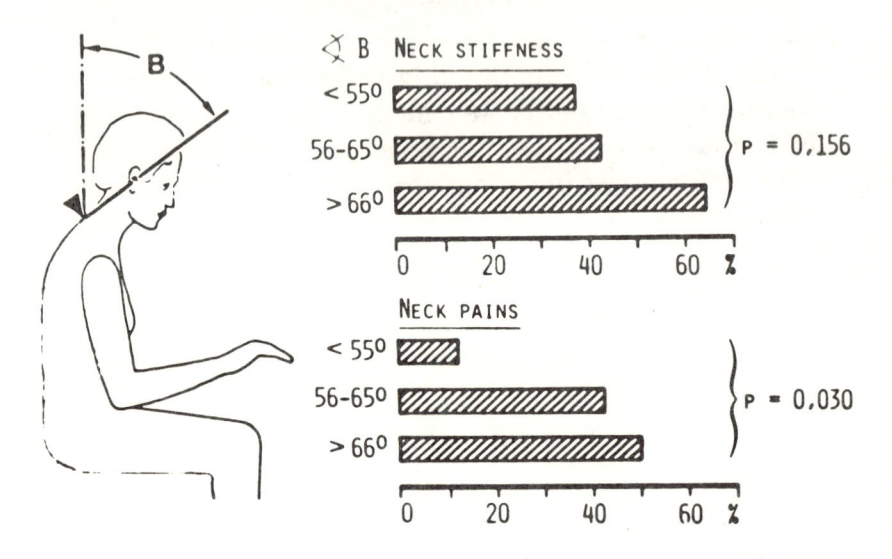

∡ B NECK STIFFNESS

< 55°
56-65°
> 66° } P = 0.156

0 20 40 60 %

NECK PAINS

< 55°
56-65°
> 66° } P = 0.030

0 20 40 60 %

100% = Subjects in each of the three "Angle-Groups"

Grandjean, E. Postural problems at office machine work station in *Ergonomics and Health in Modern Offices*. London and Philadelphia, Taylor & Francis, 1984.

The results reveal that serious impairments were observed in each group, but it is obvious that the highest figures are seen in the group operating data entry terminals and the lowest figures in the group occupied with traditional office work. These "almost daily pains" must be considered as

THERAPY, ERGONOMICS, REHABILITATION § 9-8

relevant injuries, since about 20% of the VDT operators visited a doctor because of reported troubles (entry 18).

Many recommendations for sitting desk job station designs have been made. The best designs are those with the most adaptable adjustments to the chair, desk, and VDT. See Figures 6, 7, 8 (entry 30). The sitting worker should always attempt to assume a position that minimizes the elbow distance from the body with or without arm rests (sometimes, there is no space at desk for arm rests), maintains no more than a 30-degree forward flexion of the neck while reading or typing, and prevents the head and neck from being rotated or extended for any prolonged period of time. The worker should be comfortable and be able to function with minimum strain. (Figure 9) (entry 18).

Figure 6: Adjustment Features of an Ergonomic Work Seat

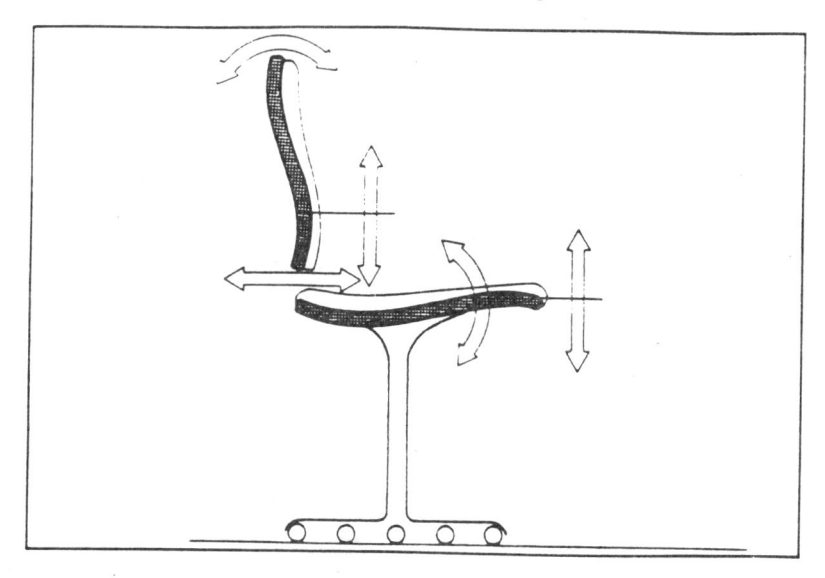

§ 9-8 NECK PAIN

Figure 7: Adjustment Features of an Ergonomic VDT Work Station

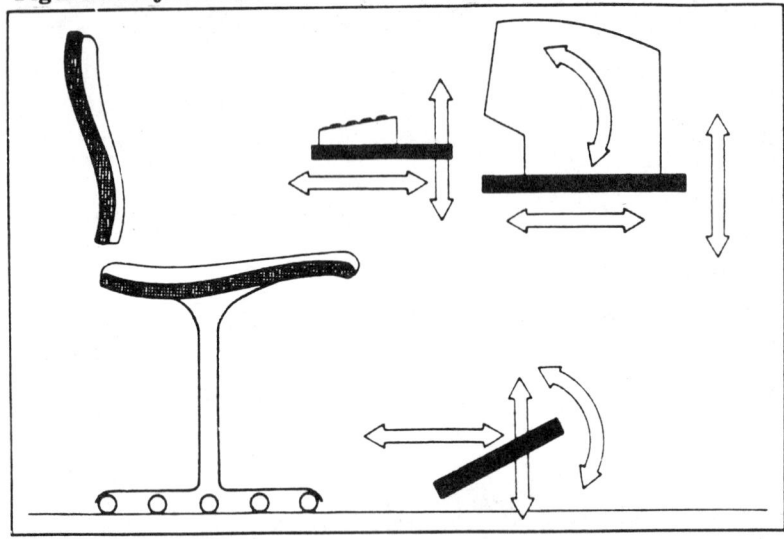

Figure 8: Recommended Approximate Dimensions (in centimeters)

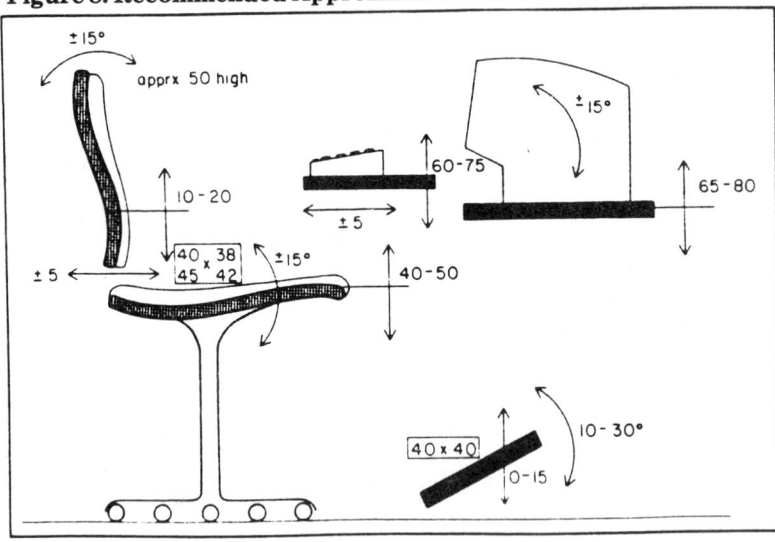

Kroemer, K.H.E. and Price, D.L. Ergonomics in the office: comfortable work stations allow maximum productivity. Industrial Engineering, July 1982.

THERAPY, ERGONOMICS, REHABILITATION   § 9-8

Figure 9

The "Mean Body Posture" Under Practical Conditions at Preferred Settings of the VDT Work Station. Results of 236 Observations on VDT operators.

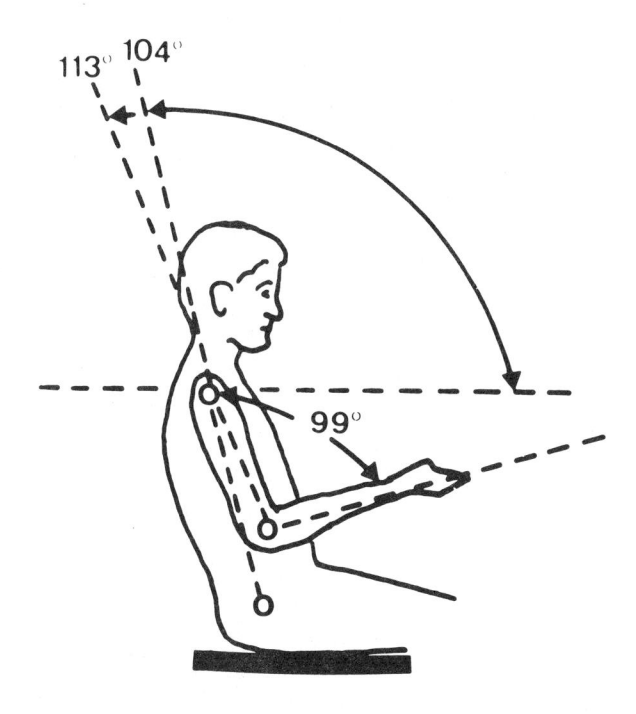

Grandjean, E. Postural problems at office machine work station in *Ergonomics and Health in Modern Offices*. London and Philadelphia, Taylor & Francis, 1984.

§ 9-9. Returning the Injured Worker to the Job.

After recovery from a painful neck syndrome and the physician has already planned for the individual to return to work, two important considerations should be made: (1) job restrictions, and (2) job description. This is another case where referral to a physical therapist would be appropriate. By consulting with the patient, the employer or the vocational rehabilitation counselor, the physical therapist can design an exercise program for the individual to best prepare for the demands of the job description. In Table IX a model for return to work and prevention of recurrence is presented.

In reviewing the job description, observations should be made of the visual tasks, hand tasks, task objectives, sequence of operations, strength and mobility, physical requirements. Different positions should be practiced to minimize energy expenditure and static muscle contractions. Any complaint of difficulty of discomfort in performing the task should be noted. Physical limitations may then be evaluated and an assessment made whether they are due to the injury and if they can be overcome with exercise, work methods and education in self-treatment, equipment adjustment, and prevention of injury. If the physical limitation cannot be resolved, then administration intervention may be needed. Light duty, a change in job classification or vocational training may all be considered.

During the recovery period progressive resistive exercises may be initiated for the legs, trunk, and arm within the individual's tolerance. This will assure performance readiness in strength and endurance and prevent debilitation. After all, it is only the neck involved and not the whole body. Exercises should be individualized and assigned by the physical therapist.

§ 9-10. Summary.

The course of rehabilitation of the individual with neck pain syndrome has been presented by a physical therapist beginning from the initial assessment and treatment to the return to gainful employment. The importance of therapeutic exercise in bodily posture and function has been stressed. A description of various physical therapy modalities has also been presented. Their effectiveness is discussed based on empirical success for lack of clinical or experimental studies in the literature.

BIBLIOGRAPHY

1. Alexander, D.D., and Smith, L.A. Evaluating industrial jobs, determining problem areas and making modifications. Industrial Engineering, June 1982.
2. Abramson, D.I. et al. Changes in blood flow, oxygen uptake and tissue temperatures produced by therapeutic physical agents. I. Effects of ultrasound. American Journal of Physical Medicine, 39:51-62, 1960.
3. Bocchi, L., and Orso, C.A. Whiplash injuries of the cervical spine, pp. 171-181.
4. Caillet, R. *Neck and Arm Pain,* 2d ed., Philadelphia, F.A. Davis Company, 1981.
5. Cantoni, S., et al. Posture analysis and evaluation at the old and new work place of a telephone company in Grandjean, E. *Ergonomics and Health in Modern Offices,* London and Philadelphia, Taylor & Francis, 1984.
6. Cloward, R. Acute Cervical Spine Injuries, Clinical Symposia, Vol. 32, No. 1, 1980.
7. Colachis, S.C., Strohm, B.R. Effect of duration of intermittent cervical traction on vertebral interspaces in the cervical spine. Arch. Phys. Med., 47:353, 1966.
8. Colachis, S.C. et al. A study of tractive forces and angle of pull on vertebral interspaces in the cervical spine. Archives Physical Med. and Rehab., Dec., 1965, 820-830.
9. DeLacerda, F.G. Effects of angle of traction pull on upper trapezius muscle activity. J. Ortho and Sports P.T., 1:205-209, 1980.

10. DePalma, A., and Rothman, R. *The Intervertebral Disc,* Philadelphia, W.B. Saunders Co., 1970.
11. Erickson, M.B.E. et al. Long term results of peripheral conditioning stimulation as an analgesic measure in chronic pain. Pain, 6 (1979), 335-447.
12. Erickson, M.B.E. *Transcutaneous Nerve Stimulation and Chronic Pain.* London, Liber Forlag, 1983.
13. Erickson, M.B.E. et al. Hazard from transcutaneous nerve stimulation in patients with pacemakers. Lancet 1, 1978, pp. 1319.
14. Frykholm, R. The clinical picture in Hirsch C. Zotterman, Y. (eds), *Cervical Pain,* Pergaman Press, Oxford, 1971.
15. Gelb, H. *Clinical Management of Head, Neck, and TMJ Pain and Dysfunction.* Philadelphia, W.B. Saunders Co., 1977.
16. Gould, J., and Davies, G. *Orthopaedic and Sports Physical Therapy,* C.V. Mosby, St. Louis, Toronto, Princeton, 1985.
17. Grandjean, E. *Ergonomics of the Home,* Taylor & Francis, London, Holstead Press, New York, 1973.
18. Grandjean, E. Postural problems at office machine work station in Grandjean, E. *Ergonomics and Health in Modern Offices.* London and Philadelphia, Taylor & Francis, 1984.
19. Grieve, G.P. *Common Vertebral Joint Problems,* New York, Churchill Livingstone, 1981.
20. Hohl, M. Soft tissue injuries of the neck in automobile accidents — factors influencing prognosis. J Bone and Joint Surgery, 56A:1675, 1974.
21. Hartman, et al. Cineradiography of the braced cervical spine. Clin Orthop, 109:97.
22. Jackson, R. *The Cervical Syndrome,* Springfield, Charles C. Thomas, 1977.
23. Jackson, R. Updating the neck. Trauma, 5:7, 1970.
24. Jette, D. et al. Effect of intermittent cervical traction on the myoelectric activity of the upper trapezius muscle in subjects with neck pain. JAPTA, 65:8, August 1985.
25. Johnson, R.M., et al. The Yale cervical orthosis: an evaluation of its effectiveness in restricting cervical motion in normal subjects and a comparison with other cervical orthoses. Physical Therapy, 58(7):865.
26. Johnson, R.M., Hart, D.L., et al. Cervical orthoses: a study comparing their effectiveness in instructing cervical motions in normal subjects. Am Bone and Joint Surg (Am), 59(3):332, 1977.

27. Kapandji, I.A. *Physiology of the Joints,* Vol. 3, New York, Churchill Livingstone, 1974.
28. Kendall, F. et al. *Posture and Pain.* Baltimore, MD, William and Wilkins Co., 1964.
29. Kopell, M.P., et al. *Peripheral Entrapment Neuropathies,* Huntington, New York, Robert E. Krieger Publishing Co., 1976.
30. Kroemer, K.H.E. and Price, D.L. Ergonomics in the office: comfortable work stations allow maximum productivity. Industrial Engineering, July 1982.
31. Kuntz, A. Relation of autonomic nervous system to physical therapy. Arch Phys Ther, 19:24-29, Jan. 1938.
32. Licht, S. *Therapeutic Heat and Cold,* Baltimore, MD, Waverly Press, Inc., 1972.
33. Licht, S. *Massage, Manipulation and Traction,* New Haven, 1968.
34. Long, D.M. et al. Electrical stimulation in the nervous system: current status for relief of pain. Pain, 1:109-123, 1975.
35. Maitland, G.D. *Vertebral Manipulation,* London-Boston, Butterworths, 1977.
36. Melzak, R. Prolonged relief of pain by brief, intense transcutaneous somatic stimulation. Pain, 1, 1975, pp. 357-373.
37. Meyerson, B.A. Electrostimulation procedures: effects presumed rationale, and possible mechanisms, in J.J. Bonica et al. (eds), *Advances in Pain Research and Therapy,* Vol. 5, New York, Raven Press, 1983.
38. NIOSH. Potential health hazards of video display terminals. U.S. Dept of Hlth and Human Services, Cincinnati, Ohio, June 1981.
39. Nyborg, W. Physical mechanism of biological effects of ultrasound. HEW Publ, 78-8062, May 1968.
40. Ong, C.N. VDT work place design and physical fatigue: a case study in Singapore in Grandjean, E. *Ergonomics and Health in Modern Offices,* London and Philadelphia, Taylor & Francis, 1984.
41. Paris, S. Seminar notes: spinal and extremity joint manipulation with notes on traction, April 1975, Wash. D.C.
42. Pain Control Letter. Let's do something about pain, #10, October 1977.
43. Rogoff, J. *Manipulation, Traction and Massage,* 2d ed., Baltimore, MD, Williams and Wilkins, 1980.
44. Rath, W.W. A Review Paper. Cervical traction: a clinical perspective. Ortho Review, 29-48, August 1984.

45. Shestach, R. *Handbook of Physical Therapy,* New York, Springer Publishing Co., 1977.
46. Smith, L.A., et al. How can an IE justify a human factors activities program to management? I.E., July 1982.
47. Starr, S.J. et al. Relating posture to discomfort in VDT use. JOM, Vol. 27, No. 4, April 1985.
48. Sternbach, R.A., et al. Transcutaneous electrical analgesia: a follow-up analysis. Pain 2, 1976, 35-41.
49. Stoddard, A. *Manual of Osteopathic Technique, 10th Impression.* London, Hutchinson and Co., 1978.
50. ter Haar, G.R. Basic physics of therapeutic ultrasound. Physiotherapy, 64, 1978, 100-103.
51. Thorsteinsson, G. et al. Transcutaneous electrical stimulation: a double blind trial of its efficacy for pain. Arch Phys Med, 58, 1977, pp 88-13.
52. Thorsteinsson, G. et al. The placebo effect of transcutaneous electrical stimulation. Pain, 5, 1978, pp 31-41.
53. Ultrasound. *Proceedings of the International Symposium on Therapeutic Ultrasound,* Sept. 1981, Winnipeg, Manitoba, Canada.
54. Wakin, K.G. et al. *Basic Fundamentals and Clinical Applications for Heat and Cold.* Medical Arts and Sciences, Vol. XIII, No. 2, 3, 4, 1959.
55. Weber, A., et al. The effects of various keyboard heights on EMG and physical discomfort in Grandjean, E. *Ergonomics and Health in Modern Offices,* London and Philadelphia, Taylor & Francis, 1984.
56. Wells, P.N.T. Absorption and dispersion of ultrasound in biological tissue. Ultrasound in Medicine and Biology I, 1975, 369-376.
57. White, A., et al. *Clinical Biomechanics of the Spine,* Philadelphia, J.P. Lippincott Co., 1978.
58. Zohn, D.A., et al. *Musculoskeletal Pain, Diagnosis, and Physical Treatment,* Boston, Little, Brown, and Co., 1976.

Table I
Limits and Representative Values of Range of Rotation of the Lower Cervical Spine

Interspace	Flexion/Extension (x-axis rotation) Limits of Ranges (degrees)	Representative Angle (degrees)	Lateral Bending (z-axis rotation) Limits of Ranges (degrees)	Representative Angle (degrees)	Axial Rotation (y-axis rotation) Limits of Ranges (degrees)	Representative Angle (degrees)
C2-C3	5-23	8	11-20	10	6-28	9
C3-C4	7-38	13	9-15	11	10-28	11
C4-C5	8-39	12	0-16	11	10-26	12
C5-C6	4-34	17	0-16	8	8-34	10
C6-C7	1-29	16	0-17	7	6-15	9
C7-T1	4-17	9	0-17	4	5-13	8

Table I (Continued)
Limits and Representative Values of Range of Rotation of the Thoracic Spine

Interspace	Flexion/Extension (x-axis rotation) Limits of Ranges (degrees)	Representative Angle (degrees)	Lateral Bending (z-axis rotation) Limits of Ranges (degrees)	Representative Angle (degrees)	Axial Rotation (y-axis rotation) Limits of Ranges (degrees)	Representative Angle (degrees)
T1-T2	3-5	4	5	6	14	9
T2-T3	3-5	4	5-7	6	4-12	8
T3-T4	2-5	4	3-7	6	5-11	8
T4-T5	2-5	4	5-6	6	4-11	8
T5-T6	3-5	4	5-6	6	5-11	8
T6-T7	2-7	5	6	6	4-11	8
T7-T8	3-8	6	3-8	6	4-11	8
T8-T9	3-8	6	4-7	6	6-7	7
T9-T10	3-8	6	4-7	6	3-5	4
T10-T11	4-14	9	3-10	7	2-3	2
T11-T12	6-20	12	4-13	9	2-3	2
T12-L1	6-20	12	5-10	8	2-3	2

Table I (Continued)
Representative Values of the Range of Rotation of the Lumbar Spine

INTERSPACE	FLEXION/EXTENSION (x-axis rotation) LIMITS OF RANGES (degrees)	REPRESENTATIVE ANGLE (degrees)	LATERAL BENDING (z-axis rotation) LIMITS OF RANGES (degrees)	REPRESENTATIVE ANGLE (degrees)	AXIAL ROTATION (y-axis rotation) LIMITS OF RANGES (degrees)	REPRESENTATIVE ANGLE (degrees)
L1-L2	9-16	12	3-8	6	1-3	2
L2-L3	11-18	14	3-9	6	1-3	2
L3-L4	12-18	15	5-10	8	1-3	2
L4	14-21	17	5-7	6	1-3	2
L5-S1	18-22	20	2-3	3	3-6	5

(White, A. A., III, and Panjabi, M. M.: The basic kinematics of the human spine. A review of past and current knowledge. Spine, 3:12, 1978.)

Table II
Mean Percentage

Mean percentage of normal flexion-extension restricted at each segmental level of the cervical spine (mean percentage flexion-extension and 95% confidence limits of mean percentage)*

Orthosis or collar	0-C1	C1-C2	C2-C3	C3-C4	C4-C5	C5-C6	C6-C7	C7-T1
Yale	53.7 ± 15.6	28.5 ± 23.6	70.8 ± 7.5	75.0 ± 5.7	69.6 ± 7.5	72.1 ± 6.9	68.4 ± 9.7	64.4 ± 14.5
Cervicothoracic	50.5 + 11.8	47.4 ± 11.8	68.3 + 5.9	75.0 ± 5.7	76.6 ± 4.0	80.4 + 4.1	81.1 + 5.4	67.8 + 6.8
Four-poster	37.2 ± 12.4	48.2 ± 16.2	69.2 ± 7.5	69.3 ± 7.4	74.1 ± 7.0	73.1 ± 6.4	66.0 ± 7.3	64.4 ± 12.0
SOMI brace	31.9 ± 14.5	40.9 ± 18.4	55.8 ± 10.1	55.1 ± 10.3	61.2 ± 8.0	59.4 ± 9.2	58.7 ± 11.7	55.9 ± 17.1
Philadelphia	59.6 ± 10.8	38.0 ± 14.0	71.7 ± 8.4	63.6 ± 8.0	48.3 ± 9.9	44.7 ± 8.7	41.3 ± 13.1	42.4 ± 13.7

Mean percentage of normal flexion restricted at each segmental level of the cervical spine (mean percentage flexion and 95% confidence limits of mean percentage)*

Orthosis or collar	0-C1	C1-C2	C2-C3	C3-C4	C4-C5	C5-C6	C6-C7	C7-T1
Yale	—	18.2 ± 30.6	73.6 ± 15.5	83.7 ± 10.3	80.6 ± 15.7	83.3 ± 9.7	79.2 ± 11.3	64.4 ± 18.1
Cerviocothoracic	—	35.1 ± 25.3	75.0 ± 11.3	70.4 ± 12.3	72.8 ± 6.9	86.0 ± 7.1	94.4 ± 4.8	77.4 ± 11.3
Four-poster	—	42.9 ± 28.0	77.8 ± 14.1	78.6 ± 11.3	82.5 ± 8.8	73.7 ± 10.6	68.8 ± 12.9	68.9 ± 15.8
SOMI brace	—	64.9 ± 24.0	87.5 ± 9.9	83.7 ± 11.3	81.5 ± 7.8	75.4 ± 10.6	76.8 ± 12.9	65.6 ± 20.3
Philadelphia	—	48.0 ± 24.0	77.8 ± 14.1	68.4 ± 11.3	55.3 ± 17.6	45.6 ± 16.8	50.4 ± 12.9	38.9 ± 20.3

Table II (Continued)

Mean percentage of normal extension restricted at each segmental level of the cervical spine (mean percentage extension and 95% confidence limits of mean percentage)*

Orthosis or collar	0-C1	C1-C2	C2-C3	C3-C4	C4-C5	C5-C6	C6-C7	C7-T1
Yale	59.7 ± 15.7	41.7 ± 27.8	66.7 ± 17.1	64.1 ± 15.7	58.2 ± 13.5	60.9 ± 15.5	52.4 ± 19.9	63.0 ± 43.7
Cervicothoracic	53.5 ± 11.8	58.3 ± 13.9	56.2 ± 15.0	79.5 ± 9.2	77.5 ± 9.3	73.3 ± 8.7	58.5 ± 13.7	37.0 ± 31.8
Four-poster	48.6 ± 12.3	46.7 ± 24.3	58.3 ± 15.0	59.0 ± 15.7	65.3 ± 13.5	72.4 ± 8.7	62.2 ± 18.7	40.7 ± 31.8
SOMI brace	49.7 ± 14.6	10.0 ± 33.0	8.3 ± 23.6	19.2 ± 18.3	38.8 ± 18.7	42.9 ± 19.3	31.7 ± 22.4	22.2 ± 43.7
Philadelphia	62.5 ± 12.3	25.0 ± 26.0	62.5 ± 19.3	56.4 ± 13.1	40.8 ± 12.4	43.8 ± 11.6	29.3 ± 24.9	51.8 ± 35.7

*Modified from Johnson, R.M., Hart, D.L., and others: The Yale cervical orthosis: an evaluation of its effectiveness in restricting cervical motion in normal subjects and a comparison with other cervical orthoses; reprinted from *Physical Therapy* 58(7):865, 1978 with the permission of the American Physical Therapy Association.

Table III
Approximate Percentage Restriction

Approximate percentage restriction of range of motion (C1-C7)*

Orthoses	Motion picture			Cineradiograph		
	Flexion/extension	Lateral bending	Axial rotation	Flexion/extension	Lateral bending	Axial rotation
Soft cervical collar	5-10	5-10	0	0	0	0
Thomas hard plastic collar	75	75	50	75	75	50
Four-poster collar	80-85	80-85	60	85	85	60
Long two-poster collar	95	90	90	90	90	90
Guilford two-poster collar	90-95	90-95	90-95	90	90-95	90
Halo device	(Essentially no motion)						

*Data modified from Hartman, J.T., Palumbo, F., and Hill, B.J.: Cineradiography of the braced normal cervical spine, Clin. Orthop. 109:97, 1975 and White, A., and Panjabi, M.: Clinical biomechanics of the spine, Philadelphia, 1978, J.B. Lippincott Co., p. 355.

THERAPY, ERGONOMICS, REHABILITATION

Table IV
Flexion and Extension

Flexion and extension allowed at each segmental level (mean degrees and 95% confidence limits of the mean)*

Test situation	Motion	Occ.-C1	C1-C2	C2-C3	C3-C4	C4-C5	C5-C6	C6-C7	C7-T1
Normal, unrestricted	Flexion	0.7 ± 0.5	7.7 ± 1.2	7.2 ± 0.9	9.8 ± 1.0	10.3 ± 1.0	11.4 ± 1.0	12.5 ± 1.0	9.0 ± 1.1
	Extension	18.1 ± 2.1	6.0 ± 1.2	4.8 ± 0.8	7.8 ± 1.1	9.8 ± 1.2	10.5 ± 1.3	8.2 ± 1.2	2.7 ± 0.7
Soft collar	Flexion	1.3 ± 1.3	5.1 ± 1.9	4.5 ± 1.2	7.4 ± 1.5	8.4 ± 2.4	9.9 ± 1.7	9.7 ± 0.9	7.7 ± 2.5
	Extension	13.7 ± 3.5	1.9 ± 1.4	3.9 ± 1.0	5.8 ± 1.7	6.8 ± 1.6	7.8 ± 1.2	7.4 ± 1.4	2.8 ± 1.9
Philadelphia collar	Flexion	0.9 ± 1.0	4.0 ± 1.8	1.6 ± 1.0	3.1 ± 1.1	4.6 ± 1.8	6.2 ± 1.9	6.2 ± 1.6	5.5 ± 1.8
	Extension	6.8 ± 2.2	4.5 ± 1.5	1.8 ± 0.9	3.4 ± 1.0	5.8 ± 1.2	5.9 ± 1.2	5.8 ± 2.0	1.3 ± 0.9
SOMI brace	Flexion	3.6 ± 1.8	2.7 ± 1.8	0.9 ± 0.7	1.6 ± 1.1	1.9 ± 0.8	2.8 ± 1.2	2.9 ± 1.6	3.1 ± 1.8
	Extension	9.1 ± 2.6	5.4 ± 1.9	4.4 ± 1.1	6.3 ± 1.4	6.0 ± 1.8	6.0 ± 2.0	5.6 ± 1.8	2.1 ± 1.1
Four-poster brace	Flexion	2.9 ± 2.0	4.4 ± 2.1	1.6 ± 1.0	2.1 ± 1.1	1.8 ± 0.9	3.0 ± 1.2	3.9 ± 1.6	2.8 ± 1.4
	Extension	9.3 ± 2.2	3.2 ± 1.4	2.0 ± 0.7	3.2 ± 1.2	3.4 ± 1.3	2.9 ± 0.9	3.1 ± 1.5	1.6 ± 0.8
Cervicothoracic brace	Flexion	1.3 ± 0.9	5.0 ± 1.9	1.8 ± 0.8	2.9 ± 1.2	2.8 ± 0.7	1.6 ± 0.8	0.7 ± 0.6	2.4 ± 1.0
	Extension	8.4 ± 2.1	2.5 ± 0.8	2.1 ± 0.7	1.6 ± 0.7	2.2 ± 0.9	2.8 ± 0.9	3.4 ± 1.1	1.7 ± 0.8

Table IV (Continued)

Normal motion allowed from the occiput to the first thoracic vertebra (mean percentage and 95% confidence limits of the mean)*

Test situation	Number of subjects (male/female)	Mean age (years)	Flexion-extension	Significance†	Rotation	Significance†	Lateral bending	Significance†
Normal, unrestricted (all subjects)	44	25.8 (20-36)	100		100		100	
Soft collar	20 10/10	26.2 (20-36)	74.2 ± 7.2	0.001	82.6 ± 4.6	0.001	92.3 ± 8.0	0.057, NS
Philadelphia collar	17 9/8	25.8 (20-34)	28.9 ± 4.7	0.001	43.7 ± 6.7	0.001	66.4 ± 10.7	0.001
SOMI brace	22 7/15	25.0 (21-31)	27.7 ± 6.6	0.772, NS	33.6 ± 6.4	0.05	65.6 ± 9.4	0.899, NS
Four-poster brace	27 11/16	25.9 (21-36)	20.6 ± 5.4	0.05	27.1 ± 3.9	0.05	45.9 ± 7.5	0.001
Cervicothoracic brace	27 11/16	25.9 (21-36)	12.8 ± 3.0	0.05	18.2 ± 3.2	0.001	50.5 ± 7.1	0.063, NS
Halo with plastic body vest	7 6/1	40.0 (20-48)	4		1		4	

*Modified from Johnson, R.M., Hart, D.L., and others: Cervical orthoses: a study comparing their effectiveness in restricting cervical motion in normal subjects, J. Bone Joint Surg. (Am.) 59(3):332, 1977.

†Significance recorded is the probability value of one brace or collar varying significantly compared with the test situation listed above, using the paired t-test. For example, flexion-extension in a soft collar was significantly different from normal unrestricted motion (P < 0.001). The Philadelphia collar was significantly better in restricting flexion-extension than the soft collar (P = 0.772).

Table V

Human Factors and Task Redesign

Indicators of the Need for Human Factors Engineering Evaluation

☐ Is absenteeism on this task too high?
☐ Is turnover on this task too high?
☐ Is production efficiency on this task too low?
☐ Do employees complain frequently about this task?
☐ Is personnel assignment on this task limited by age, sex or body size?
☐ Is the training time for this task too long?
☐ Is product quality too low?
☐ Have there been too many accidents on this job?
☐ Have there been too many visits to medical?
☐ Does this task result in too much material waste?
☐ Is there excessive equipment damage on this job?
☐ Does the worker make frequent mistakes?
☐ Is the operator frequently away from his or her work place?
☐ Is this work place utilized on more than one shift per day?

Indicators of the Need for Task Redesign

☐ Is the worker required to lift and carry too much weight?
☐ Is the worker required to push or pull carts, boxes, rolls of material, etc., that involve large break-away forces to get started?
☐ Is the worker required to push or pull carts and hand trucks up or down ramps and inclines?
☐ Does the task require the worker to apply pushing, pulling, lifting or lowering forces while the body is bent, twisted or stretched out?
☐ Is the work pace rapid and not under the operator's control?
☐ Does the worker's heart rate exceed 120 beats per minute during task performance?

Table V (Continued)

Indicators of the Need for Task Redesign (Continued)

☐ Do workers complain that their fatigue allowances are insufficient?
☐ Does the task require that one motion pattern be repetitively performed at a high frequency?
☐ Does the task require the frequent use or manipulation of hand tools?
☐ Does the task require both hands and both feet to continually operate controls or manipulate the work unit?
☐ Is the worker required to maintain the same posture, either sitting or standing, all the time?
☐ Is the worker required to mentally keep track of a changing work situation particularly as it concerns the status of several machines?
☐ Is the rate at which the worker must process information likely to exceed his capability?
☐ Does the worker have insufficient time to sense and respond to information signals that occur simultaneously from different machines?

Alexander, D.D., and Smith, L.A. Evaluating industrial jobs, determining problem areas and making modifications. Industrial Engineering, June 1982.

Table VI

Work Place Redesign Considerations

Indicators of the Need for Work Place Redesign

☐ Does the work surface appear to be too high or too low for many operators?
☐ Do workers frequently sit on the front edge of their chairs?
☐ Must the worker assume an unnatural or stretched position in order to see dials, guages or parts of the work unit and in order to reach controls, materials or parts of the work unit?
☐ Is the worker required to operate foot pedals while standing?
☐ Does the operation of foot pedals or knee switches prevent the worker from assuming a natural, comfortable posture?
☐ Are foot pedals too small to allow foot position changes?
☐ Is a footrest necessary?
☐ Do workers frequently attempt to modify their work chair by adding cushions or pads?
☐ Are workers required to hold up their arms or hands without the assistance of armrests?
☐ Are dials and equipment controls difficult to operate or poorly labeled?
☐ Is the design and layout of equipment a hindrance to cleaning and maintenance activities?
☐ Does the work place appear unnecessarily cluttered?
☐ Is the worker required to use a non-adjustable chair?
☐ Can the worker be relieved of static holding work by providing clamps or supports for the work units?

Indicators of Special Considerations in the Working Environment

☐ Does process noise interfere with the reception of speech or auditory signals?
☐ Is process noise of an irritating nature so that it interferes with the worker's attention to his task?

Table VI (Continued)

> ### Indicators of Special Considerations
> ### in the Working Environment (Continued)
>
> ☐ Is process noise loud enough to cause hearing loss?
> ☐ Do the work tasks contain significant visual components, thus necessitating careful attention to lighting?
> ☐ Does the worker's eye have to move periodically from dark to light areas?
> ☐ Are there any direct or reflected glare sources in the work area?
> ☐ Do lights shine on moving machinery in such a manner as to produce stroboscopic effects or distracting flashes?
> ☐ Does task background coloration interfere with the color codes on knobs, handles or displays?
> ☐ Is the air temperature uncomfortably hot or cold?
> ☐ Is the relative humidity uncomfortably high?
> ☐ Are radiant heat sources located near an operator's work station?
> ☐ Is the worker exposed to rapid thermal or visual environmental changes?
> ☐ Do hand tools or process equipment vibrate the worker's hands, arms, or whole body?
> ☐ Does process dust settle on displays, making them difficult to see?

Alexander, D.D., and Smith, L.A. Evaluating industrial jobs, determining problem areas and making modifications. Industrial Engineering, June 1982.

Table VII

Postural Efforts at VDT Work Stations

In another field study, 159 VDT operators and 133 other office employees were examined. The results of reported "almost daily" pains are shown for all examined groups.

Incidence of "almost daily" pain in five office jobs.

Groups	n	neck %	shoulder %	r. arm %	r. hand %
Data entry terminals	53	11	15	15	6
Accounting machine operators	119	3	4	8	8
Conversational terminals	109	4	5	7	11
Typists	78	5	5	4	5
Traditional office work	55	1	1	1	0

Grandjean, E. Postural problems at office machine work station in *Ergonomics and Health in Modern Offices.* London and Philadelphia, Taylor & Francis, 1984.

Table VIII

Medical Findings in a VDT field study: painful pressure points at tendons, joints and muscles in the shoulder area. r = right, l = left.

Palpation findings in shoulders

Painful pressure points at tendons, joints and muscles

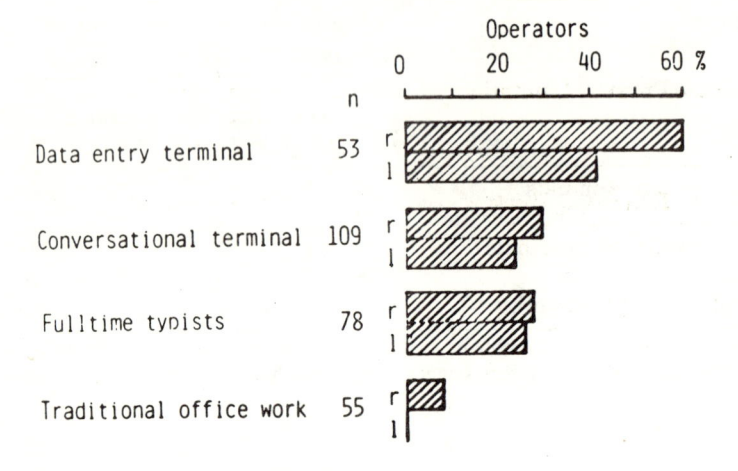

Work type	n	r/l	Operators % (0, 20, 40, 60)
Data entry terminal	53	r	~60
		l	~50
Conversational terminal	109	r	~25
		l	~20
Fulltime typists	78	r	~20
		l	~25
Traditional office work	55	r	~5
		l	~2

Grandjean, E. Postural problems at office machine work station in *Ergonomics and Health in Modern Offices.* London and Philadelphia, Taylor & Francis, 1984.

Table IX

Model for Prevention and Return to Work

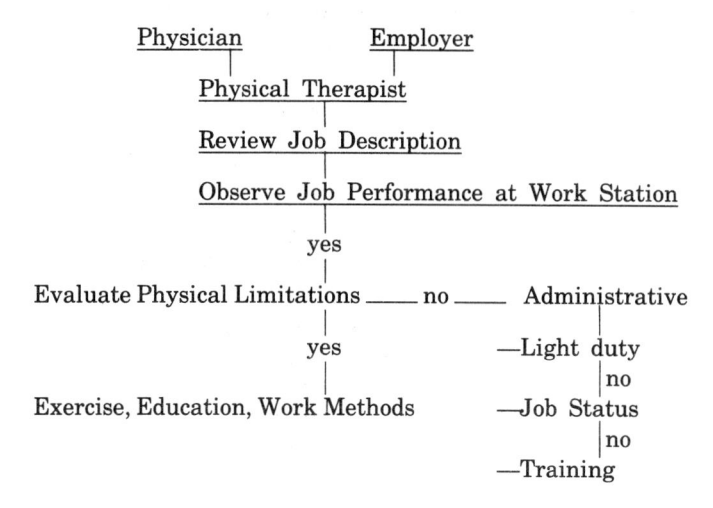

```
        Physician            Employer
            |                    |
          Physical Therapist
            |
          Review Job Description
            |
          Observe Job Performance at Work Station
            |
           yes
            |
Evaluate Physical Limitations ―― no ―― Administrative
            |                              |
           yes                            —Light duty
            |                              | no
Exercise, Education, Work Methods         —Job Status
                                           | no
                                          —Training
```

421

CHAPTER 10

STANDARDIZED CERVICAL SPINE EVALUATION FOR IMPAIRMENT RATING

Henry L. Feffer, M.D.

§ 10-1. The Cervical Spine Evaluation Problem.
§ 10-2. Standardized Neck Evaluation Guidelines.
Bibliography.
Table I. Industrial Back Injury Work Restriction Classification.
Table II. Disability Evaluation of the Cervical Spine.

The assignment of a permanent partial impairment for neck injuries is not consistent at the present time (entry 5). No official set of guidelines has been established (entry 4). Each physician learns by trial and error and he/she has usually reached senior citizen status before becoming functionally competent. This chapter will first present an overview of the problem for currently determining impairment and conclude with a standardized system for the neck based on diagnosis.

§ 10-1. The Cervical Spine Evaluation Problem.

Physical disability and physical impairment are not synonymous. The physical impairment rating is the objective assessment of body dysfunction. Physical disability, on the other hand, is very complex. It is affected by culture, socioeconomic background, education, experience, and the psychological makeup of the individual. While a physician should be able to objectively rate physical impairment, and can have a valid opinion concerning disability, a full assessment of disability is not strictly a medical matter, and is best done by non-medical people.

These non-medical people are rehabilitation specialists who have been trained as vocational experts. They are trained to take a physician's objective physical impairment rating and translate it into a disability rating. In essence, this assessment reflects an individual's ability to procure employment generally and is called *Residual Occupational Access*. It is an evaluation system conceived on the premise that all individuals, based on their age, education, and previous work experience, qualify for a certain percentage of the jobs found in the labor force. Personal injury, when it results in permanent impairment and functional restrictions, reduces that percentage. Therefore, by comparing an individual's pre-injury access to the labor force with the post-injury access to the same labor force, one has a measure of reduced employability or reduced occupational access, and accordingly, a measure of loss of earning power. Thus, if these vocational experts could get a consistent impairment rating they could calculate a consistent disability.

Unfortunately, there are no standardized guidelines to aid the physician in determining a physical impairment rating for the neck. The best available is the American Medical Association's *Guide to the Evaluation of Permanent Impairment* (entry 1). However, most experienced evaluators have given up on this text for guidance on neck injuries because these tables consider motion as the sole criteria of impairment and do not consider pain in the determination of neck impairment except when associated with peripheral nerve injury or when "substantiated by clinical findings." As happens so often chronic neck pain is often associated with little or no objective clinical signs and these, or the lack thereof, frequently are unrelated to the injury or disability in question. In addition, accurate measurement of cervical spine motion, even in the most experienced of hands, is often just about impossible. In effect, the facts that are utilized by most physicians, such as motivation, age, education, personality, I.Q., and social environment, strongly suggest that evaluators often rate disability rather than impairment.

The *AMA Guides* do, however, present one very useful concept. This is the "whole man" idea. Each part of the body is considered to represent only a part of the whole; the percent each part contributes is based on a notion of function. Since the spine (low back and neck) is important to many functions, it contributes a maximum of sixty percent of the whole man. Thus, once the impairment for the given part is estimated, the whole man impairment can be determined easily.

The only other reference for rating impairment with any credibility in this field is the *Manual for Orthopaedic Surgeons in Evaluating Permanent Physical Impairment* (entry 2) published by the American Academy of Orthopaedic Surgeons. However, this text for the neck relies on subjective symptoms for the most part and is of little practical value to the examining physician. The problem is that information regarding bending and twisting of the neck simply does not furnish the answers. The patient twists as far as he wants to and certainly there is a wide discrepancy among individuals with normal necks. In evaluating one extremity it can be compared to the other but unfortunately the neck stands alone in this respect. Some attempt must be made to correlate the objective symptoms available with the subjective complaints to achieve a consistent impairment rating system.

§ 10-2. Standardized Neck Evaluation Guidelines.

To try to establish a standardized impairment rating system, a questionnaire was circulated among 53 American members of the Cervical Spine Research Society. They were asked to fill out the impairment ratings they use in

§ 10-2   NECK PAIN

33 specific clinical situations. As would be expected, the responses from these experts were anything but consistent. However, they could be handled statistically so that in most cases a medium range was obvious. The figures spread from a zero percentage in the completely recovered acute neck sprain to 20% following failed neck surgery. The overall goal was to establish a valid linkage between a specific diagnosis, impairment rating, and physical exertion requirement.

The physical exertion requirements that will be related to a specific impairment rating are those defined by the Social Security Administration (entry 3). They are relatively simple and easy to use since the terms have the same meaning as they have in the *Dictionary of Occupational Titles* published by the Department of Labor. Even though the Social Security Administration does not use the permanent partial physical impairment rating system, it is relatively easy to modify their classification to conform to a compensation/litigation setting in the following way:

Very Heavy Work is that which involves lifting objects weighing more than 100 pounds at a time, with frequent lifting or carrying of objects weighing 50 pounds or more.

Heavy Work involves lifting of no more than 100 pounds at a time, with frequent lifting or carrying of objects weighing up to 50 pounds.

No one with any neck related permanent partial physical impairment can be expected to perform safely within either of the above two categories. If a patient cannot possibly be qualified to do anything lighter, he would have to be approved for social security.

Medium Work is defined as involving the lifting of no more than fifty pounds at a time, with frequent lifting or carrying of objects weighing up to twenty-five pounds. Workers with five percent or less back related permanent partial physical impairment can qualify in this category, but those with higher ratings cannot.

Light Work is described as involving lifting of no more than twenty pounds at a time with frequent lifting or carrying of objects weighing up to ten pounds. Applicants with between ten and fifteen percent permanent partial physical impairment because of a low-back problem should be able to do this type of work.

Sedentary Work is described as that involving no more than the lifting of ten pounds at a time and occasional lifting or carrying of articles like docket files, ledgers, or small tools. Applicants with twenty or twenty-five percent permanent partial physical impairment should be capable of this type of work.

Those people with more than twenty percent neck related permanent partial physical impairment will rarely qualify for any type of productive occupational activity unless they have special sedentary qualifications which can be done part time or at home. These work restriction classifications are summarized in Table I.

Table II presents neck pain impairment ratings in a standardized set of diagnostic situations. It also matches physical exertion requirements with each diagnostic category. Some of the more common diagnostic entities will be briefly presented.

An Acute Neck Sprain is defined as a soft tissue injury of an otherwise normal neck. X-rays are negative and there is no radiating pain. Patients should be able to return to their normal activity within two to three weeks. If recovery is delayed, some non-traumatic medical or psycho-social problem should be suspected.

Most patients who have a herniated nucleus pulposus will rarely fully recover without some degree of residual physical impairment. In the vast majority of cases it can be assumed that none of them will ever get back to very heavy work. No surgical procedure should be expected to return a patient to heavy work. Surgery is indicated to relieve an unacceptable level of pain. As a rule, a patient who has had a discectomy in their cervical spine may be expected to end up with anywhere between a 10% and 20% permanent partial physical impairment. A perfect operative result will rate at least 10% whereas a patient with a painful neck and a substantial neurological deficit will rate 20%.

Finally, one of the more difficult situations to evaluate relates to on-the-job injuries incurred by workers with pre-existing osteoarthritis. Neck sprains under these circumstances can be slow to respond. The symptoms from the osteoarthritis tend to be perceived as being more disabling than they were before the compensable injury. In spite of this, the spinal experts surveyed were in favor of awarding a 5% permanent partial physical impairment rating to those who were subjectively worse and a 10% rating to those who were both subjectively and objectively worse. In either situation light work was the most that could be required of these patients.

BIBLIOGRAPHY

1. American Medical Association: *Guides to the Evaluation of Permanent Impairment,* 1977.
2. American Academy of Orthopaedic Surgeons: *Manual for Orthopaedic Surgeons in Evaluating Permanent Physical Impairment,* 1962.
3. Anonymous: Social Security Rulings. Title 20 — Employees' Benefits, 404.1567 — Physical Exertion Requirements.
4. Brand, R.A., Lehmann, T.R. Low-back impairment rating practices of orthopaedic surgeons. Spine, 8:75-78, 1983.
5. Ziporyn, Terra: disability evaluation — a fledgling science? JAMA, 250:873-4 - 879-80, 1983.

Table I
Industrial Back Injury
Work Restriction Classification
(As Adapted From Social Security Regulations)

Work Classification	Work Restrictions	PPPI	Relevant Diagnoses
VERY HEAVY WORK	Occasional lifting in excess of 100 pounds Frequent lifting of 50 pounds or more Overhead work	Zero	Recovered neck strain Recovered hyperextension injury
HEAVY WORK	Occasional lifting of 100 pounds Frequent lifting of up to 50 pounds Overhead work	Zero	Herniated nucleus pulposus treated conservatively with complete recovery Recovered neck strain on top of pre-existing degenerative disease or cervical canal stenosis
MEDIUM WORK	Occasional lifting of 50 pounds Frequent lifting of 25 pounds Restricted overhead work	5%	Chronic neck strain Degenerative cervical intervertebral disc disease under reasonable control Herniated nucleus pulposus treated by surgical discectomy and completely recovered Hyperextension injury with residual pain Healed odontoid & hangman's fracture treated nonoperatively Pre-existing radiologically evident degenerative disease with secondary hyperextension injury with moderate pain and restriction

Table I (Continued)
Industrial Back Injury
Work Restriction Classification
(As Adapted From Social Security Regulations)

Work Classification	Work Restrictions	PPPI	Relevant Diagnoses
LIGHT WORK	Occasional lifting of no more than 20 pounds Frequent lifting of up to 10 pounds No overhead work	10% to 15%	Degenerative cervical disc disease with chronic pain and restriction Herniated nucleus pulposus treated conservatively or operatively, but left with discomfort, restriction, and neurological deficit Hyperextension injury with chronic pain and restriction Cervical canal stenosis Moderately severe osteoarthritis accompanied by instability Hangman's fracture treated with fusion Odontoid fracture treated with fusion Burst/compression fracture of lower cervical spine with no neurological deficit treated with fusion or external fixation
SEDENTARY WORK	Occasional lifting of 10 pounds No overhead work		Multiply operated neck (constant pain) Pre-existing cervical stenosis with neck injury treated by surgery with patient subjectively and objectively worse

Table II

Disability Evaluation of the Cervical Spine

Note: Compensable injuries are underlined. Please indicate percentage of permanent impairment for each sub-heading.

Work Permitted		(PPPI) % Impairment
	(1) Acute neck sprain ♦ conservative care ✧	
Very Heavy Work	(a) complete recovery	0
Medium Work	(b) chronic neck strain (no x-ray findings)	5
	(2) Pre-existing, radiologically evident degenerative disease ♦ acute neck sprain ♦ conservative care ✧	
Heavy Work	(a) complete recovery	0
Medium Work	(b) acceptable level of discomfort and restriction	5
Light Work	(c) chronic pain and restriction	10
	(3) Herniated nucleus pulposus ♦ conservative care ✧	
Heavy Work	(a) complete recovery	0
Light Work	(b) acceptable level of discomfort and restriction, with or without neurologic deficit	10
	(4) Herniated nucleus pulposus ♦ surgical discectomy, with or without fusion ✧	

Table II (Continued)

Work Permitted		(PPPI) % Impairment
Medium Work	(a) complete recovery	5
Light Work	(b) acceptable level of discomfort, with or without neurologic deficit	10
Light Work	(c) pain and restriction without neurologic deficit	15
Sedentary Work	(d) pain and restriction with neurologic deficit	20

(5) <u>Herniated nucleus pulposus</u> ♦ surgical discectomy (x times), with or without fusion ↻

Medium Work	(a) complete recovery	10
Light Work	(b) moderate pain and restriction (employable)	15
Sedentary to No Work	(c) failed neck (constant pain)	20

(6) <u>Hyperextension injury</u> (no objective findings) ♦ conservative care ↻

Very Heavy Work	(a) complete recovery	0
Medium Work	(b) moderate pain and restriction (employable)	5
Light Work	(c) chronic pain and restriction	10

(7) Pre-existing, radiologically evident degenerative disease ♦ <u>hyperextension injury</u> ♦ conservative care ↻

Heavy Work	(a) complete recovery	0

EVALUATION FOR IMPAIRMENT RATING

Table II (Continued)

Work Permitted		(PPPI) % Impairment
Medium Work	(b) moderate pain and restriction (employable)	5
Light Work	(c) chronic pain and restriction	10
	(8) Pre-existing cervical canal stenosis ♦ acute neck strain ♦ conservative care ⟡	
Heavy Work	(a) status quo	0
Light Work	(b) subjectively worse	10
Light Work	(c) subjectively and objectively worse	15
	(9) Pre-existing cervical canal stenosis ♦ acute neck strain ♦ decompression, with or without fusion ⟡	
Medium Work	(a) status quo	5
Light Work	(b) subjectively worse	15
Sedentary to no Work	(c) subjectively and objectively worse	20
Medium Work	(10) Acute neck strain ♦ conservative care ♦ NL no objective residuals ♦ confirmed neurosis ⟡	0
Medium Work	(11) Odontoid fracture ♦ external fixation ⟡	10
Light Work	(12) Odontoid fracture ♦ fusion ⟡	20

Table II (Continued)

Work Permitted		(PPPI) % Impairment
Medium Work	(13) Hangman's fracture ♦ external fixation ◊	10
Light Work	(14) Hangman's fracture ♦ fusion ◊	15
Light Work	(15) Burst/compression fracture, lower cervical spine, with no NL neurologic deficit ♦ external fixation ◊	15
Light work	(16) Burst/compression fracture, lower cervical spine, with no NL neurologic deficit ♦ fusion ◊	15

Index

A

ADVERSE EFFECT OF PAIN TREATMENT.
Disruption of social and family situations, §8-12(D).
Experiencing loss of future sense, §8-12(C).
Inappropriate surgery and hospitalization, §8-12(E).
Loss of ability to work, §8-12(B).
Polypharmacy and overutilization of analgesics, §8-12(A).

AGE.
Frequency of injury affected by, §1-9.

ALGORITHM.
Diagnosis and treatment, §3-1.

ANATOMY.
See NECK ANATOMY.

ANEURYSMAL BONE CYST.
Clinical findings, §4-4(D)(2).
Course, §4-4(D)(8).
Differential diagnosis, §4-4(D)(6).
Etiology, §4-4(D)(1).
Laboratory findings, §4-4(D)(4).
Outcome, §4-4(D)(8).
Physical findings, §4-4(D)(3).
Prevalence, §4-4(D)(1).
Radiographic findings, §4-4(D)(5).
Treatment, §4-4(D)(7).

ANKYLOSING SPONDYLITIS.
Clinical features, §4-2(C)(2).
Course, §4-2(C)(8).
Differential diagnosis, §4-2(C)(6).
Etiology, §4-2(C)(1).
Laboratory findings, §4-2(C)(4).
Outcome, §4-2(C)(8).
Physical examination, §4-2(C)(3).
Prevalence, §4-2(C)(1).
Radiologic findings, §4-2(C)(5).
Treatment, §4-2(C)(7).

INDEX

APOPHYSEAL JOINTS.
Introduction to neck anatomy, §2-1(D).
ASSESSMENT OF DISORDER, §9-4.

B

BASIC SCIENTIFIC KNOWLEDGE OF CERVICAL SPINE, §2-3.
Biochemistry, §2-3(B).
Biomechanics and stability, §2-3(C).
Immunology, §2-3(E).
Kinematics, §2-3(A).
Nociceptive factors, §2-3(F).
Nutrition, §2-3(D).
BIOCHEMISTRY.
Basic scientific knowledge of cervical spine, §2-3(B).
BIOMECHANICS.
Basic scientific knowledge of cervical spine, §2-3(C).
BLOOD SUPPLY.
Introduction to neck anatomy, §2-1(E).
BRACHIAL PLEXUA.
Introduction to neck anatomy, §2-1(G).

C

CERVICAL DEGENERATIVE DISC DISEASE.
Clinical condition, §2-4(C).
CERVICAL DISC DISTENTION TEST, §6-13.
CERVICAL HYPEREXTENSION INJURIES.
Introduction, §5-1.
Management, §5-4.
Pathophysiology, §5-2.
Return to work, §5-6.
Symptoms, §5-3.
Treatment, §5-5.
CHORDOMA.
Clinical findings, §4-4(H)(2).
Course, §4-4(H)(8).
Differential diagnosis, §4-4(H)(6).
Etiology, §4-4(H)(1).
Laboratory findings, §4-4(H)(4).

INDEX

CHORDOMA—Cont'd
  Outcome, §4-4(H)(8).
  Physical findings, §4-4(H)(3).
  Prevalence, §4-4(H)(1).
  Radiographic findings, §4-4(H)(5).
  Treatment, §4-4(H)(7).
CLINICAL CONDITION, §2-4.
  Acute herniated disc, §2-4(B).
  Cervical degenerative disc disease, §2-4(C).
    Cervical spondylosis, §2-4(C)(1).
    Cervical spondylosis with myelopathy, §2-4(C)(2).
  Neck sprain, §2-4(A).
  Rheumatoid arthritis, §2-4(D).
COMPUTERIZED AXIAL TOMOGRAPHY, §6-10.

D

DIAGNOSIS AND TREATMENT.
  Algorithm, §3-1.
  Arm pain predominant, §3-4.
  Drug therapy, §3-7.
  Exercises, §3-11.
  Immobilization, §3-6.
  Manipulation, §3-10.
  Neck pain predominant, §3-3.
  Protocol, §3-2.
  Traction, §3-8.
  Treatment modalities, §3-5.
  Trigger point injection, §3-9.
DIAGNOSTIC PROCEDURES.
  Cervical disc distention test, §6-13.
  Computerized axial tomography, §6-10.
  Discography, §6-12.
  Electromyogram, §6-9.
  History, §6-1.
  Injury to upper cervical segment, §6-4.
  Laboratory tests, §6-6.
  Lower cervical segment, §6-5.
  Magnetic resonance imaging, §6-14.
  Myelography, §6-8.
  Occipitocervical segment, §6-3.

INDEX

DIAGNOSTIC PROCEDURES—Cont'd
  Physical examination, §6-2.
  Thermography, §6-11.
  X-ray, §6-7.
DIFFUSE IDIOPATHIC SKELETAL HYPEROSTOSIS.
  Clinical findings, §4-2(G)(2).
  Course, §4-2(G)(8).
  Differential diagnosis, §4-2(G)(6).
  Etiology, §4-2(G)(1).
  Laboratory findings, §4-2(G)(4).
  Outcome, §4-2(G)(8).
  Physical findings, §4-2(G)(3).
  Prevalence, §4-2(G)(1).
  Radiographic findings, §4-2(G)(5).
  Treatment, §4-2(G)(7).
DISCOGRAPHY, §6-12.
DRUG THERAPY.
  Standardized approach to diagnosis and treatment, §3-7.

E

ECONOMIC IMPACT, §1-14.
ELECTROMYOGRAM, §6-9.
EMOTIONAL FACTORS, §1-12.
ENDOCRINOLOGIC AND METABOLIC DISORDERS, §4-5.
ENTEROPATHIC ARTHRITIS.
  Clinical features, §4-2(F)(2).
  Course, §4-2(F)(8).
  Differential diagnosis, §4-2(F)(6).
  Etiology, §4-2(F)(1).
  Laboratory findings, §4-2(F)(4).
  Outcome, §4-2(F)(8).
  Physical findings, §4-2(F)(3).
  Prevalence, §4-2(F)(1).
  Radiographic findings, §4-2(F)(5).
  Treatment, §4-2(F)(7).
EOSINOPHILIC GRANULOMA.
  Clinical findings, §4-4(F)(2).
  Course, §4-4(F)(8).
  Differential diagnosis, §4-4(F)(6).

INDEX

EOSINOPHILIC GRANULOMA—Cont'd
    Etiology, §4-4(F)(1).
    Laboratory findings, §4-4(F)(4).
    Outcome, §4-4(F)(8).
    Physical findings, §4-4(F)(3).
    Prevalence, §4-4(F)(1).
    Radiographic findings, §4-4(F)(5).
    Treatment, §4-4(F)(7).

ERGONOMICS AND PREVENTION, §9-8.

ESTIMATES OF WHIPLASH INJURIES, §1-3.

EXERCISES.
    Standardized approach to diagnosis and treatment, §3-11.

F

FIBROSITIS.
    Clinical findings, §4-2(I)(2).
    Course, §4-2(I)(8).
    Differential diagnosis, §4-2(I)(6).
    Etiology, §4-2(I)(1).
    Laboratory findings, §4-2(I)(4).
    Outcome, §4-2(I)(8).
    Physical examination, §4-2(I)(3).
    Prevalence, §4-2(I)(1).
    Radiographic findings, §4-2(I)(5).
    Treatment, §4-2(I)(7).

G

GIANT CELL TUMOR.
    Clinical findings, §4-4(C)(2).
    Course, §4-4(C)(8).
    Differential diagnosis, §4-4(C)(6).
    Etiology, §4-4(C)(1).
    Laboratory findings, §4-4(C)(4).
    Outcome, §4-4(C)(8).
    Physical findings, §4-4(C)(3).
    Prevalence, §4-4(C)(1).
    Radiographic findings, §4-4(C)(5).
    Treatment, §4-4(C)(7).

INDEX

H

HEAD RESTRAINTS, §1-7.

HEIGHT.
Correlation between height and neck injuries, §1-10.

HEMANGIOMA.
Clinical findings, §4-4(E)(2).
Course, §4-4(E)(8).
Differential diagnosis, §4-4(E)(6).
Etiology, §4-4(E)(1).
Laboratory findings, §4-4(E)(4).
Outcome, §4-4(E)(8).
Physical findings, §4-4(E)(3).
Prevalence, §4-4(E)(1).
Radiographic findings, §4-4(E)(5).
Treatment, §4-4(E)(7).

HEMATOLOGIC DISORDERS, §4-6.

HERNIATED DISC.
Clinical condition, §2-4(B).

HERNIATED NUCLEUS PULPOSUS.
Patient factors, §7-2(F).
Progressive neurologic deficit, §7-2(C).
Recurrent episodes of arm pain, §7-2(E).
Selection of operation for acute disc herniation, §7-2(G).
Surgery.
  Neck pain, §7-2(A).
  Profound spinal cord impingement, §7-2(B).
  Unrelenting radicular arm pain, §7-2(D).

I

IMMOBILIZATION.
Standardized approach to diagnosis and treatment, §3-6.

IMMUNOLOGY.
Basic scientific knowledge of cervical spine, §2-3(E).

IMPAIRMENT OF FUNCTIONAL ABILITY, §9-3.

IMPAIRMENT RATINGS.
Standardized cervical spine evaluations.
  Cervical spine evaluation problem, §10-1.
  Standardized neck evaluation guidelines, §10-2.

INDEX

INCIDENCE, §1-2.
INFECTIONS, §4-3.
Introduction, §4-3(A).
Meningitis, §4-3(C).
Paget's disease of bone, §4-3(D).
Vertebral osteomyelitis, §4-3(B).
INFILTRATIVE LESIONS.
See TUMORS AND INFILTRATIVE LESIONS.
INNERVATION.
Introduction to neck anatomy, §2-1(F).
INTEVERTEBRAL DISC.
Introduction to neck anatomy, §2-1(B).
INTRASPINAL NEOPLASM.
Clinical features, §4-4(K)(2).
Course, §4-4(K)(8).
Differential diagnosis, §4-4(K)(6).
Etiology, §4-4(K)(1).
Laboratory findings, §4-4(K)(4).
Outcome, §4-4(K)(8).
Physical findings, §4-4(K)(3).
Prevalence, §4-4(K)(1).
Radiographic findings, §4-4(K)(5).
Treatment, §4-4(K)(7).

K

KINEMATICS.
Basic scientific knowledge of cervical spine, §2-3(A).

L

LABORATORY TESTS, §6-6.
LIGAMENTS.
Introduction to neck anatomy, §2-1(D).
LITIGATION.
Effect of, §1-11.
LYMPHOMAS.
Clinical findings, §4-4(I)(2).
Course, §4-4(I)(8).
Differential diagnosis, §4-4(I)(6).

INDEX

LYMPHOMAS—Cont'd
  Etiology, §4-4(I)(1).
  Laboratory findings, §4-4(I)(4).
  Outcome, §4-4(I)(8).
  Physical findings, §4-4(I)(3).
  Prevalence, §4-4(I)(1).
  Radiographic findings, §4-4(I)(5).
  Treatment, §4-4(I)(7).

M

MAGNETIC RESONANCE IMAGING, §6-14.

MANIPULATION.
  Standardized approach to diagnosis and treatment, §3-10.

MENINGITIS.
  Clinical findings, §4-3(C)(2).
  Course, §4-3(C)(8).
  Differential diagnosis, §4-3(C)(6).
  Etiology, §4-3(C)(1).
  Laboratory findings, §4-3(C)(4).
  Outcome, §4-3(C)(8).
  Physical findings, §4-3(C)(3).
  Prevalence, §4-3(C)(1).
  Radiographic findings, §4-3(C)(5).
  Treatment, §4-3(C)(7).

MODALITIES.
  Treatment modalities, §3-5.

MULTIPLE MYELOMA.
  Clinical findings, §4-4(G)(2).
  Course, §4-4(G)(8).
  Differential diagnosis, §4-4(G)(6).
  Etiology, §4-4(G)(1).
  Laboratory findings, §4-4(G)(4).
  Outcome, §4-4(G)(8).
  Physical findings, §4-4(G)(3).
  Prevalence, §4-4(G)(1).
  Radiographic findings, §4-4(G)(5).
  Treatment, §4-4(G)(7).

MUSCLES.
  Introduction to neck anatomy, §2-1(H).

INDEX

MYELOGRAPHY, §6-8.

N

NECK ANATOMY.
Blood supply, §2-1(E).
Brachial plexua, §2-1(G).
Innervation, §2-1(F).
Intevertebral disc, §2-1(B).
Introduction to, §2-1.
Ligaments and apophyseal joints, §2-1(D).
Muscles, §2-1(H).
Occipito-atlanto-axial articulation, §2-1(C).
Osseous anatomy, §2-1(A).
  Atlas, §2-1(A)(2).
  Axis, §2-1(A)(3).
  Lower cervical vertebrae, §2-1(A)(4).
  Occiput, §2-1(A)(1).

NECK SPRAIN.
Clinical condition, §2-4(A).

NOCICEPTIVE FACTORS.
Basic scientific knowledge of cervical spine, §2-3(F).

NON-MECHANICAL CAUSES.
Endocrinologic and metabolic disorders, §4-5.
Hematologic disorders, §4-6.
Infections of the lumbosacral spine, §4-3.
Introduction, §4-1.
Rheumatologic disorders, §4-2.
Tumors and infiltrative lesions, §4-4.

NUTRITION.
Basic scientific knowledge of cervical spine, §2-3(D).

O

OCCIPITO-ATLANTO-AXIAL ARTICULATION.
Introduction to neck anatomy, §2-1(C).

OCCIPITOCERVICAL SEGMENT, §6-3.

ORGANIZED APPROACH.
Implementation of, §1-13.

OSSEOUS ANATOMY, §2-1(A).

INDEX

OSTEOBLASTOMA.
    Clinical findings, §4-4(B)(2).
    Course, §4-4(B)(8).
    Differential diagnosis, §4-4(B)(6).
    Etiology, §4-4(B)(1).
    Laboratory findings, §4-4(B)(4).
    Outcome, §4-4(B)(8).
    Physical findings, §4-4(B)(3).
    Prevalence, §4-4(B)(1).
    Radiographic findings, §4-4(B)(5).
    Treatment, §4-4(B)(7).

P

PAGET'S DISEASE OF BONE.
    Clinical findings, §4-3(D)(2).
    Course, §4-3(D)(8).
    Differential diagnosis, §4-3(D)(6).
    Etiology, §4-3(D)(1).
    Laboratory findings, §4-3(D)(4).
    Outcome, §4-3(D)(8).
    Physical findings, §4-3(D)(3).
    Prevalence, §4-3(D)(1).
    Radiographic findings, §4-3(D)(5).
    Treatment, §4-3(D)(7).

PASSENGER POSITION IN CAR, §1-5.

PATHOPHYSIOLOGY OF NECK PAIN, §2-2.

PHYSICAL THERAPY.
    Cervical collar, §9-6.
    Exercise.
        Therapeutic, postural and preventive, §9-7.
    Introduction, §9-1.
    Modalities.
        Cold, §9-2(B).
        Electrical stimulation, §9-2(C).
        Heat, §9-2(A).
        Joint mobilization, §9-2(F).
        Traction, §9-2(E).
        Ultrasound, §9-2(D).
    Nerve root pain, §9-5(C).
    Postural pain, §9-5(D).

PHYSICAL THERAPY—Cont'd
Spondylosis, §9-5(B).
Summary, §9-10.
Temporo-mandibular joint dysfunction, §9-5(E).
Whiplash, §9-5(A).
  Ligament sprain, §9-5(A)(1).
  Muscle strain, §9-5(A)(2).

POLYMYALGIA RHEUMATICA.
Clinical findings, §4-2(H)(2).
Course, §4-2(H)(8).
Differential diagnosis, §4-2(H)(6).
Etiology, §4-2(H)(1).
Laboratory findings, §4-2(H)(4).
Outcome, §4-2(H)(8).
Physical examination, §4-2(H)(3).
Prevalence, §4-2(H)(1).
Radiologic findings, §4-2(H)(5).
Treatment, §4-2(H)(7).

PREVENTION OF INJURY, §1-4.

PROTOCOL.
Cervical spine protocol, §3-2.

PSORIATIC ARTHRITIS.
Clinical features, §4-2(E)(2).
Course, §4-2(E)(8).
Differential diagnosis, §4-2(E)(6).
Etiology, §4-2(E)(1).
Laboratory findings, §4-2(E)(4).
Outcome, §4-2(E)(8).
Physical findings, §4-2(E)(3).
Prevalence, §4-2(E)(1).
Radiologic findings, §4-2(E)(5).
Treatment, §4-2(E)(7).

PSYCHOSOCIAL PROSPECTIVES.
Acute and chronic pain, §8-4.
Are chronic pain patients depressed?, §8-9.
Complications of treatment, §8-10.
Doing and not doing, §8-16.
Failure of traditional treatment, §8-11.
Illness and disease, §8-3.
Importance of the meaning of pain, §8-15.

INDEX

PSYCHOSOCIAL PROSPECTIVES—Cont'd
  Introduction, §8-1.
  Is chronic pain really a variant of depression?, §8-8.
  Pain and the American worker, §8-2.
  Pain as a four component system.
    Implications for the treatment of pain, §8-14(E).
    Nociception, §8-14(A).
    Pain behavior, §8-14(D).
    Pain message, §8-14(B).
    Suffering, §8-14(C).
  Patient in pain versus pain patient, §8-7.
  Psychosocial effects of chronic pain, §8-6.
  Understanding the pain complaint, §8-13.
  What is chronic pain?, §8-5.

R

REITER'S SYNDROME.
  Clinical findings, §4-2(D)(2).
  Course, §4-2(D)(8).
  Differential diagnosis, §4-2(D)(6).
  Etiology, §4-2(D)(1).
  Laboratory findings, §4-2(D)(4).
  Outcome, §4-2(D)(8).
  Physical findings, §4-2(D)(3).
  Prevalence, §4-2(D)(1).
  Radiologic findings, §4-2(D)(5).
  Treatment, §4-2(D)(7).

RETURNING INJURED WORKER TO JOB, §9-9.

RHEUMATOID ARTHRITIS.
  Clinical condition, §2-4(D).
  Clinical symptoms, §4-1(B)(2).
  Course, §4-2(B)(8).
  Differential diagnosis, §4-2(B)(6).
  Etiology, §4-2(B)(1).
  Laboratory findings, §4-2(B)(4).
  Physical findings, §4-2(B)(3).
  Prevalence, §4-2(B)(1).
  Prognosis, §4-2(B)(8).
  Radiographic findings, §4-2(B)(5).
  Treatment, §4-2(B)(7).

INDEX

RHEUMATOLOGIC DISORDERS.
Ankylosing spondylitis, §4-2(C).
Diffuse idiopathic skeletal hyperostosis, §4-2(G).
Enteropathic arthritis, §4-2(F).
Fibrositis, §4-2(I).
Introduction, §4-2(A).
Polymyalgia rheumatica, §4-2(H).
Psoriatic arthritis, §4-2(E).
Reiter's syndrome, §4-2(D).
Rheumatoid arthritis, §4-2(B).

S

SCOPE OF PROBLEM, §1-1.
SEAT BELTS, §1-6.
SEX.
Frequency of injury as affected by, §1-8.
SHOULDER RESTRAINTS, §1-6.
SKELETAL METASTASES.
Clinical findings, §4-4(J)(2).
Course, §4-4(J)(8).
Differential diagnosis, §4-4(J)(6).
Etiology, §4-4(J)(1).
Laboratory findings, §4-4(J)(4).
Outcome, §4-4(J)(8).
Physical findings, §4-4(J)(3).
Prevalence, §4-4(J)(1).
Radiographic findings, §4-4(J)(5).
Treatment, §4-4(J)(7).
SPINAL FUSION.
Indications for, §7-4.
Neck and arm pain, §7-4(B).
Neck pain and myelopathy, §7-4(C).
Neck pain only, §7-4(A).
STENOSIS.
Surgery.
Selection of operation for cervical spinal stenosis, §7-3(A).
SUMMARY OF PROBLEMS, §1-15.
SURGERY.
Cervical spinal stenosis, §7-3.

INDEX

SURGERY—Cont'd
  Cervical spine fusion, §7-4.
  Complications.
    During operation.
      Complications as a result of position, §7-6(A)(1).
      Neural element injuries, §7-6(A)(4).
      Vascular injuries, §7-6(A)(2).
      Visceral injuries, §7-6(A)(3).
    Immediate postoperative complications.
      Intestinal illeus, §7-6(B)(3).
      Pulmonary atelectasis, §7-6(B)(1).
      Spinal cord compression, §7-6(B)(6).
      Thrombophlebitis and pulmonary embolus, §7-6(B)(4).
      Urinary retention, §7-6(B)(2).
      Wound problems, §7-6(B)(5).
    Technical complications resulting in persistent symptoms.
      Disc space infection, §7-6(C)(3).
      Foreign bodies, §7-6(C)(6).
      Illiac crest pain, §7-6(C)(4).
      Inadequate nerve root decompression, §7-6(C)(1).
      Inadequate spinal cord decompression, §7-6(C)(2).
      Late instability and degenerative changes, §7-6(C)(5).
  Herniated nucleus pulposus.
    Surgical indications, §7-2.
  Introduction, §7-1.
  Results of operative treatment, §7-5.
  Summary, §7-7.

T

THERMOGRAPHY, §6-11.

TRACTION.
  Standardized approach to diagnosis and treatment, §3-8.

TREATMENT.
  Assessment of cervical musculoskeletal disorders and treatment plan, §9-4.
  Diagnosis and treatment.
    See DIAGNOSIS AND TREATMENT.

TRIGGER POINT INJECTION.
  Standardized approach to diagnosis and treatment, §3-9.

TUMORS AND INFILTRATIVE LESIONS.
  Aneurysmal bone cyst, §4-4(D).

INDEX

TUMORS AND INFILTRATIVE LESIONS—Cont'd
Chordoma, §4-4(H).
Eosinophilic granuloma, §4-4(F).
Giant cell tumor, §4-4(C).
Hemangioma, §4-4(E).
Intraspinal neoplasm, §4-4(K).
Introduction, §4-4(A).
Lymphomas, §4-4(I).
Multiple myeloma, §4-4(G).
Osteoblastoma, §4-4(B).
Skeletal metastases, §4-4(J).

V

VERTEBRAL OSTEOMYELITIS.
Clinical findings, §4-3(B)(2).
Course, §4-3(B)(8).
Differential diagnosis, §4-3(B)(6).
Etiology, §4-3(B)(1).
Laboratory findings, §4-3(B)(4).
Outcome, §4-3(B)(8).
Physical findings, §4-3(B)(3).
Prevalence, §4-3(B)(1).
Radiographic findings, §4-3(B)(5).
Treatment, §4-3(B)(7).

W

WEIGHT.
Correlation between weight and neck injuries, §1-10.

X

X-RAY, §6-7.